Pra

MW00366151

HERBAL MEDICINE OF THE AMERICAN SOUTHWEST

"For anyone interested in botanical medicine, Herbal Medicine of the American Southwest is a valuable addition to your library."
—*Alternative Medicine Review*

"If you want to know more about these precious and in some cases powerful medicines, check out Kane's book..."
—*Herbal Bookworm*

"The comprehensive field guide to plants from Acacia to Yucca instructs on collection, preparation and use of the Southwest's botanical bounty."
—*Arizona Highways*

"Kane explains how to dry the plants and to make teas and tinctures. He includes a glossary, a therapeutic index and an extensive bibliography."
—*Book News*

"Herbal Medicine of the American Southwest is highly recommended to all naturalists living in the southwest of America, as well as organic studies students, however especially recommended to all inhabitants of the featured area."
—*Mid West Book Review*

"Useful as both a field guide and a reference source, the plants are carefully identified and include the chemistry of active ingredients, medicinal uses, and collection and preparation suggestions. The author has a functional belief in self-healing; the approach here is to offer non-pharmaceutical, "green" alternatives to standard medical therapeutics, promoting a do-it yourself functional philosophy."
—*The Bloomsbury Review*

HERBAL MEDICINE
OF THE
AMERICAN SOUTHWEST

A GUIDE TO THE
MEDICINAL AND EDIBLE PLANTS
OF THE SOUTHWESTERN
UNITED STATES

Charles W. Kane

LINCOLN TOWN PRESS

Herbal Medicine of the American Southwest
Lincoln Town Press

Book design and cover by Charles W. Kane

Library of Congress Control Number: 2005906551

ISBN 0-9771333-0-3

Printed in the United States of America

CONTENTS

THE PLANTS

{ vii }

CONTENTS

CONTENTS

{ ix }

CONTENTS

ACKNOWLEDGMENTS

I am fortunate that my formative years were filled with what they were. My father, Walter Kane and mother, Peggy Kane raised us well; my grandparents, Charles and Florence Kane added greatly to that – for those times and what was passed on words can not express. Thanks goes out to my brother, Adam Kane for his advice as an author and his inexhaustible supply of Burdock, his wife, Andrea Kane for her generosity and kind words, Lisa Kane for her practicality, and Nick Wyatt for his stories of travel, war, and transcendence. Valued is the assistance from Peter Gierlach, Chuck Rahang, Joe Billings, and Nancy Reid, particularly in their knowledge of native plant botany and horticulture. Desert Survivors and the Arizona Desert Museum deserve acknowledgment for providing several plant models for Frank Roses' paintings.

A warm thanks to Diane Jimenez, Jon Helleson, Jessie Emerson, Phyllis Hogan, and Peter Bigfoot for their medicinal plant influences early on, and particularly to Michael Moore whose teaching style, knowledge, and unpretentiousness stand unequaled. Both he and Francis Brinker lent a critical eye in reviewing the manuscript; for that I am grateful. Appreciation goes out to the University of Arizona for their research materials and to J.J. Lamb, Pam Hyde-Nakai, Donna Chesner, Robert Cauble, Adam Seller, and John and Donna Albertsen for their support. Frank and Louise Rose's editing skills are well regarded, and I am indebted to Frank Rose whose timeless art will remain long after these words become obsolete. I only have the greatest love and appreciation for my wife Christy; her support for this project was unwavering. As an infantryman's wife, her patience, faith, and hope served as a deliverance.

To all who have remained unmentioned, who have shaped this book in some way, I thank you.

FOREWORD

The drawing of comparisons is integral to the literary process. You might think that gathering your herbs in the wild is like growing your own corn, and buying them in the store is like buying some ears of corn from the produce section. Actually a better comparison is your garden corn to the dehydrated corn in an instant soup cup.

The majority of bulk herbs are gathered in the third world or at least Eastern Europe. They may be gathered and dried with care...more likely they are crudely garbled by exporters to remove rocks, clods of dirt and the more lavish adulterants. Further, the American herbs may, as in Black cohosh, be harvested by backhoes, followed by the removal of the roots from the excavated dirt. Yet some, too, may be gathered with care.
Echinacea was formerly harvested by crews of six, riding in flatbed trucks, digging every plant along smaller roadsides in Missouri and Arkansas...until outlawed as a traffic hazard. Some Echinacea, also, is harvested with care.

Buying bulk herbs in the co-op or health food store is a crapshoot. Buying herbal preparations, like capsules, teabags, even tinctures, is still further from the source, and is playing at even lower odds.

The picker picks, sells to the buyer, who sells to the broker, who sells to the bulk wholesaler, who sells to the retailer, who sells to you. If the plant is labeled somewhere along the road as "Arnica montana" (a European medicinal plant) it can be sold to the wholesaler, manufacturer, retailer...and you, as Arnica montana. The plant is usually Heterotheca, a Mexican wildflower, and often called locally, "Arnica Mexicana". No laws are broken...just faith.

Then again, Yarrow is almost always Yarrow. But contemporary commerce calls for Yarrow Flowers. Yarrow often grows in humid mountains; the only practical way for a Croat wildcrafter to dry them is to lay them out in the sun until they are dry. Sunlight seriously deteriorates herbs. The buyer in steamy northern Florida, faced with tons of freshly gathered Passionflower herb, resorts to retooled pottery kilns to dry the herb quickly...at temperatures of 400 degrees or higher. The dried herb is green and pretty, but the active alkaloids in the Passionflower are destroyed by the high desiccating heat.

So is the herb industry a cheat? Not exactly. No more so than nearly every aspect of Commercial America.

The supplement manufacturer receives a 55-gallon barrel of powder labeled "60% citrus flavonoid complex", and they can happily label a bottle of 800-milligram capsules as containing 480 mg citrus flavonoid complex per capsule. In fact, the bulk powder may contain any actual amount of actual flavonoids...from 1% to 60%. If it was also labeled 5% rutin, etc., then it legally must contain those actual numbers. "Complex" means zilch.

Enlarge the picture. Does anyone REALLY expect the exercise machine advertised on TV to work as well as claimed? Does anyone REALLY think that the car dealer is selling below invoice? Does anyone REALLY think that the credit card has a fixed interest rate? Does anyone REALLY believe the government? the pentagon? the bank? the hospital billing office? the 9 minutes with the actual M.D.? the "buy" recommendation from your financial adviser?

So, faced with an increasingly callow and morally bankrupt society, more and more of us are adopting the simple attitude: "If it's in my hands, I can trust it."

For years I have had the realization that what Green Herbalists do is one of the most profoundly subversive activities to be found. We believe that, excluding major diseases, we can actually LEARN enough about anatomy and physiology to make sensible self-diagnostics and use naturally occurring substances we gather ourselves to treat ourselves. I use the term Green Herbalist to describe folks that know a bit of medicine, know a bit of botany, know a bit of pharmacy, and are capable of identifying a plant, preparing it properly, and knowing what physical conditions it is useful for and what it is inappropriate for. Each part is equally important.

There are British Medical Herbalists, beautifully trained in medicine, often sadly lacking in actual plant knowledge. Naturopaths know medicine, but prescribe sophisticated and expensive herbal supplements...they don't know plants. The Doctor of Oriental Medicine or acupuncturist usually only knows patent medicines and herbal tablets.

What Charles Kane is writing about here, and as I, too, have written, is how to identify plants, prepare plants, have reasonable understanding of the mild disorders and subpathologies they can be used for, and those occasions where they are inappropriate.

Nice and simple. Most disorders are self-limiting and self-treatable. Medicines derived from plants you can gather yourself can be used to modify discomfort. If things get worse, see a doctor. Most won't get worse.

Charles has written an impeccable book. Based on personal experience, trial and error, well-researched and tidy.

How to find the plant.

How to prepare it.

What it can be used for, what side effects may occur.

What resources, if needed, will further define the plant.

You are lucky to have it...there are few like it.

Michael Moore
Bisbee, Arizona

INTRODUCTION

I navigate my old truck down a winding dirt road. The morning sun has just started to peek over some rimrock to the east. If I squint directly at it, the rays fill my eyes and appear as a shooting halo. The road becomes more of a two-lane trail, no longer accessible by passenger car, and given the amount of Popcorn flower and Filaree growing in the middle burm, even more robust vehicles seldom come here – maybe an occasional rancher checking on a stock tank. This basin is vast; small, volcanic, craggy mountain chains can be seen in all directions, pushing seasonal rainwater dropped from above nearly to the middle, where I am now. Funneled by the mountains and hills, canyons and gulches, the water ends up slowing, where over time it has formed a huge flood plain. On it, the reason I have come here today, grows Creosote bush, thick and abundant.

I stop the truck next to an expansive wash. The morning spring air is cool here and prompts me to keep my long sleeved shirt on. I gather my gear from the truck bed – paper bags, water, and some fruit and jerky that I stuff in a shoulder bag. A knife and pistol I feed through my belt. As I start moving southward down the wash I stay to the compacted sand, some is still moist from when the rains petered out a week or two ago. The Mesquites that line the wash are almost fully leafed-out and dapple the ground underneath with shade. Wolfberry, Graythorn, and some Hackberry bushes are close by as well. I look forward to the Hackberries ripening in the summer; they have sweet fruits. Mule deer are also in the area. Their bedding areas are notable. I cross over the wash, ascend the small embankment, continue through the Mesquites, and pass through several smaller draws. Here lies a vast plain of Creosote bush; I like to think they are ancient, some hundreds, maybe thousand of years old, many from the same genetic stock. From the silty earth the plants form in circular clumps; their grayish stems issuing forth from slightly raised mounds. The plant's new leaf growth is verdant, and with accompanying yellow flowers and fuzzy seeds, it is a perfect time to collect. Most of the leaves group themselves on the outer branch ends. I grab a branch between my thumb and forefinger and pull. The leaves, flowers, and seeds strip from the plant leaving the woodier stems intact – a simple method. If both hands are used several pounds of the leaf can be gathered in 20-30 minutes. I move around, as not to take too much from one plant, no need with a sea of it around.

After a couple of hours of collecting, I look at my hands. They are green with resin build-up that even the most vigorous of scrubbing will be hard pressed to remove. I have enough of the plant to last a year. The smell of the collected leaf is like a good rain in the summertime desert. I place the gathered Creosote bush under a Mesquite tree, as I will pick it up on the way back to the truck. For now I trek further south, enjoying the desert, the land, creation.

A small jagged rock out-cropping catches my eye, as I make towards it signs of activity from an earlier time abound – pottery shards, grinding holes, and even an old desert tortoise shell. Less subtle are the signs of recent activity. They become more apparent as I walk further south. Discarded water bottles, shirts, towels, bras, food wrappers, plain and simple trash from thousands of illegal aliens on the move north. I stop at a little makeshift encampment occupied briefly and left hurriedly. Ashes from a campfire still are intact. I poke it with my boot as I ponder the larger ramifications. The buzzards high above are coming from the south too this time of year; several ravens fly low overhead, the sun glistening off their black-as-night feathers. I try to mimic their throaty call – never was good at that. They seem to be laughing.

After circling back north I find the Mesquite tree with the bagged Creosote bush underneath. I sit, eat and drink a little of what I have brought. It is simple food, for a simple place. The peace of the natural world enters my mind as I lay down on years of dropped Mesquite leaves and ephemeral plants that have lived and died, making the tree's shelter comfortable. I doze for a short time and awake refreshed. As I head back to the truck, I take it all in with my eyes as if this were my last day here.

Several weeks later, I sit in my office, not entirely comfortable with the surroundings, but knowing they are necessary. I greet Jim at the receptionist's desk and led him to where we sit. He tells me his story, his medical history, and other subtleties surrounding his medical condition most MDs would think were frivolous. I take his pulse, look at his tongue and skin, and along with other observations, discern his constitutional make-up. Jim's main complaint is rheumatic pain in his hands and wrists. He has chronic skin rashes around his scalp, and as a child, he suffered from asthma. Jim has never used herbs before but is willing to try something new. I dispense Creosote bush, along with other supportive herbs. Within a week his pain is greatly reduced; he is getting better results than when he took pharmaceuticals.

Helping people or helping yourself with plants that come from the land around you is what regional herbal medicine is all about. Always has been, always will be.

You hold in your hands a resource that will enable you to properly use the plants of the southwest for healing. The majority of plants discussed within are found throughout the lower-lying deserts; others have a wider western range, and then some are found countywide. Use this book to find out what the plants look like, where to find them, how to gather and prepare them, and why to take them. If you like to do things yourself and value a no-nonsense, coherent approach to herbal medicine, then this book is for you.

Part folk medicine, part well-researched scientific findings, the information contained within these pages is a combination of personal experience, contributions of others in the field, and conclusions found in the latest scientific literature. It is a working model on how to use many plants of the American Southwest, in real situations, to positively affect health – an herbal for today.

FORMAT EXPLANATION

Plant Names: Common and scientific names are given for both the plant and family. Each profile is headed by the main common name, followed by a current scientific name and synonyms. Secondary common names follow. The majority of main common names assigned to the plants are generally accepted as the most common, i.e. Yellowdock, Passionflower, Dandelion, etc. One notable exception to this is Creosote bush, popularly known in the medicinal herb world as Chaparral. Even though Chaparral has name recognition, it adds no descriptiveness to the plant; on the contrary, it is misleading, as it refers to a vegetation zone found throughout the mid-mountain southwest. Arctostaphylos and Ceanothus are typical inhabitants, not Larrea. Creosote bush fits; anyway that is its local name to people who live around it. Many of these plants have popular Spanish names. With several exceptions, I have opted for the English name because this book is obviously written in English, for English readers. With all of that said, do not get stuck in the name game. Most common names as well as many scientific names for any given plant change from generation to generation. No name is set in stone and botanical classifiers can be as fickle in applying and reapplying nomenclature depending on the classifying politics of the day as any leaf in the wind. When you know the plant, you know the plant, names be damned.

Description and Distribution: Look to these sections for the plant's botanical description and growth tendencies. All measurements are in standard, not metric. Pertinence is placed on where the plant grows in this country. Its elevation ranges, topographies, and environments are discussed.

Chemistry: A sometimes general, sometimes specific compilation of chemical constituents for each plant.

Medicinal Uses: The plant's effect on organ systems, tissue groups, and occasionally symptoms are described. Application to disease syndromes has been keep to a minimum but occasionally it is pertinent – how the plant affects stress patterns and its mechanisms of action are preferred. This may make for slow reading but the reward is a deeper understanding of the plants and how they work.

Plants are multi-directional; rarely do they affect just one area of the body. They influence the body by how an organ or tissue group eliminates or detoxifies the compounds comprising them. It is not the plant that is the remedy for the ailment or discomfort, but it is what the plant does to the body, organ system or group of tissues that then affects the manifested problem. Only after knowing that an aromatic-bitter herb stimulates secretion and dilates vasculature of the stomach lining will its effect on quieting indigestion make sense.

Indications: A synopsis of medicinal uses. The indicated medicinal use for the plant.

Collection: Depending on the plant, virtually any part can be medicinally potent. Mostly though roots, bark, leaves, flowers, seeds, and sap or exudate provide the strongest medicines. Stems, branches, and core wood are the least likely parts to give benefit. The former parts are functional, having an array of chemical processes taking place within them. The latter parts are structural, serving mainly as a skeletal support for the functional parts – much like our bodies.

There are two main polarized attitudes encountered concerning the collection of wild plants for medicine. The ideologies that these attitudes spring from have an affect on our perspectives concerning nature, and society as well. Whether it is the big-money, corporate-consumption mentality or the tendencies that go along with most environmental groups out to "save" the natural world through litigation, neither world-view is helpful to the respectful wildcrafter who takes only what he needs…which may not be what he desires. The first attitude: take all that you can if it is of any value regardless of environmental impact. This tendency and its effects are noticeable on a number of medicinal plants in commerce. This same attitude enables consumption for its own sake at many levels of our society. No need to go into our voracious appetites for all things new and environmentally burdensome. The second attitude is the exact opposite – it is one of containment and cordoning nature off with red tape, charging to get in, leaving no trace, and then exiting back to the city or suburbs. One sees the natural world existing soley to be exploited, the other sees the same as godlike and as more important than people. Ironically both attitudes are opposite sides of the same coin. They alienate and remove us from meaningful interaction with our natural surroundings. Meaningful interaction hinges on having something to do in the natural world. Want to save nature? Then interact with her; know her through involvement – hunt, fish, build a log cabin, collect some plants. These activities foster common-sense respect.

Guidelines:
- Have positive identification of the plant.
- Collect away from roadsides, inner city areas, industrial sites, agricultural areas, and heavily traveled foot trails – explaining yourself to every busy-body hiker gets to be tiresome, although visibly packin' heat usually limits conversation to furtive glances.
- Become familiar with the overall plant populations in your area. If only a small stand of a particular plant exists in one area, move on and collect where it is more abundant.
- Do not collect more than 10% of any stand of plants.
- Clean up before leaving; fill in holes and if preparing medicines in the field then spread around core wood and other unusable plant materials to lessen visual impact of your activities.
- Have respect; if done right, without greed, you are supported by the plants – the natural world, and they are supported through your understanding of them.

Drying Plants:
- Dry plant materials out of the direct sunlight. Small bundles of leafing tops, with the topmost portions of the plant hanging down (see pictures of Bricklebush) are secured from ceiling rafters until dry.
- Herbage can also be placed loosely in paper bags or laid well-spaced on cardboard flats or similar material for drying.
- After fully dried garble the leaves and flowers from the stems; discard the stems.
- Chop roots into ¼-½ inch pieces or longer longitudinal strips. Both these and bark strips dry adequately if well spaced.

♦ For quicker drying or to ensure no mold growth occurs if in a humid environment a dehydrator can be used.

Preparations: The herb can be of the highest quality and collected in a pristine environment, but if the delivery method is inferior, the quality will not amount to much. The best way internally to get the medicinal benefits of a plant is to eat it, preferably fresh. For most of us, this is cumbersome, if not impractical. Generally speaking the simpler the preparation, the more potent the end result. Here are the main preparations:

Teas

Tea preparations are best applied to plants that have a large array of water-soluble compounds. Plants that are being used for their tannins, starches, minerals and other polar compounds are best taken as teas. All plants are dried first then infused or decocted. Making tea with a fresh plant is a waste. Intact, living plant cells are adept at holding on to their vital cellular compounds, not giving them up to water. Through drying this force is disrupted – cell walls are broken making the plant's various constituents permeable to water. Make tea or any water-based preparation fresh daily.

Infusion

Bring 1 quart of water to a boil. Turn off heat. Stir in 1 ounce of dry fragile plant materials – leaves, flowers, thin stems, etc. Cover and steep for 15 minutes. Uncover and strain. Make fresh daily. *Ratio: 1 part herb (weight) to 32 parts water (volume)*

Decoction

Bring 1 quart of water to a slow simmer. Stir in 1 ounce of thicker dried plant materials – bark, roots, stems, pods, etc. Cover and simmer for 15 minutes. Turn heat off. Steep for 15 minutes. Uncover and strain. Make fresh daily. *Ratio: 1 part herb (weight) to 32 parts water (volume)*

Cold Infusion

Suspend in a mesh tea bag or colander 1 ounce of dried plant materials in 1 quart of water. Let this stand over night at room temperature. Strain. Make fresh daily. *Ratio: 1 part herb (weight) to 32 parts water (volume)*

Tinctures
- Plants that are high in volatile oils, complex starches, and other non-polar constituents are best prepared through tincturing.
- A 1:2 FPT (fresh plant tincture) means 1 part of fresh herb to 2 parts of menstruum. A 1:5 DPT (dry plant tincture) means 1 part of dried herb to 5 parts of menstruum.
- A 1:2 FPT is equal in strength to a 1:5 DPT. Since the dried plant lacks water it is being added back into the menstruum to properly extract the plant's constituents.
- The alcohol percentage of the FPT is high. What is being relied upon in this tincture preparation is the hydroscopic activity of alcohol. The alcohol literally dehydrates the fresh plant, pulling all of its constituents/cytoplasm, into itself. The result is a highly potent, intact representation of the fresh plant. FPTs with lower alcohol contents are inferior; water limits the pulling activity of alcohol.
- 1:2 for a FPT and 1:5 for a DPT are standard ratios originated by chemists in western medicine's past when plants were the main medicines.
- Depending on the plant, lower tincture and extract ratios (1:1 or 2:1, etc.) are not necessarily better or stronger. One characteristic of a good quality tincture is its lack of particulate matter, or sediment. Often many plants respond poorly to a 1:1 or more concentrated preparation because their constituents are not able to remain in suspension and "salt out" through being too concentrated. This limits the body's ability to properly absorb the preparation and ultimately its effectiveness.
- All tinctures are made with 190 proof ethyl alcohol, commonly called Everclear. Look to liquor stores or the liquor section of grocery stores. Availability varies from state to state.

Fresh Plant Tincture
Place 2 ounces of fresh, chopped plant material in a glass jar. Add 4 ounces of alcohol. Secure the lid. There is no need to shake the mixture. After 10-14 days, press or squeeze the tincture from the herb. Discard the marc (spent herb), bottle the tincture. A simpler method is as follows: Place 5½ ounces of fresh, chopped plant material in a pint mason jar. Fill to the top with alcohol. Secure the lid and follow the instructions mentioned previously. Filling the jar

to the top with alcohol will not amount to exactly 11 ounces (or 2 parts), but is close enough. *Ratio: 1 part fresh herb (weight) to 2 parts 190 proof ethyl alcohol (volume)*

Dry Plant Tincture
Place 2 ounces of dried and powered plant material in a glass jar. Add 10 ounces of alcohol/water mixture – see each plant's preparation/dosage for the correct alcohol/water percentages. If a plant calls for 60% alcohol then add 6 ounces of grain alcohol and 4 ounces (40%) of water. Combine together with the powdered herb in a glass jar. Secure lid and then shake well for several minutes. Let stand for 2 weeks – shaking everyday for 5 minutes. Squeeze or press the tincture from the marc with a piece of cloth. Discard the marc. Bottle the tincture. When using this tincture method with high tannin-content plants the menstruum should consist of 10% glycerin. This inhibits the tannins from binding together and with other constituents. *Ratio: 1 part dried herb (weight) to 5 parts menstruum (volume)*

Bath
Draw a hot bath; add 1 gallon of tea to water; soak.

Capsules
Capsules come in various sizes with '0', '00', and '000' being the most common. To fill simply immerse the two halves in an herbal powder, then fit the capsule together, enclosing the herbal powder. Encapsulation machines speed up the process. They are available in various designs.

Cough syrup
Method 1: Take 5 ½ ounces of finely chopped, fresh plant material; pack into a pint mason jar and fill to the top with honey. Secure lid and set aside for several weeks. Squeeze or press the honey from the herb and bottle the infused honey. *Ratio: 1 part herb (weight) to 2 parts of honey (volume)*
Method 2: Mix together 8 ounces of appropriate tincture(s) with 4 ounces of honey and 2 ounces of glycerin; bottle. *Ratio: 4 parts tincture (volume) to 2 parts honey (volume) to 1 part glycerin (volume)*

Douche
Make a half-strength tea; cool until warm; add ½ teaspoon of table salt per pint of tea. Use as directed. Make fresh daily.

Eyewash
Method 1: Make 1 pint of tea with distilled or filtered water through the properly designated method (infusion, decoction, etc.); strain well through a paper towel or cloth. Add ½ teaspoon of table salt. Stir until dissolved. Apply as needed. Make fresh daily.
Method 2: Add 10 drops of appropriate tincture to two ounces of isotonic water (¼ teaspoon of table salt to 1 cup of distilled or filtered water). Apply as needed. Make fresh daily.

Fluidextracts
Unlike FPTs that are 1:2 in strength and DPTs that are 1:5 in strength fluidextracts use dried materials and are 1:1 in strength. Not all plants lend themselves well to fluidextracts, but the ones that are well suited for this preparation are mentioned in each plant profile. Fluidextracts are complicated to prepare; for one, the base tincture is made through percolation (another method of making DPTs entirely) and then concentrated to a 1:1. Essentially fluidextracts enable a lower, more concentrated dose, and can prove necessary if making formulas. Unfortunately, the procedure does not lend itself well to words. This preparation is best taught in person by someone experienced in the process. Find an herbalist local to your area, learn it from him; if he does not know how, then move on and find someone who does. In fact, an herbalist's depth can often be gauged by whether or not he makes and uses fluidextracts.

Fomentation
Soak a cloth or towel in a warm herb tea; squeeze excess tea from the cloth, and apply the cloth to the affected area. Re-soak and apply as needed.

Liniment
An externally applied tincture. Isopropyl alcohol can be used instead of ethyl alcohol for this preparation. Do not use isopropyl alcohol internally.

Herbal Oil

Powder 1 ounce of dried herb. Add one ounce of 190 proof ethyl alcohol to the herb and stir in. Cover and let stand for about an hour. Pour 5 ounces of olive oil into a blender. Add the alcohol-saturated herb. Blend on high for 15 minutes or until blender container is very warm. Strain the oily mass through a piece of cloth. Discard the marc, bottle the oil. *Ratio: 1 part herb (weight) to 1 part 190 proof ethyl alcohol (volume) to 5 parts olive oil (volume)*

Poultice

Method 1: Moisten the needed amount of dried and powdered herb with warm water until a porridge-like consistency is reached. Apply directly to the affected area, or cover the area first with muslin cloth, then apply. Secure poultice with a covering and/or bandage. Change 2-3 times daily, or when cool.

Method 2: Bruise and/or puree the fresh plant; apply to affected area and secure. Change 2-3 times daily. A "spit poultice" can be quickly made by chewing the intended herb (make sure it is internally non-toxic) and applying it to the affected area.

Powders

Depending on the part of the plant some materials are harder than others to powder. Roots, bark, and stems are more difficult than leaves, flowers, and lightweight parts. For lighter materials an average blender with a metal or glass container is adequate; for tougher materials a vita-mix works well, or an industrial grinder/mill. Once the plant is powdered it can then be used as a dust, or as a starting point for DPT's, poultices, etc.

Salve

While slowly heating 5 ounces of herbal oil add 1 ounce of bee's wax. Let wax slowly dissolve. While still hot, pour into containers. As the salve cools, it will solidify. *Ratio: 5 parts herbal oil (volume) to 1 part bee's wax (weight)*

Sitz Bath

Using ½ strength or full strength tea apply/soak until tea is cool.

Wash

Topically apply an herb tea to the affected area.

Dosage: The preparation is given with suggested dosage. This dosage is a good starting point – depending on weight and sensitivity, it may be decreased or increased slightly. All percentages apply to the alcohol content.

Cautions: If the following general precepts are adhered to when using medicinal plants there will be little to fear from potential adverse reactions.
- Quantity: a little will help, a lot may harm. Any plant properly dosed in small amounts can be medicinal. The same plant may be toxic in larger amounts.
- As a society, we are over medicated. If taking pharmaceuticals for a particular problem, throwing an herb or two into the mix to affect the same organ or tissue group may be OK...or not. Do some homework first, or see a professional versed in such matters.
- If any herb makes you sick, causes a headache, diarrhea, nausea, dizziness, or other unwanted sensations then lessen the dose or discontinue the herb.
- If an herb affects the mother to be, then it is affecting the fetus. The herb's activity is usually delivered to the baby through breast milk as well. While pregnant or nursing limit herbs that have strong physiologic activities. In these times think of food as medicine.
- Aside from the fundamental social and moral wrong of abortion, and the medical procedures' link to breast cancer, a number of herbs discussed in this book have abortifacient potential. As a rule, they are unreliable and if used in sufficient quantity are apt to cause harm to the mother as well.

A Note on Formulas
This book is lacking formulas for a reason – one size does not fit all. If you think the situation calls for a formula instead of one herb then keep it simple. A formula comprised of over six herbs (some will argue four to five) is likely to cause more physiologic chatter than therapeutic direction. This is largely due to inexperienced practitioners playing guessing games or formulators combining as many herbs "for" high blood pressure, constipation, depression, etc. as possible – the "more is better" approach. Having a formula comprised of a dozen or more herbs is laughable. The desire to do this stems from man's inherent ability for complicating things. A well-formulated mixture should be direct, elegant, and unfettered. Keep in consideration the multi-systemic

nature of herbs; they usually affect more than one organ system. Excessive polypharmacy is rampant in the natural supplement industry. Look at the label of most herbal supplement combinations; if the ingredient list is filled with numerous herbs then that formula has absolutely no direction, and only can help someone through placebo or by creating a little physiologic "noise" in the body by its elimination through various pathways.

ACACIA

Acacia greggii
Catclaw acacia

Acacia constricta
White thorn acacia

Acacia angustissima
Fern acacia

Description: Acacia greggii is a large shrub or multi-trunked small tree occasioning 15-20 feet in height. Like many Acacias, A. greggii has a bipinnate leaf pattern; each leaf has 2-4 sets of leaflets comprised of 4-6 pairs of secondary leaflets or pinnae. The thorns are recurved, solitary, and alternately spaced along the branches. The small flowers form dense, yellowish cylindrical clusters, which are 1-2 inches long. The pods, which follow, are 2-5 inches long, ½-¾ of an inch wide, ribbon-like, and slightly twisted. The green pods and seeds have a distinctive onion-like smell.

At maturity, Acacia constricta is a large shrub, reaching 6-8 feet tall by the same dimension wide. At branch nodes there are 2 large white thorns; these diminish in size and eventually disappear as the branch or trunk ages and increases in girth. The leaves are composed of 1-7 sets of primary leaflets and 6-16 pairs of secondary leaflets; each of these are very small, usually no more than ½-inch long. The small yellow flowers form into ball-like clusters that are between ½-1 inch in width; they are very fragrant and sweet smelling. The seedpods that develop in June are light reddish-brown, smooth, and 1½-4 inches long. The small black and gray seeds are mottled and between ½-¼ of an inch long.

Out of the three plants profiled here, Acacia angustissima tends to be the most herbaceous. The plant is rarely woody and typically is no more than 4 feet tall by 4 feet wide. The branch stems are deeply grooved and wooly. Each large-bipinnate leaf has 2-14 sets of primary leaflets and 9-33 sets of secondary leaflets. The white, ball-like flower clusters are arranged in racemes originating from leaf axils. The brown seedpods are 1½-3 inches long and up to ½-inch wide. The seeds are small and dark brown.

Distribution: Acacia greggii is found in a large array of zones throughout the southwest. From sea level to 5,000 feet, the plant ranges extensively throughout the Mojave, Sonoran, and Chihuahuan Deserts. In low elevation, arid areas look for A. greggii along gullies and washes; the higher in elevation the plant is found the more common it is encountered in Desert Grasslands, open areas, and among rocky hillsides and slopes.

From much of the southern half of Arizona, Acacia constricta is found east to southern New Mexico's Gila River, Rio Grande, and Pecos River Drainages to Trans-Pecos Texas. A. constricta is typically found from 2,000-6,000 feet in many areas where A. greggii is present. The plant is commonly found along drainages and on slopes and hillsides.

Westward from southern Florida Acacia angustissima has a patchwork-like distribution. The plant is found through Arkansas, Missouri, and much of eastern Texas, skipping most of New Mexico except for an isolated pocket east of the southern expanse of the Rio Grande Drainage. Although the plant does not occur in California, below the Mogollon Rim it is common throughout much of southeastern and south-central Arizona.

Chemistry: legume-type condensed and hydrolyzable tannins

Medicinal Uses: Acacias are simply mild astringents, nothing more, nothing less. Their best use is as a topical wash or powder for redness and skin irritation from insect bites, sunburn, scrapes, and abrasions. Along with Mesquite this ubiquitous genus is easily accessed throughout the southwestern part of the country.

Indications:
♦ Burns, scrapes, abrasions (external)

Collection: From mid-spring through early fall clip the small leafing branch ends. Dry, and then garble the leaves from the branches. Discard the branches.

Preparations and Dosage:
♦ Leaf infusion/powder/poultice: topically as needed

Cautions: None known.

Other Uses: Acacia seeds can be eaten raw in small quantities. The biggest limiting factor is the pseudo onion-like scent that becomes repugnant rather quickly. Dried, the seeds can be cooked like any other legume, or ground into a meal and eaten alone or mixed with other flours.

ALOE
Liliaceae – Lily family

Aloe barbadensis (Aloe vera, A. vulgaris, A. perfoliata var. vera)
True aloe

Aloe ferox
Cape aloe, Bitter aloe

Description: Aloe barbadensis or A. vera, as it is more commonly referred to, is a succulent plant standing between 2-4 feet tall. The thickened lance-shaped leaves form in large rosettes at the plant's base. A well-hydrated mature leaf may reach 30 inches in length and weigh 2-3 pounds. The leaf skin is smooth, rubbery, and grayish-green with recurved teeth lining its margins. Tall flower spikes originate from the center of the plant; individual flowers are arranged in branched spike-like clusters. They are tubular, yellow, and droop downwards. The lower flowers mature and open first.

Aloe ferox in many respects is similar to A. barbadensis. It is a larger plant, reaching 6-10 feet at maturity. Its central stem crown bares a rosette of thick, succulent green leaves. Older plants can develop impressive trunks and if left unpruned older leaves can cover it like a skirting. The leaves also have reddish-brown teeth along their margins and occasionally on both the top and bottom of the leaf. Flower stalks stand several feet tall, can be branched, and support clusters of reddish-orange tubular flowers. Like A. barbadensis, the bottom-most flowers are the first to mature and open. Although somewhat similar in appearance, Aloe is unrelated to Agave and Yucca.

Distribution: Aloe barbadensis appears to be originally from the eastern Mediterranean area, but like Cupressus sempervirens, it has been cultivated and transported for thousands of years making the exact location of its native region difficult to ascertain. Now though, the plant is widely distributed throughout the Middle East, northern Africa and peninsular India. Here in the west it is found throughout Central America, Mexico, Florida, Texas, and throughout the low-elevation southwest where it is grown with some extra care. In the United States, the plant is widely cultivated for its commercial value in Texas and Florida. A. ferox is a South African native, but like A. barbadensis, it is extensively grown as an ornamental. In the past, it was widely cultivated for its dried exudate.

Chemistry: anthraquinones: barbaioin (aloin), which breaks down into aloe-emodin-9-anthrone; isobarbaloin; lignins, saponins, and sterols

Medicinal Uses: There are two essentially different medicines derived from Aloe. Both have somewhat diverging physiologic activities, modes of action, and collection techniques. Aloe leaf juice, which is yellowish-brown when fresh, is mainly held within a layer of specialized cells positioned between the rind and inner leaf. Collected as an exudate and dried it is the historical Bitter aloe of the old drug trade, and even up until 2002 comprised some over-the-counter and pharmaceutical preparations. This dried or fresh juice is primarily a stimulant laxative. Internally use it for short periods if constipated. Like other stimulant laxatives, Aloe can be habit forming if taken for lengthy periods. Address liver health, stress patterns, and diet before relying on Aloe or any stimulant laxative for regular bowel movements. Aloe juice stimulates peristalsis and fluid secretion by the large bowel; interestingly these activities are largely achieved only after the anthraquinone aloin is transformed by colonic bacteria into an active metabolite, aloe-emodin-9-antrone. Similarly to Senna the addition of carminative herbs such as Dogweed or Chinchweed will offset potential griping caused by Aloe alone. Arthritis that is dependent upon poor bowel health and constipation will improve under the use of Aloe leaf juice. Topically it is significantly inhibiting to fungi, yeast, and bacterial strains. Therefore, as a paint or dust it is well applied to various infections and inflammations from non-resolving external conditions.

Aloe's internal leaf material or leaf pulp is used topically for wound healing as well, but its modes of action differ from the leaf juice. The inner leaf pulp diminishes inflammation through its inhibitory effect on bradykinin breakdown and thromboxane, both mediators of inflammation. Skin repair as well as connective tissue synthesis is enhanced by Aloe's polysaccharide content. A fresh leaf poultice applied to burns is one of the best applications of the plant. Its speed in diminishing pain and redness verges on remarkable.

Secondarily the inner leaf pulp facilitates wound healing by its absorbent quality. Like all succulent plants, Aloe's internal structure is hydrophilic; it absorbs polar fluids and holds on to them. Placing an open leaf poultice on a damaged area facilitates the absorption of disorganized fluids in surface tissues, speeding injury resolution. Change leaf poultice often to fully take advantage of Aloe's absorbent qualities. Fresh Prickly pear pad will prove as efficacious as Aloe in this respect.

The inner leaf pulp taken internally has a lowering effect of blood glucose levels. It is reasonable to assume its mode of action is similar to Prickly pear's. The plant's array of hydrophilic constituents slows simple carbohydrate breakdown and absorption. Take several tablespoons before meals for its blood sugar lowering effect. Internally, the inner leaf pulp is soothing to stomach inflammation; also, it is healing to peptic ulcers.

Indications:
Leaf juice:
♦   Chronic constipation, dry feces
♦   Infections, bacterial and fungal (external)
Inner leaf pulp:
♦   Burns from heat and sun
♦   Wounds, injuries (external)
♦   Hyperglycemia
♦   Peptic ulcers

Collection: To begin, first clip a number of large hydrated leaves from the lower main stem. Place the clipped leaves with the cut ends facing down in a large strainer or colander; pack enough leaves into the strainer as to keep them upright. Place the strainer in a large bowl or pot. Let the exudate drain from the leaves until the flow has ceased. Larger yields will occur if the leaves are well hydrated from recent rains or watering. The collected leaf juice is then preserved with 20% alcohol or it can be slowly heated until it has thickened considerably, then dried and stored. It can be reconstituted or powdered as needed.

The internal pulp of the leaf is simply scraped out after an incision has been made. This mucilaginous pulp can then be stored in a refrigerator for 1-2 weeks at a time, unpreserved for use. Refined Aloe vera gel and juice are derived from the internal leaf and are processed to remove most of the anthraquinones, cellulose, and leaf material, but also have preservatives. Preparing your own is always preferable. Aloe has the greatest anthraquinone content throughout the summer months.

Preparations and Dosage:
♦ Leaf juice: 10-20 drops 1-2 times daily or externally as needed
♦ Inner leaf pulp: 1-2 tablespoons 2-3 times daily or externally as needed

Cautions: As with any anthraquinone containing plant, too much of the leaf juice can cause intestinal cramping and diarrhea. Do not take the leaf juice while pregnant due to the plant's sympathetic stimulation on uterine contractions, although in small amounts the inner leaf pulp is fine. Nursing babies may experience a laxative effect through the anthraquinone's transmission through breast milk.

Other Uses: Aloe is one of a number of herbs that has a cult-like following. It joins the ranks of Wild oregano, Olive leaf, Essiac tea, Noni juice, and others as being endowed with extraordinary powers. Although these herbs or formulas do have intrinsic value they have a window of 5-10 years of trendy use, and then they fall to the wayside. Aloe though has kept a tenacious foothold in the public's mind mainly through exaggerated claims by multi-level marketers.

ANTELOPE HORNS   *Asclepiadaceae* – Milkweed family

Asclepias asperula
Spider milkweed, Inmortal

Description: Antelope horns is a low-growing perennial, 1-2 feet tall, by 2-3 feet wide. The herbaceous stems radiate outward from a central taproot forming rounded mounds. The leaves, which are creased at the mid-vein, are 3-4 inches long and lance-shaped. They have wavy margins, are pointed at the tip and are alternately spaced but can form in groupings of 2 or 3 around the stems. The globe-like flower clusters are large, solitary, and form at stem ends. The individual flowers are 2-toned in their appearance; they are a mixture of greenish-white lobes and purple hoods. The slightly spiny, 2-4 inch long, seedpods stand upright and contain tufted, light brown, flat seeds.

Distribution: Antelope horns is found over a wide array of elevations. Look for the plant on dry plains, rocky slopes, and openings in Pinyon, Juniper, and Oak habitats from Kansas and Arkansas, west to Nevada and California. There is concern that in some traditional picking grounds in Colorado and

New Mexico it is becoming scarce. In these areas, collect the plant with a light hand or go further east to Texas where the plant is in greater abundance.

Chemistry: at least four cardenolide-type cardiac glycosides: calotropin, coroglaucignin, uscharidin, and uzarin; preganane glycosides and most likely the flavonoids rutin and quercetin

Medicinal Uses: Use Antelope horns when upper and lower respiratory tract tissues are dry due to lack of secretion. When it hurts to breath, the lungs feel stuffy and hot, and bronchial mucus is impacted and difficult to expectorate Antelope horns fits the picture. It is well used in episodes of dry bronchitis with a hacking cough, dry, non-spasmodic asthma, and in pleuritic conditions. Through Antelope horns' vagus nerve stimulation, similar to Pleurisy root's, bronchial tissue is moistened because of enhanced mucus secretion. This serves to soothe inflamed membranes. Antelope horns works well by itself or in formula for individuals with the above bronchial conditions that tend to exhibit adrenaline stress patterns. The plant's parasympathetic stimulation can be found by these people to be quite sedating. The effect Antelope horns has here is appropriate; often what a sick person needs most is time in bed.

Antelope horns has a moderate cardiac glycoside content, making its use as a mild heart stimulant practical. The plant slows and strengthens the heartbeat, as do the majority of properly dosed cardiac affecting plants, such as Convallaria and Selenicereus. It is best used when the pulse is weak and fast and cardiac output is diminished. Traditionally Antelope horns is used in heart weaknesses accompanying age, "tobacco heart", and heart enlargement. When constrictive breathing is dependent upon heart weakness Antelope horns can often seem bronchial dilating, when it is in fact improving tissue oxygenation through its cardiac stimulation. Also fluid retention, if dependent on heart weakness, is reduced.

Because of Antelope horns' parasympathetic stimulation and the effect the root constituents have on the intestinal walls, moderate to large doses of the plant can prove laxative – an attribute of this plant and most Milkweeds that is greatly reduced in drying. Although not very predictable, Antelope horns can stimulate menses if the period is stop and start or is late due to chronic stress or intense episodes of fear or anger. The plant has been put to use by Hispanic New Mexicans and Coloradoans for several hundred years to stimulate labor and to assist in the body's full separation and expulsion of the postnatal placenta.

Antelope horns' white-milky sap is antifungal and moderately antibacterial, as is the sap from most other Milkweeds. Although sticky, the fresh latex, when applied daily, is useful in treating athlete's foot, ringworm and other topical fungal infections. The latex, which is also high in proteolytic enzymes, is an effective wart treatment. Apply it fresh daily until the tissue softens enough so the wart can easily be picked off, or falls off by itself.

Indications:
- Asthma, dry, non-spasmodic
- Bronchitis, with non-productive cough
- Pleurisy
- Cardiac weakness, from age or tobacco use
- Amenorrhea
- Labor, slowed
- Fungal infections/warts (external)

Collection: When the foliage of the plant is visible, so it can serve as a locator, dig a hole about 1 foot across and 1-2 feet deep on one side of the plant. The soils that this plant is found in are typically dry, rocky, and calcrete-laden (at least in the southwest), so it is usually not an easy root to procure. The taproots of older plants can be several inches thick and up to 2 feet deep. They usually descend vertically with some secondary smaller roots coming off the main root. The outside root bark is brownish-tan; the inside is porous and cream-colored. The last 6-8 inches is the most difficult part to collect; it is the deepest part and it has narrowed considerably. Make sure to finish the job by getting the entire root. Discard the foliage. Use the roots within a year, shortly after the oils can become rancid, making the medicine tedious on the gut and liver.

Preparations: Spilt the porous roots several times length-wise. If living in an arid environment the roots will dry sufficiently. Chop the roots width-wise, every ¼-½ inch if environmental humidity is a factor or use a dehydrator.

Dosage:
- Root decoction/cold infusion: 2 ounces 2-3 times daily
- DPT (50% alcohol): 5-30 drops 3 times daily
- Fluidextract: 5-10 drops 3 times daily

- Latex pellets or '00' capsules: 1-2, 3 times daily
- Latex: externally as needed

Cautions: Do not use Antelope horns internally during pregnancy or while nursing. It is also unwise to mix the plant with heart effecting pharmaceuticals. In fact, Antelope horns best fits "old coots" with aging hearts who abhor doctors, pharmaceuticals, and the intrusive nature of that sector. Antelope horns is not recommended in cardiac excess: slow, bounding, forceful pulse, and strong determination of blood.

BACCHARIS   *Compositae* – Sunflower family

Baccharis glutinosa (Baccharis salicifolia)
Seepwillow, Batamote, Jarilla, Juatamote, Vara dulce

Baccharis pteronioides
Yerba del pasmo

Baccharis sarothroides
Desert broom, Rosin brush

Description: The Baccharis' profiled here have resinous leaves and male and female flowers on separate plants making them dioecious. Baccharis glutinosa is a large, fast-growing bush. Its branches are straight and vertical; they become woody and tan with age. The plant's lance-shaped, green leaves are serrated and when crushed are sticky and resinous. B. pteronioides, not nearly as dense as B. glutinosa, is a 3-6 foot tall bush. The lance-shaped leaves are variable in shape, but generally are toothed and form in clusters along the stems. The leaves and young stems have visible resin glands, which if crushed become sticky. The flowers develop at branch ends.

   Baccharis sarothroides being a pioneer plant starts cycles of flora and soil stabilization. It does this by being an advantageous grower in disturbed earth. The plant lives an average 10-20 years. After B. sarothroides dies, other longer-lived perennials establish themselves in the recently stabilized ground. If the plant receives adequate water, sizes of 9 feet by 9 feet are not uncommon. B. sarothroides' small linear leaves are easily overlooked; the plant has a twiggy, broom-like appearance.

Distribution: Baccharis glutinosa is a plant of watercourses and streamsides. Up to 5,000 feet, in the western United States, it frequently can be seen growing among Cottonwoods and Sycamores. Its extensive range stretches south from isolative pockets found in central Colorado. Being a riparian area plant, it often grows in dense thickets where environmental factors are optimal. B. pteronioides is found from 3,000-5,000 feet from northwestern Arizona east through southern New Mexico and southwestern Texas. Look for the plant growing on rocky hillsides and along drainages throughout Desert Grasslands and Oak Woodlands.

Baccharis sarothroides is commonly encountered in fallow fields, along roadsides, in drainage areas, and other disturbed soils. At elevations between 1,000-5,000 feet, it is found from northern Arizona along the Colorado River, south to include much of the lower part of the state, and west to southern California.

Chemistry: diterpenoids, lactones, coumarins, and saponins

Medicinal Uses: Use Baccharis when there is spasmodic diarrhea. It lessens intestinal cramping by inhibiting smooth muscle depolarization. Peristaltic waves are diminished, as is transit time of intestinal contents. Baccharis works well to limit intestinal excesses that have inflammatory overtones be it from functional or organic causes. Used in combination with Tree of heaven, its application in intestinal protozoal infections is worthwhile.

Baccharis diminishes stomach acidity. This has particular value in healing duodenal ulcers. Whether using Baccharis or other plants, such as Bird of paradise, an acidity lowering approach is primary in resolving duodenal ulcers. Establishment of healthier eating habits and stress management is needed in long-term resolution.

Externally applied to acute physical injuries Baccharis is analgesic and antiinflammatory. As a fresh plant poultice or liniment, the plant applied to an injured area diminishes pain noticeably. It is also mildly antimicrobial.

Indications:
- Spasmodic diarrhea with intestinal cramping
- Gastritis
- Duodenal ulcers
- Intestinal inflammation
- Cuts/scrapes (external)

Collection: With pruners, collect the top 4-6 inches of new leaf growth from the branch ends.

Preparations: The leaf infusion, the traditional preparation, is preferable to the fresh and dried plant tinctures, but they too still have value.

Dosage:
♦ Leaf infusion: 4-8 ounces 3-4 times daily
♦ FPT/DPT (60% alcohol): 30-60 drops 3-4 times daily

Cautions: Baccharis can potentate phenobarbital. It is unwise to use Baccharis with other anticholinergic therapies. Do not use during pregnancy due to the plant's menses stimulating potential.

BEARGRASS   *Agavaceae* – Agave family

Nolina microcarpa
Sacahuista

Description: Like other Agave family plants, Beargrass's dense, leafy mass is one of its most notable characteristics. This perennial has numerous, long, narrow leaves with minutely serrated margins. Dense thickets of the plant are possible due to underground stem growth and the development of numerous above ground leaf rosettes. Given ample size, nutrients, and water Beargrass flowers in the spring sending 1 or more 3-6 foot long stalks into the air. The open inflorescence is approximately 3 feet long. The compartmentalized seed capsules contain up to 6 small light brown seeds.

Distribution: From several isolated patches in Texas, west of the Pecos River, Beargrass spreads west through central New Mexico along the Rio Grande and Gila River Drainages. Through Arizona, Beargrass's range cuts a diagonal swath from the Colorado River area, below the Mogollon Rim to Pima and Cochise Counties. The plant is found on rocky slopes and hillsides, in canyons and along drainages. From 3,000-6,000 feet Beargrass inhabits several diverging vegetation zones making it a common plant in varying areas.

Chemistry: saponins: nolinospiroside, ruscogenin, and doubtlessly others

Medicinal Uses: Through a comparable saponin content, Beargrass' medicinal effect is similar to Butchers broom's (Ruscus aculeatus). Initially cued to the plant by Michael Moore, I have observed several cases where venous laxity in the leg and trunk area has improved. Applying the oil or salve tends to improve varicosities, spider veins, associated leg heaviness, and edema. The effects on vasculature of these Butchers broom-Beargrass saponins are well documented. Apparently, they have an adrenergic-like effect on veins and venules of the lower body, subsequently providing a tightening effect. There is reason to believe that taken internally Beargrass diminishes arthritic joint pain, similarly to other Agave family plants.

Indications:
- Venous stasis/varicosities/spider veins (internal and external)
- Leg heaviness, fatigue, and fluid retention (internal and external)
- Rheumatoid arthritis

Collection: Collect Beargrass's new leaves throughout the spring and summer. The newer leaves originate from the center of the plant and tend to rise vertically from this point. These are long, flexible, and sharp-edged. Paper-type cuts are easily received when harvesting.

Preparations: Dry the long leaves intact then cut them into 1-½ inch pieces for storage.

Dosage:
- Oil/salve: as needed
- Leaf decoction: 2-4 ounces 3 times daily
- '00' capsules: 2-3, 3 times daily

Cautions: Do not use during pregnancy.

Other Uses: The young, immature, 1-2 foot high flower stalks can be clipped at their bases, peeled and eaten either cooked or raw. Being slightly bitter and soapy, they are not the best edible fare, but are at least interesting.

BIRD OF PARADISE   *Leguminosae* – Pea family

Caesalpinia gilliesii (Poinciana gilliesii)
Yellow bird of paradise

Caesalpinia mexicana (Poinciana mexicana)
Mexican holdback, Mexican bird of paradise, Mexican poinciana

Caesalpinia pulcherrima (Poinciana pulcherrima)
Red bird of paradise, Pride of barbados, Peacock flower

Description: Caesalpinia gilliesii is a large perennial bush usually between 4-6 feet tall. The leaves form on stout many-branched stems. They are bipinnate; the secondary leaflets are ¼-½ inch in length and oblong. The most distinguishing characteristic is the plant's large, yellow flowers, which form in racemes at branch ends. The sepals are larger than the petals. The long red stamens are 2-4 inches long and out reach the other flower parts. The flattened pods are several inches long. When the seeds mature, the pods pop open, sending them many feet. In the summer, they can often be heard flying into windows and aluminum siding.
   Caesalpinia pulcherrima is an ungainly, large perennial bush. In areas throughout the southwest, the plant usually dies back to the ground in response to colder temperatures, but if protected it is only deciduous. In warmer areas, the plant reaches 4-10 feet in height. It is much larger in the tropics. The leaves are bipinnate, feathery, and composed of small leaflets. The plant's stems are lined with weak spines. The showy flowers are red-orange and form at branch ends; they are composed of 5 petals, 5 sepals, and 10 stamens.
   Caesalpinia mexicana tends to be similar in structure to the others, although the plant's foliage is denser due to its larger leaflets. This plant can sometimes reach tree-like proportions in protected areas, but is more typically 4-6 feet tall and bush-like. The showy yellow flower clusters form at branch ends. The plant, like C. pulcherrima, is cultivated extensively as an ornamental.

Distribution: All three plants are non-natives from Subtropical or Tropical America. Now though they are planted as ornamentals in warmer locales throughout the southwest. Caesalpinia gilliesii originally from Argentina and

Chile is well established in drainage areas and along roadsides from southeastern Arizona, southern New Mexico, to central Texas.

Chemistry: for Caesalpinia pulcherrima: peltogynoids, homoisoflavonoids, caesalpins, diterpenoids, pulcherrimin, bonducellin, and galactomannans; ellagitannin

Medicinal Uses: Bird of paradise tea is mainly a gastrointestinal tract medicine. Like many other desert Pea family plants, this plant is astringent and antiinflammatory. Internally the tea has use in irritative conditions such as gastritis and intestinal inflammation. The plant will also prove lessening to diarrhea and dysentery. The plant's range of flavonoids tends to be supportive to tissue structure and healing.

Externally the wash or poultice is soothing to rashes, bites, and stings. The plant has promise in relieving Poison ivy and chemical sensitivity rashes. In combination with internal use of Canyon bursage or Brittlebush, it can limit systemic outbreaks.

Indications:
- Gastritis
- Intestinal inflammation
- Diarrhea/dysentery
- Rashes/bites/stings (external)

Collection: Gather flowers, leaves, and stems. Dry for tea.

Preparations and Dosage:
- Herb infusion/decoction: 4-6 ounces 2-3 times daily
- Wash or poultice: as needed

Cautions: Several varieties of Caesalpinia have traditional use as emmenagogues, so it is best not to use this plant during pregnancy.

BRICKLEBUSH

Compositae – Sunflower family

Brickellia californica
Prodigiosa, Hamula, Peston

Description: Bricklebush is a semi-herbaceous bush of moderate stature. Normally it is 3-4 feet tall by the same dimension wide. The leaves, which are more or less triangularly shaped and covered with small rough hairs, are arranged alternately along the stem. With an oppositely arranged leaf pattern, new herbaceous growth can look deceivingly mint-like. During the winter, at middle and high elevations, the plant loses its leaves entirely; at lower elevations some may remain only to be released as new growth forms in the spring. The slender flower heads are interspaced with smaller leaves at the branch ends. The whole plant is sticky and it is not uncommon for the lower leaves to be dust and debris covered. After crushing a leaf between your fingers, the plant's potency can be partly determined by its sweet smell and stickiness.

Distribution: Bricklebush is a common plant of the west. From coastal California it ranges eastward through southern Idaho to the panhandles of Oklahoma and Texas, and south through Arizona and New Mexico. Throughout Bricklebush's lower-elevation habitats, it is usually found in canyons and ravines where at least some seasonal water flows. In areas of higher altitude and longitude, Bricklebush becomes a plant of open grasslands and Ponderosa pine forests.

Chemistry: phenylpropanoid: caffeic acid; sesquiterpenes: caryophyllene, caryophyllene epoxide, costunolide, β-farnesene, d germacrene, α-humulene, kauniolide, spathulenol, and zaluzanin c; flavonoids and pyrrolizidine alkaloids

Medicinal Uses: Firstly, the tea is a good hypoglycemic agent, being most useful for individuals with NIDDM (non-insulin dependent diabetes mellitus). Bricklebush is best suited for the thin and easily stressed Type 2 diabetic who is not on insulin and responds well to newer generation hypoglycemic pharmaceuticals such as Metformin. Among other unknown mechanisms, Bricklebush is presumed to diminish blood glucose levels by inhibiting the activity of norepinephrine on glycogen breakdown, therefore reducing stress mediated blood sugar elevations. Bricklebush taken before meals can reduce blood sugar concentrations by 15-20%, and potentially more with proper dietary adherence.

As with most bitter herbs, Bricklebush stimulates saliva production, hydrochloric acid and mucin, all necessary for proper upper gastrointestinal function and food breakdown. Bricklebush suits individuals who are under constant, low-grade adrenaline, fight or flight responses. Existing in this state tends to shift activity and blood movement away from digestion and assimilation to skeletal muscles and the brain. This pattern is useful if running away from or fighting a mugger, but not necessarily when stuck in gridlock traffic. Use Bricklebush before meals when long-term stress has caused indigestion, gastritis, and loss of appetite.

Bricklebush, like many other bitters, also has a stimulatory effect on the liver and is a useful cholagogue, increasing the quantity of bile released into the small intestine. Traditionally Bricklebush is used to lessen diarrhea with associated stomach pain and intestinal cramps.

Indications:
♦ Asecretory gastritis
♦ Dyspepsia form overwork and stress
♦ NIDDM
♦ Hepatic congestion
♦ Diarrhea with stomach pain and intestinal cramps

Collection: Before the plant flowers and when the leaves are verdant and sticky to the touch, prune the herb portion from Bricklebush's upper stems. After drying the herbage, strip the leaves from the stems and discard the latter.

Preparations and Dosage:
♦ Leaf infusion: 4-6 ounces 2-3 times daily
The leaf infusion is the best preparation. Drink between meals for its hypoglycemic action, before meals for its digestive properties and as needed for diarrhea.

Cautions: Bricklebush is not to be used by individuals with IDDM (insulin dependent diabetes mellitus) or Type 1, juvenile onset diabetes. Like many other Sunflower family plants in the Eupatory tribe, Bricklebush contains various pyrrolizidine alkaloids, but of small quantities. Given the plant's traditional non-toxic history and that the leaves are used, not the flowers (which typically have higher PA levels), consider Bricklebush a short to intermediate use herb. Do not use during pregnancy, while nursing or if there is a liver/gallbladder blockage. Although several ounces here and there for children with diarrhea are fine, consistent use with little ones is not recommended.

BRITTLEBUSH   *Compositae* – Sunflower family

Encelia farinosa
Incienso, Yerba del vaso

Description: Depending on the surrounding environment, Brittlebush has differing growth habits. Among rocks and boulders in mid-elevation desert foothills Brittlebush becomes upright, stretching out for the sun. Lower in elevation the plant appears as a semicircle mound of leaves hugging the ground. Leaf characteristics can vary depending on water availability. When produced in drier times, they are grayish-white, compact and hairy; the leaves' solar reflective ability increases making the plant more resilient to the intense sun. With rain, the leaves become large and green, enabling the plant to fully utilize the incoming solar energy. When in bloom radiant yellow flowers are suspended over the mounded body of the plant. The flower stems are narrow and long, giving the inflorescences a unique suspended look. The floral display can usually be seen in early to mid-spring, but it is not unknown for the plant to occasion an off-season bloom if enough water and proper temperatures are present. The fragile branches of Brittlebush are easily broken. Upon this a fine sap weeps from the damaged area; after drying the exudate hardens into crystallized, yellow bead-like droplets.

Distribution: Sub-freezing temperatures limit Brittlebush in elevation and northward expansion. The plant tops out at about 4,000 feet. Here it maintains itself with the help of sun-charged, heat radiating boulders, which help sustain the plant on cold winter nights. At lower elevations, pure stands of Brittlebush can be found growing in huge expanses on open flats and basins. Brittlebush is widespread throughout the Mojave and Sonoran Deserts. It can be found from the interior valleys of southern California to the southern tip of Nevada, westward through low elevation Arizona.

Chemistry: sesquiterpene lactone: farinosin; chromenes: encecalin and demethylenceclin; benzofuran: euparin

Medicinal Uses: The fresh plant tincture works quickly to diminish hayfever reactions. Its drying and antiinflammatory nature is expedient in its effect on sinus and ocular membranes. Use when allergic reaction has caused watery eyes and runny nose. The plant can also limit isolated Poison ivy outbreaks from transmuting into systemic reactions. Brittlebush tends to be diaphoretic and traditionally has been used in treating arthritic conditions aggravated by cold and damp weather. External preparations of the leaves or resin tend to be pain relieving as well. They can be used in accordance with the internal tea or tincture.

Indications:
♦ Rhinitis
♦ Poison ivy reactions, systemic
♦ Arthritis (internal and external)

Collection: Collect the hydrated and grayish-green leaves before the plant flowers after seasonal winter-spring rains.

Preparations and Dosage:
♦ FPT/DPT (50% alcohol): 30-60 drops 3-4 times daily
♦ Leaf infusion: 4-6 ounces 2-4 times daily
♦ External preparations: as needed

Cautions: Occasionally Brittlebush can elicit a caffeine-like nervous system excitability, so it is not recommended before bed. Moreover do not take the plant during pregnancy or while nursing.

Other Uses: In the past, the collected resin was used as a patching material, similar to Pine pitch, and as a regional incense in colonial era churches.

BURROBRUSH

Compositae – Sunflower family

Hymenoclea monogyra
Romerillo, Jecota

Hymenoclea salsola
White burrobrush, Jecota

Description: Hymenoclea monogyra is a large upright bush reaching 3-12 feet in height. The alternating thread-like leaves, which are elongated and 1-3 inches long, are delicate in appearance. Contrastingly, they are borne on vertical, grayish, stout branches. Both male and female flowers develop on the same plant and typically form in intermingled clusters on the branch ends. The developed fruit is surrounded by a whorl of winged bracts; this fan shape makes wind and water highly successful at seed dispersal. H. salsola is a smaller, more mound-forming plant. Its flowers are slightly larger and tend to be more densely arranged.

Distribution: Both Hymenoclea species are found primarily in wash beds where soil is sandy and loose. Also, look to the edges of these areas where the ground is slightly higher, banked, and equally exposed to rainwater. Hymenoclea monogyra is mostly found in drainages throughout the Sonoran and Chihuahuan Deserts. From central-eastern Arizona, the plant is found eastward to the Rio Grande Drainage, to southern Texas. H. salsola practically starts where H. monogyra leaves off. From western Arizona's Sonoran and Mojave Deserts, the plant is found further north into Mineral County, Nevada and through much of inland California.

Chemistry: sesquiterpene lactones: hymenin, hymenolin, salsolin, ambrosin, neoambrosin, coronopilin, dihydrocoronopilin, ilicic acid, psilostachyin, psilostachyin c, costunolide, and b-eudesmol

Medicinal Uses: Chemically, Burrobrush and Canyon bursage are closely allied and contain many of the same constituents. Medicinally there is not a great difference between the two. Traditional use in Mexico indicates the plant is used in reducing sensitivity and pain in joint inflammations. Use Burrobrush as you would Canyon bursage leaf. See Canyon bursage for a full discussion.

Collection: Prune the upper new leaf growth from the plant and wrap using string or rubber bands into small bundles or dry loosely in a flat out of direct sunlight.

Preparations and Dosage:
♦ FPT/DPT (60% alcohol): 20-60 drops 3 times daily
♦ Leaf infusion: 2-4 ounces 3 times daily

Cautions: Do not use during pregnancy.

BUTTONBUSH   *Rubiaceae* – Madder family

Cephalanthus occidentalis
Buttonwillow, Buttonball, Riverbush

Description: Buttonbush is a large, deciduous shrub that forms dense thickets. In rare instances, it grows as a small tree, 30-40 feet in height, usually in isolative pockets in southern Arkansas and eastern Texas. As the plant ages the blackish-brown trunk bark becomes deeply fissured. Like other Madder family plants, Buttonbush's leaves are situated in wholes of 3 or 4, although sometimes they are found in oppositely arranged pairs. The leaves are shiny, leathery, and oblanceolate. The small trumpet-shaped, cream-colored flowers are arranged densely in ball-like clusters terminating at branch ends, hence the name Buttonbush.

Distribution: Look for Buttonbush along streamsides, pond and marsh borders, and river bottoms, or at least in places where the earth stays consistently moist. From sea level to approximately 6,000 feet, Buttonbush is found throughout North America.

Chemistry: cephalanthin, cephaletin, cephalin, and tannin, among other constituents

Medicinal Uses: Although not used extensively in present-day herbalism, Buttonbush still has the same value today as it did in the past. It is effective in strengthening the gastrointestinal tract in weakened and atonic states. It is a useful bitter tonic that can be used with success in chronic states of indigestion. After a meal if stomach secretions are deficient, bloating, oppressive feelings of fullness, and general dyspepsia can ensue; in these situations Buttonbush stimulates proper digestive responses.

Living a harried lifestyle (particularly, worry and rumination while eating) is a quick way to set up harmful digestive patterns. Buttonbush redirects digestive emphasis back where it belongs, to the belly. Buttonbush, as is the case with most bitters, combines well with aromatic herbs such as Ginger, Peppermint, or Fennel. The plant's stimulatory effect on the liver and gallbladder make it of use in relieving mild constipation, especially if there is difficulty digesting fat.

Indications:
- ♦ Indigestion
- ♦ Intestinal distress, in response to meals high in fat
- ♦ Constipation, dependent on stress and worry
- ♦ Liver/gallbladder congestion, non-organic causes

Collection: Collect the leaves in the spring before the plant flowers, or the inner bark in colder seasons.

Dosage and Preparations:
- ♦ Leaf infusion/bark decoction: 4-6 ounces before meals 3 times daily
- ♦ FPT/DPT (50% alcohol): 30-40 drops before meals 3 times daily

Cautions: Because Buttonbush is a gastric stimulant do not use if there is an over production of hydrochloric acid (which tends to be rare), or if there is an existing duodenal ulcer. Because there are still unknowns concerning Buttonbush's physiologic effects, it is best not to use in pregnancy or while nursing. Moreover, do not use if there is an active biliary blockage.

CALIFORNIA POPPY   *Papaveraceae* – Poppy family

Eschscholtzia californica
Copa de oro

Eschscholtzia mexicana (Eschscholtzia aliena, E. arizonica, E. jonesii, E. paupercula)
Mexican poppy, Gold poppy

Description: Eschscholtzia californica is a small, clump-forming annual or short-lived perennial. Its bluish-green 5-20 inch long stems weaken and droop with age. They are smooth and covered with a fine, white-waxy coating that is easily rubbed off. The leaves are finely dissected. Most are basal but some are attached alternately along the stems. The showy 4-petaled flowers are generally orange but are occasionally yellow and even white. The seed capsules are 1-celled, narrow, ribbed, and slender; contained within are numerous small, dark seeds. Although some botanists do not consider E. mexicana a separate species, there are some general differences: mainly the plant is smaller and the flowers tend to be predictably yellow-gold in color.

Distribution: Eschscholtzia californica is found throughout California, usually below 5,000 feet, and in parts of Oregon and Washington. The densest populations occur west and south of the Sierra Nevadas to the Mojave Desert. E. mexicana has a sporadic occurrence across Arizona, Nevada, Utah, southern New Mexico, and southwestern Texas. Both species are dependent upon winter-spring rains and if given sufficient moisture will carpet hillsides and rocky slopes in color.

Chemistry: pavine alkaloids: eschscholtzine and californidine; benzophenantridine alkaloids: sanguinarine and chelerythrine; protopine alkaloids: protopine and allocryptopine; berberine and other compounds

Medicinal Uses: Consider California poppy a sub-opiate, meaning its effect is broadly opiate-like, although much weaker than popularly used isolated substances. California poppy is distinctly sedative and spasmolytic. Use the plant when sleep is difficult from anxiousness and particularly from acute pain. It is lessening to both nerve centered and muscular pain. California poppy is useful in diminishing a spasmodic cough when the face and chest are flushed, there is a strong, bounding pulse, and even fever. It is a rather chemically complex plant with diverging effects on adrenergic neurotransmitters. However California poppy is explained to work, it does work in unchanging ways. Topically, the plant is antimicrobial and can be used on a wide array of bacterial conditions that also respond well to Berberis-Mahonia plants.

The plant can be useful to highly motivated individuals in diminishing or eliminating stronger opiate habits or other similar non-opiate pharmaceutical habits used for pain relief. California poppy is particularly useful combined with Golden smoke. To some sensitive individuals the plant can exhibit very subtle euphoric properties. Consider the plant child-safe.

Indications:
- Pain, from acute injury
- Insomnia/anxiety
- Spasmodic cough
- Cuts/scrapes (external)

Collection: When California poppy is fully mature having both flowers and seed capsules, pull the whole plant from the ground, tap root and all.

Preparations and Dosage:
- FPT/DPT (50% alcohol): 60-90 drops 3 times daily
- Whole plant infusion: 4-8 ounces 3 times daily
- Topical preparations: as needed

Cautions: California poppy may potentate analgesic-sedative pharmaceuticals. Do not use during pregnancy. Long-term use is acceptable, as the plant is generally not considered habit forming.

Other Uses: Eschscholtzia mexicana has a peculiar ability of growing in copper rich soils and has been used as an adjunct indicator of the mineral.

CALTROP   *Zygophyllaceae* – Caltrop family

Kallstroemia grandiflora
Orange caltrop, Arizona poppy

Kallstroemia californica
California caltrop

Kallstroemia parviflora
Warty caltrop

Description: Caltrop is an herbaceous annual that commonly grows prostrated on the ground. Large plants can reach 3-4 feet in length. The small leaves are pinnate and are arranged in pairs. The flowers are 5-petaled and are greenish-yellow to bright orange. The mature fruit is small and breaks up into 8-12 nutlets. Caltrop superficially resembles Puncturevine.

Kallstroemia grandiflora is the largest Caltrop of the three species profiled here. Its many branched stems can reach lengths of 4 feet. They have stiff, prominent yellow hairs as do the leaves (although they are smaller and are isolated mainly to the outer margins). The leaves are 1-3 inches long and have 3-7 sets of smaller leaflets. The large orange flowers are prominent and are between 2/3-1¼ inches long. They are solitary and attached to smaller stems originating from the leaf axils. The oval seedpods split into 8-12 nutlets or carpels.

Kallstroemia californica is smaller in stature than K. grandiflora. The stems and leaves are almost completely lacking hairs. The ¼-½ inch long leaflets are arranged into 3-7 sets. The orange-yellow flowers have small petals; the seedpods separate into 8-12 wedge-shaped nutlets. K. parviflora is a 1-3 foot long plant with few white stem hairs. The leaves are composed of 3-5 sets of leaflets. The flowers, like K. californica, are small; the petals are typically a ¼-inch long. The small fruits are similar to the others.

Distribution: In southern California Kallstroemia grandiflora is found along with Creosote bush around 900 feet in elevation. In central and southern Arizona, the plant is encountered below 5000 feet, often in disturbed soils, but generally on open slopes, flats, and mesas. It is also found in similar areas in New Mexico and east to Texas. K. parviflora enjoys a wider range; from 5,000-6,000 feet in southern California it is found east to Mississippi. K.

californica is found throughout most of Arizona, between 100-7,000 feet, throughout southeastern California, and north to southern Colorado.

Chemistry: flavonoids: quercetin, isorhamnetin, and tricin

Medicinal Uses: Caltrop is an interesting mix of mild astringent and alterative. Internally the tea is lessening to diarrhea and is mildly sedating to gastrointestinal tract inflammation. Passive hemorrhaging of the urinary tract as well as menorrhea is lessened. Caltrop's relation to other alterative plants in the same family such as Creosote bush and Guaiacum suggest that it is well used in low-grade, chronic inflammatory conditions. Traditional use supports the notion that the plant is indicated internally (externally as well) for hive outbreaks, rashes, and fevers. Think of the plant as a diminutive Creosote bush and because of its mildness it can be used longer-term for many of the same conditions. The isotonic tea used as an eyewash is soothing to conjunctivitis and allergy induced eye irritation.

Indications:
♦ Diarrhea
♦ GI tract inflammation
♦ Menorrhea
♦ Hives/rashes (internal and external)
♦ Conjunctivitis (eyewash)

Collection: Gather and dry the entire plant, small taproot included.

Preparations and Dosage:
♦ Herb infusion: 4 ounces 3 times daily
♦ Eyewash: 2-3 times daily

Cautions: To err on the side of caution, do not use during pregnancy or while nursing.

CAMPHORWEED

Compositae – Sunflower family

Heterotheca subaxillaris
Telegraph plant, Arnica

Description: When this annual (occasionally bi-annual) is young, its basal leaves point up from the ground. This identifying characteristic is very different from other herbaceous plants whose initial leaf growth radiates out flattened against the ground's surface. Later in the season when the stalk develops, it becomes many branched at the top, giving credence to another common name for Camphorweed – Telegraph plant. The leaves on the lower stems are petioled, whereas the upper leaves clasp the stem. Generally, they are ovoid, irregularly toothed, wavy, and arranged alternately along the stem. In mass, the common looking yellow composite flowers appear disorganized; they are approximately ½-inch wide by ¼-inch high. The whole plant is sticky to the touch due to its gland tipped leaf and stem hairs. The camphor-like odor given off affords the plant a level of respect its weedy appearance tends to detract from.

Distribution: Camphorweed, like many other weedy plants, does extremely well around disturbed soils. It is found along roadsides, trails, and the margins of fields. Look for Canadian fleabane and Tobacco, if found Camphorweed is not far away. From 1,000-5,000 feet the plant's range is quite extensive – and still expanding – in the United States. From mid-east coast states, such as Delaware, it extends to Florida and west to Arizona. Heterotheca grandiflora, its flowers being slightly larger, can be found from New Mexico to southern California.

Chemistry: Heterotheca general: flavonoids: galangin, kaempferol, and quercetin; monoterpenoids, sesquiterpenoids, and triterpenoids

Medicinal Uses: Externally applied Camphorweed is diminishing to pain, inflammation, and the fluid build-up of acute injury. The plant's medicinal qualities lend themselves well in treating numerous acute accidents – sprains, contusions, etc. Specifically, Camphorweed inhibits inflammatory mediators within injured tissues, diminishing subsequent edema and pain.

There are qualitative differences in how to properly use Camphorweed versus true Arnica (Arnica montana and others). At first glance, they seem slight, because both are used topically for painful episodes, but the differences are marked. Camphorweed is a tissue sedative, lessening the reactive process that brings about inflammation. Arnica actually heightens the body's response locally by increasing white blood cell activity. This is why conventional herb wisdom calls for Arnica to be applied "when it hurts to move", not "when it hurts to be still". Use Arnica when the condition is subacute and not when the problem is hot, fiery, and throbbing. Use Camphorweed when the injury is acute and painful, particularly if the pain does not stop when the injured part is at rest.

Indications:
♦ Acute injury with pain, swelling, and fluid build-up (external)

Collection: From late spring through summer, collect the whole herb portion. Use the leaves, stems, and flowers alike, fresh or dry.

Preparations and Dosage:
♦ Leaf infusion/liniment/oil: as needed

Cautions: None known for external use.

CANADIAN FLEABANE   *Compositae* – Sunflower family

Conyza canadensis (Erigeron canadensis)
Horseweed, Colt's tail, Pazotillo

Description: This annual or occasional biennial grows tall and upright. At maturity it can reach upwards of 5-6 feet. From spring through early summer, the plant appears as an up-turned feather duster. Its leaves, which are several inches long, are clustered along the main stems and spread outward. As time passes, nutrient dynamics are shifted to the small inconspicuous whitish flower heads that form in staggered masses at the plant's top. At this point, the leaves on the lower central stem lose their vitality and often yellow. The achenes are scattered by wind and many will surely sprout the following year.

Distribution: Look for this advantageous weed in disturbed places such as roadsides, irrigation ditches, and other moist areas where water tends to collect and linger. Unlike looking for some annuals, Canadian fleabane is predictable in where it will be found. If you know where to find it, chances are it will be found there year after year provided ground moisture is the same. Originally indigenous to the eastern part of the country, Canadian fleabane is now found throughout the west. Since the early eighteenth century, Canadian fleabane has even crossed the Atlantic Ocean and is now ubiquitous in parts of Europe.

Chemistry: sesquiterpenes: trans-α-bergamotene, delta-cadenol, α-curcumene, α-farnesene, and farnesol; monoterpenes: carvone and α-thujene; lipids: enoic and diynoic acids; miscellaneous lactone: furanone; flavonoid: syringic acid

Medicinal Uses: An infusion of Canadian fleabane is highly useful in chronic inflammatory states of the intestines where there is diarrhea, attending mucus, and tissue disruption. This preparation is well used in ulcerative colitis. Canadian fleabane's overall astringency and tightening effect on mucus membranes is not derived wholly from the plant's tannins, but from its volatile oil content, which is locally, and in the case of the essential oil, systemically hemostatic. The plant's tonic effect on intestinal walls has use in "leaky gut syndrome", where immune responses and inflammatory mediators are wreaking havoc in the area, resulting in malabsorption, digestive discomfort and food allergies.

The essential oil of Canadian fleabane or oil of Erigeron as it is commonly called is a systemic hemostatic. In times when modern coagulate pharmaceuticals were non-existent, various herbal preparations did (and still do) work to quell mild to moderate hemorrhaging. Today, the use of oil of Erigeron to staunch internal bleeding is considered antiquidated, but there is merit to the principle. Use oil of Erigeron internally to quell mild hemorrhaging from the lungs, particularly if severe coughing is a contributing factor. Likewise, if there is mild uterine bleeding after childbirth or blood in the urine from acute injury to the kidneys, the essential oil will prove useful. Mild bleeding from the stomach and intestines, most likely from ulcerative conditions, acute physical injury, or the aftermath of viral or microbial espousers can be stopped or at least lessened.

Indications:
♦ Chronic intestinal inflammation
♦ Diarrhea with mucus and blood

♦   Malabsorptive syndromes with intestinal debility
♦   Passive hemorrhaging from the lungs, kidneys, uterus, stomach, and intestines (essential oil)

Collection and Preparations: Collect the upper half of the plant before it flowers. After drying the entire portion, garble the leaves from the stems. Discard the woody stem portions since the majority of volatile oils are held within the leaf. The leaf infusion is the superior preparation.

Dosage:
♦   Leaf infusion: 4-6 ounces 3-4 times daily
♦   Essential oil: 3-10 drops 3 times daily

Cautions: The main problem with Canadian fleabane use is developing an over-confidence of its sphere of influence. If there is injury resulting in serious blood loss the emergency room is the best place to start. Avoid during pregnancy; the plant may exert an unwanted vasoconstricting effect on uterine lining.

CANYON BURSAGE   *Compositae* – Sunflower family

Ambrosia ambrosioides
Canyon ragweed, Chicua, Yerba del sapo

Description: Canyon bursage is a moderately sized, perennial shrub. Its deciduous leaves are serrated and grow into elongated triangles, 1-2 inches wide by 6-8 inches long. In the spring, the pistillate flowers mature into burs resembling a small cocklebur, and similarly they stick to clothing and animal fur. Of all the Ambrosias, Canyon bursage is the most tropical in appearance and requirements. It is dependent on summer monsoon rains and warm temperatures to survive in the southwest deserts. The name Ambrosia refers to the fragrance the leaf aromatics emit when the plant is crowded in canyons and the summer air moves through. It may not be the nectar of the gods, but it certainly is not rank as described by many botanical authors.

Distribution: Look for Canyon bursage growing along washes, canyons, and draws where rainfall deeply saturates the ground. From central Arizona, it ranges south.

Chemistry: the foliage contains sesquiterpene lactones: damsin, damsinic acid, franserin, parthenolide, and psilostachyin c; flavonoid: hispidulin

Medicinal Uses: Canyon bursage root is a valuable remedy in relieving menstrual cramps. In addition to being a reliable menstrual stimulant, the root is also useful when menses has become sluggish and there are corresponding pelvic feelings of inertia and congestion. Root preparations are also quieting to stomach and intestinal cramps. Its spasmolytic activity is especially well suited in diminishing rapid intestinal movement from acute viral or stress initiated diarrhea.

Although not an entirely different medicine, the leaves of Canyon bursage elicit other therapeutic responses. They tend to diminish allergic reactions that are head centered. Rhinitis from pollen, dust, and animal hair is abated. Whole body allergic reactions that manifest as general itchiness or even hive breakouts are diminished. It is proposed that Canyon bursage is broadly antiinflammatory and specifically is diminishing to IgE antibody responses that play a central role in the allergy process.

Indications:
- Menstrual cramps with pelvic congestion
- Tardy menstruation with stop and start bleeding
- GI tract cramps
- Rhinitis and sinusitis, allergy derived
- Allergic reactivity, body-wide

Collection: Harvest Canyon bursage leaves when they are dark green and aromatic, usually in mid-spring or during summer monsoon rains. Collect the roots throughout the winter or spring when available moisture has enlivened them, rather then in the fall when they are apt to be in a dry stupor. The plant's taproots reach downward 3-4 feet so it is wise to collect in a wash where digging is easier. Even though Canyon bursage is regionally abundant, it is a wise practice not to take the entire root mass one plant has, subsequently killing the plant. When the side roots are exposed, trim several here and there while leaving the main large taproots in place. Doing this you will be able to collect a pound or two from an older plant with little harm. When you have the roots in your hands, smell them; they are aromatic and earthy. Several other species, namely Ambrosia deltoidea, A. artemisiifolia, and A. trifida have similar leaf uses. In comparing root qualities, these species are woody and less aromatic, therefore less therapeutic.

Preparations and Dosage:

♦ FPT/DPT (60% alcohol): 20-60 drops 3 times daily
♦ Leaf infusion/root decoction: 2-4 ounces 3 times daily

Cautions: Individuals who are allergic to ragweed should be mindful of this plant. Although the pollen containing flowers are not collected for use, some extremely sensitive people may have reactions to Canyon bursage's lactone content, present in the entire plant. If you feel this may be the case personally, start with small doses and monitor yourself to see how this plant affects you. Considering Canyon bursage's stimulating effect on the uterus, it is not an herb to use during pregnancy. Because of this plant's weak drug-like action consider it a short-term use medicine, not a long-term tonic.

CANYON WALNUT   *Juglandaceae* – Walnut family

Juglans major (*Juglans microcarpa var. major*)
Arizona walnut, Arizona butternut, Black walnut, Nogal

Description: Canyon walnut is a hard wood deciduous tree, not unlike in form and character Black walnut (Juglans nigra) of the east. The mature tree can reach 50 feet in height and develop an impressively broad canopy. The trunk can span several feet in width; the bark is dark and becomes deeply fissured with age. Canyon walnut's leaves are composed of 5-7 pairs of large, lanceolate, serrated leaflets with one terminating the bunch. This monoecious tree has male and female flowers separated into different groupings. The staminate flowers hang catkin-like, while the pistillate flowers, once pollinated, form into the fruits. As the fruit or walnut matures the skin around the hull turns from green to brownish-black. The whole plant has a unique pungency, particularly when the leaves or fruits are bruised. In the spring, when Canyon walnut is young and is beginning to leaf out, it looks very similar to Smooth sumac (Rhus glabra). Often the two plants can be found growing next to each other in mountainous drainages. The typical walnut family smell is a definite give away, helping plant people ascertain what plant is what.

Distribution: Canyon walnut is found along waterways and in canyons throughout central and southeastern Arizona. In New Mexico, it is predominant along the Gila River and southern Rio Grande Drainages; it is also found in isolative pockets in the southern part of the state. The tree as well can be found in southwestern Texas. Juglans californica, a closely allied species is found in drainage areas among foothills and valleys in warmer coastal-inland California.

Chemistry: juglone, α-hydrojuglone and β-hydrojuglone, ellagic acid, gallic acid, caffeic acid, neochlorogenic acids, and germacrene d

Medicinal Uses: In small, therapeutic doses, Canyon walnut is tonifying and soothing to the gastrointestinal tract, particularly to the large and small intestines. It quiets gastritis, irritative diarrhea and intestinal inflammation with associated ileocecal irritation. Use the tea or tincture where through chronic intestinal derangement there is nutrient malabsorption, particularly of fats, creating an overall deficient intestinal state. Canyon walnut is moderately antispasmodic, which calls for its use when there are intestinal cramps with flatulence. Internal use of the plant also clears the skin of acne-like eruptions particularly when there is fat malabsorption dependent on consuming rich foods to excess.

In larger doses, Canyon walnut is laxative and is indicated in constipation where there is liver sluggishness. Equally, there is need for the plant if constipation easily ensues if attention is not diligently maintained in keeping the bowels regular. Constrictive respiratory disturbances and chronic inflammatory issues sometimes are benefited by Canyon walnut through its tonifying effect on intestinal walls.

Although not systemically useful in limiting Candida infections, Canyon walnut can be helpful in abating the issue if limited to the gastrointestinal tract. Even though this plant is somewhat antifungal, berberine-containing plants such as Desert barberry or Oregon grape are more so, making Canyon walnut or Black walnut over-rated in this area.

Sometimes recommended in diminishing fungal infections, the fresh plant applied topically, as a poultice, whether from the green hulls, bark or leaves is rather caustic and can cause redness and blistering in even short exposures. Canyon walnut's juglone content is largely responsible for this. When the fresh plant is crushed larger juglone-like complexes are oxidized and broken down to juglone, which is responsible for the resulting brown pigmentation and characteristic smell.

Indications:

- GI tract inflammation with attending diarrhea or constipation
- Nutrient/lipid malabsorption
- Intestinal cramps
- Candida albicans infection, GI tract involvement

Collection: Collect the green leaves when available; the hulls of the fruit should be harvested when they are just starting to turn brown. Depending on the locale and elevation of the tree, this can take place anywhere from May to August. Collect the bark in long strips from secondary branches with little thickened-outward bark. Be aware that juglone makes a nice, brown stain, that when on the skin does not remove well with soap and water.

Preparations and Dosage:
- FPT/DPT (50% alcohol): 30-60 drops 3 times daily
- Leaf infusion/bark, rind decoction: 4-6 ounces 3 times daily

Cautions: Do not use during pregnancy or topically on abraded or sensitive tissues.

Other Uses: The kernels of the ripe fruits, although smaller than English and Black walnut, are tasty. As a stain or dye, the tincture or tea may be only rivaled by Desert rhubarb in its impermeability.

CHASTE TREE

Verbenaceae – Vervain family

Vitex agnus-castus
Monk's pepper, Indian spice, Safe tree

Description: Chaste tree is a large, deciduous bush or small tree capable of obtaining 20-25 feet in height. The plant's 5-7 lance shaped leaflets are palmately arranged and are supported on long leaf stems. Each leaflet is dark green above and much lighter beneath. Like other Vervain family plants the leaves are oppositely arranged along ridged upper stems. The flower spikes form at branch ends and are of a variety of colors. Lavender, blue, and white are typical. Each flower is tubular with 5 fused petals, which curl under at the flower's opening. The fruits are surrounded by a hardened layer and resemble peppercorns. They are green when young but dry to a purplish-grey. When crushed they are aromatic and spicy smelling.

Distribution: Originally a plant of the Mediterranean region of southern Europe, northern Africa, and western Asia, Chaste tree is now found throughout warmer parts of the United States. The plant is extensively naturalized through the southeast and is found as a thriving ornamental throughout warmer southwestern regions. Moreover, Chaste tree can be purchased at nurseries and found planted along roadsides.

Chemistry: iridoid glycosides: agnuside, aucubin, agnucastoside a, b, and, c, and mussaenosidic acid; flavonoids: casticin, orientin, isovitexin, luteolin, luteolin, artemetin, and isorhamnetin; diterpenes: vitexilactone, vitexlactam, and rotundifuran; phenylbutanone glucoside: myzodendrone; α-pinene and β-pinene, limonene, cineole, and sabinene

Medicinal Uses: Chaste tree is best used by women who suffer from premenstrual breast tenderness and heavy menstrual bleeding associated with longer than 28-day menstrual cycles; if lifestyle stress and moderate to heavy caffeine use is present then the plant is doubly indicated. Chaste tree supports proper corpus luteum function and therefore progesterone levels, while inhibiting excess prolactin levels. Chaste tree is effective in rectifying anovulatory cycles, corresponding infertility, secondary amenorrhea, uterine fibroids, and excessive menstrual bleeding dependent upon excessive cellular proliferation of the endometrium. These are all essentially issues of progesterone deficiency.

Because of Chaste tree's alignment with the Vervain family the plant tends to be a mild sedative, even outside of its diminishing effect on stress mediated prolactin release. This makes Chaste tree useful in premenstrual discomforts with associated anxiety, mood swings, and irritability. The plant is equally useful in beginning stages of menopause. It combines well with Motherwort in reducing hot flashes and associated irritability.

Chaste tree is of use in reestablishing coherent menstrual cycles after prolonged estrogen based contraception. Moreover, an important distinction between Chaste tree and oral or topical pharmaceutical grade progesterone use is necessary here. Progesterone, as it naturally occurs, is a reproductive hormone that is dependent upon a healthy corpus luteum and proper levels of FSH (follicle stimulating hormone) and LH (lutenizing hormone). Chaste tree supports correct corpus luteum function and therefore is pro-progesterone. Oral or topical use of progesterone does nothing for the corpus luteum but only for tissues that respond to that hormone. Use of progesterone for PMS or associated corpus luteum deficiency issues is like putting a new stereo in an old beat up truck; great tunes but still the same old truck.

Traditionally Chaste tree, as its name implies, has been used as an anaphrodisiac. I personally have seen several men use Chaste tree to curb libido because of their wives unavailability. One man became somewhat frightened after observing practically all penile sensation had left him. After discontinuing Chaste tree normal functioning returned after 2-3 weeks. Lastly Chaste tree has been found to increase milk production in lactating women and is safe for breast feeding infants.

Indications:
♦ Premenstrual discomforts with breast tenderness, agitation, and anxiety
♦ Heavy menstruation
♦ Anovulatory cycles
♦ Uterine fibroids, subserous
♦ Perimenopause
♦ Insufficient lactation

Collection: Strip the mature fruits from the branch ends. Lay out to dry.

Preparations and Dosage:

♦   DPT (60% alcohol): 30-40 drops 3 times daily

It is important to note that the effect of Chaste tree may not be noticed immediately. Often several months of use is needed to notice the benefit of therapy.

Cautions: Do not use during pregnancy.

CHICKWEED   *Caryophyllaceae* – Pink family

Stellaria media
Common chickweed

Stellaria nitens
Shiny starwort, Shining chickweed

Description: Stellaria media is a small herbaceous annual. Occasionally the plant can be found standing upright, but more often it is seen prostrated, rooting at stem nodes. The newer leaves are normally stemless; mature leaves have petioles, are opposite and ovate in shape. Each stem has a column of small hairs traversing its length. Flowers arises individually out of leaf axils; they are borne on long, slender pedicels. These small white flowers have 5 petals; each petal is 2-parted giving individual flowers a 10-petaled appearance. The fruit matures into an ovoid capsule with very small, reddish-brown seeds.

Stellaria nitens is also an annual, but is upright and stout. The leaves tend to be lanceolate. The plant's hairs are spread over the entire stem. The flowers form in cymes and are very inconspicuous owing to the very small petals and larger sepals.

Distribution: Stellaria media is a common plant. Owing to its European origin, it can be found in lawns, gardens, fields, and other moist and disturbed soils. S. nitens is largely native to the western half of the country; from Montana and British Columbia it ranges south to California, Arizona, and to parts of New Mexico. It is found in rocky crevices, next to drainages, and under shrubs and trees where it gathers protection from the sun.

Chemistry: plastocyanin, c-glycosylflavones, hentriacontane, hexacosanyl palmitate, methylstearate, pentacosanol, triacontanol, triacontanoic acid, sitosterol, and its β-d-glucoside

Medicinal Uses: All Chickweeds in the Stellaria and Cerastium genuses can be used alike. The plant is easily overlooked because of its unassuming appearance and mild nature. Externally it is best used for hot, eruptive skin afflictions in the form of a fresh plant poultice, oil, salve, or juice. The plant's cooling and soothing influence sedates itchiness from bites and rashes. Applied to sunburn and heat burns Chickweed lessens surface redness and inflammation and slightly diminishes pain. The infusion taken internally is a soothing diuretic, useful in sporadic urinary tract pain, and in combination with Canadian fleabane or Canyon walnut, it is a useful adjunct in treating low-grade intestinal inflammation.

Indications:
♦ Painful urination
♦ Intestinal inflammation
♦ Sunburn and other burns (external)
♦ Rashes/hives/bites (external)

Collection: In early to mid-spring collect the upper herb portion before it dies back. In the arid southwest with high temperatures and lack of rainfall, the plant bolts quickly.

Preparations: To make Chickweed oil wilt the plant by 50% of its weight. Chop into ½-inch sections and add 5 parts of olive oil. Steep in a warm place, but not in the direct sun, for 10-12 days. Strain the oil from the herb but do not squeeze the marc. Remove any water from the oil before storing.

Dosage:
♦ Poultice/wash/oil/salve/juice: as needed
♦ Herb infusion: 4-8 ounces 3 times daily

Other Uses: The tender, new leaves can be added to salads and used as a garnish. They have an interesting cucumber-like taste.

CHINCHWEED

Compositae – Sunflower family

Pectis papposa
Fetid marigold, Pague

Description: This small, mounding annual is no more than a foot high; often it is splayed circularly with its outward stems resting on the ground forming tidy circles. Its leaves are verdant in relation to the tan-yellowish sandy soils in which it grows. The opposite leaves have prominent oil glands, are linear, and 1-2½ inches long by ¼-½ of an inch wide. The small yellow flowers form at stem ends and are comprised of both disk and ray flowers with the latter being most prominent. They are also dotted with oil glands. The small seeds are wind carried. When crushed the whole plant is strongly aromatic; it has a peculiar odor not at all unpleasant. The plant's growth is signaled by summer rains and can be expected to be seen from mid-summer to early fall.

Distribution: Look for Chinchweed from 6,000 feet and lower. The plant is common on sand and clay rich soils, mostly occurring on desert flats with Creosote bush and Joshua tree yucca. The plant is found from Utah to southeast California through to Arizona and New Mexico.

Chemistry: specific constituents not known but at least: flavonoids and volatile oils

Medicinal Uses: Chinchweed is closely allied with Deerweed, Dogweed, and Mountain marigold; often medicinal uses overlap. The tea or tincture of Chinchweed is of use in relieving a stomachache. Through Chinchweed's carminative effect it expels stomach gas and is an efficient remedy for hiccups. The plant diminishes intestinal cramps and will lessen diarrhea in associated conditions. Several teaspoons of the tea are soothing to colicky babies. Chinchweed's volatile oils, when in contact with gastrointestinal smooth muscle coats, tend to sedate, lessen spasm, and therefore provide relief. Mixed with a bitter tonic herb such as Tarbush or Rayweed it will enhance gastric stimulation by bringing more blood to the stomach walls through topical vasodilation.

Indications:
♦ Stomachache

- Hiccups
- Gastrointestinal cramps with diarrhea

Collection: Pull the entire plant up from its base, small taproot included.

Preparations: If using for tea, after drying, garble the leaves and flowers from the stems; discard the stems and roots.

Dosage:
- Herb infusion: 4-6 ounces 3 times daily
- FPT/DPT (60% alcohol): 30-60 drops 3 times daily

Cautions: None known.

Other Uses: Rubbed on the body the Zuni used Chinchweed as an aromatic perfume. It is a traditional dye plant of the Hopi. The Zuni and Hopi both used the plant as a seasoning.

CLEMATIS   *Ranunculaceae* – Buttercup family

Clematis drummondii
Texas virgin's bower, Drummond's Clematis, Old man's beard

Clematis ligusticifolia
Western virgin's bower, Western clematis

Clematis pauciflora
Ropevine clematis

Clematis hirsutissima
Leatherflower, Sugar bowls, Hairy clematis

Description: Clematis is a perennial climbing vine, often exceeding 40 feet in length. It is frequently seen clambering over trees, bushes, and fences. The older stem sections, closest to the ground, are woody and often have thin and fissured bark. Clematis climbs by its tendril-like petioles, which wrap around supporting plants or structures. The leaves can be opposite and deeply cleft, entire, pinnate, or bipinnate. With the exception of Clematis hirsutissima, which has purple flowers, the flower sepals are petal-like and typically cream-colored. The mature fruits are small and have long feathery tails attached to them, actually converted styles, which lends descriptiveness to one of the plant's common names: Old man's beard.

Clematis drummondii can reach upwards of 30 feet in length. Its lower stem bark is striated and tawny or light gray. The leaves are composed of sets of 3-5 leaflets; they are cleft, lance shaped, or ovoid. They are grayish-green and covered with an ashy pubescence. C. ligusticifolia has 5-7 toothed leaflets per leaf. The green leaves are hairless, except in southern California where the plant has wooly leaf surfaces. C. pauciflora has 3-5 roundish leaflets that are toothed or lobed and sparsely hairy. C. hirsutissima, another woody-stemmed climber has 7-13 compound leaflets that are generally lanceolate. The flower sepals are bell-shaped, purple, and droop downwards very distinctively against its green foliage background.

Distribution: From 3,000-4,000 feet look for Clematis drummondii along washes, canyons, and streamsides. This plant is found from Arizona eastward to southern New Mexico and central-southern Texas. At various elevations C. ligusticifolia is wide spread throughout the west. From British Columbia and North Dakota it ranges southward through much of the coastal and interior west. Look for the plant in moist places, bottomlands, and along streams. C. pauciflora is largely found throughout southern California. From Los Angeles County to the Little San Bernardino Mountains, it ranges south. It is found, as are most of the species here, in moist drainage areas, and along canyon sides, streams, and gullies.

From Montana and Washington, Clematis hirsutissima is found south to northern Arizona and New Mexico. Look for the plant in Mixed Conifer Belts (Ponderosa pine, Douglas fir, etc.). There is some botanical disagreement on the plant's designated nomenclature in Arizona and New Mexico. Whether it is C. hirsutissima or C. hirsutissima var. arizonica really does not matter, what does is that the biotype is on the edge of its range and is not fairing well because of poor forest health. The plant should not be collected in this region.

Chemistry: anemonin, protoanemonin, β-sitosterol, campesterol, chlorogenic acid, caffeic acid, and other compounds

Medicinal Uses: A most telling use of Clematis is a Nez Perce application: a peeled section of Sugar bowls root (Clematis hirsutissima) was placed in a horse's nostril after it had collapsed from exhaustion from being raced too hard. This would quickly revive the horse. It would then be led to water, bathed and a short time after appear to suffer no ills from the experience – an herbal smelling-salt. The medicinal potency of Clematis can be largely rated by its causticness. It is in these acrid Buttercup family aromatics that Clematis musters its array of effects.

Worldwide, geographically disconnected groups of people have traditionally used different varieties of Clematis in relieving headaches. These days the fresh plant tincture or leaf infusion is used in congestive-type headaches, particularly migraines. Since Clematis has a relaxing and dilating effect on brain lining vasculature, it is useful in aborting migraine headaches. Use Clematis when visual and auditory disturbances are first noticed, before the intense pain of the episode descends. If a strong cup of coffee or caffeine pills have no effect on the migraine or make it worse, try Clematis.

Second to Clematis' dilatory effect, the plant is moderately antiinflammatory when taken internally. It provides cyclooxygenase and interleukin inhibition. Certainly, this plays a role in its effect on headaches, but it is of value also in its application to rheumatoid arthritis, especially if aggravated by cold and damp weather. The freshly crushed plant or fresh plant tincture applied topically is rubefacient. Use it as a counter-irritant applied specifically to areas where the above description of joint pain fits.

Indications:
♦ Migraines and migraine-like headaches, as an abortive
♦ Rheumatoid arthritis
♦ Arthritis, as a counter-irritant (external)

Collection: After finding a sizable stand of the plant, chew a leaf. If it is hot and acrid then it is good medicine, if it is not then move on (new spring growth is usually the most acrid). Prune and collect the leafing vine ends, with or without flowers.

Preparations: Drying diminishes Clematis' potency. The recently dried herb has some value, but even sealed it degrades quickly. The fresh plant tincture is the preferable preparation.

Dosage:
♦ FPT/DPT (50% alcohol): 10-40 drops 2-3 times daily

♦ Leaf infusion: 2-4 ounces 2-3 times daily
♦ Fresh plant poultice: use as needed, remove when skin begins to redden

Cautions: As with most Buttercup family plants, do not use Clematis during pregnancy. Although Clematis is useful in its inflammatory mediating effects on the autoimmune heat of rheumatoid arthritis, the plant is contraindicated in vasculitis, immunologically derived or otherwise. For some individuals even chewing a leaf can paradoxically usher in a headache. If this is the case, due to idiosyncratic vascular dynamics, Clematis is not for you.

COCKLEBUR   *Compositae* – Sunflower family

Xanthium strumarium (Xanthium saccharatum)
Common cocklebur

Xanthium spinosum
Spiny cocklebur

Description: Xanthium strumarium is a stout stemmed, 2-3 foot tall annual. The plant's reddish-purple stem blotches are distinctive. The leaves are suspended on long petioles; they are heart shaped, sometimes triangular, lobed, and irregularly toothed. The stout hairs on the leaves make them rough to the touch. Both male and female flowers emerge from the upper leaf axils. The male flowers are small, inconspicuous, and situated above the bur-like female flowers. After being pollinated 2 flattened seeds mature inside the bur. These brown, oblong, spiky burs have 2 prominent spines that because of their size stand apart from the other 400+ smaller spines. Each spine is recurved making the burs extremely efficient at attaching to anything – clothes, hair, and fur – assisting in habitat expansion.

Xanthium spinosum is distinguishable from X. strumarium by its large, 3-pronged, stiff spines protruding from the base of each leaf. The leaves are deeply lobed, narrow, covered with small white hairs, and have a distinctive white mid-vein.

Distribution: Although in the past Xanthium strumarium was limited in distribution it is now found throughout many parts of the world. In our area, it is commonly found in moist soils of drainages, roadsides, fields, and other areas where water tends to stand and is slow to drain. Although less common, X. spinosum is found in areas similar to where X. strumarium is encountered.

Chemistry: sesquiterpene lactones: xanthinin, xanthatin, xanthanol, isoxanthanol, xanthinosin, and tomentosin

Medicinal Uses: Cocklebur is primarily a plant affecting the urinary tract. It is a soothing diuretic as well as being astringent to the area. It is particularly useful in painful urination with corresponding mucus and blood tinged urine. Michael Stone, a Tucson Chiropractor, has used Cocklebur tea with success in astringing urinary tract bleeding in a patient recovering from surgery and chemotherapy to the area. Internally the plant also checks diarrhea and can be useful in diminishing sweating with attending weakness in non-infectious states (called colliquative sweating). Topically Cocklebur is moderately antimicrobial. Applied to cuts, scrapes, and like it will retard bacterial growth, therefore facilitating the healing process. Like Canyon bursage and Brittlebush, Cocklebur tends to be drying to the sinuses, so is used in allergic conditions affecting this area.

Indications:
♦ Cystitis
♦ Diarrhea
♦ Colliquative sweating
♦ Rhinitis/sinusitis
♦ Cuts/scrapes (external)

Collection: When the burs have finished maturing, usually between mid to late summer collect them from the plant; be sure to wear gloves, as the burs are spiny. Fortunately, where there is one plant there are others, so finding an adequate amount of burs is usually not a problem. In the spring, the young bur-forming, leafing tops are collected. Both parts of the plant are then dried.

Preparations and Dosage:
♦ Herb infusion/bur decoction: 2-3 ounces 3 times daily
♦ DPT (60% alcohol): 20-30 drops 3 times daily
♦ Oil/salve/wash: topically as needed

Cautions: Cocklebur should not be used continuously over 7-10 days. Large doses tend to be overtly toxic, particularly to the liver. Do not use during pregnancy or while nursing.

COPPERLEAF   *Euphorbiaceae* – Spurge family

Acalypha lindheimeri
Three seeded mercury

Acalypha neomexicana
Copperleaf, New Mexican copperleaf

Description: Depending on growth characteristics, species of Acalypha are either shrub-like or herbaceous. The leaves are petioled and are arranged alternately along the stem branches. These plants are monoecious with either male and female flowers arranged separately in shorts spikes or staminate flowers in groupings above the pistillate ones, both grouped on the same flower spike. The small seeds are contained in 3-celled capsules.

Acalypha lindheimeri is low-growing, deciduous, and shrub-like. The plant's weak branches often lay prostrated on the ground, only to be terminated by perky, upright red flower spikes. The leaves are wedge-shaped, toothed, hairy, and are folded along their mid-veins. Stem growth can be reddish-brown and is ridged and hairy.

Acalypha neomexicana is a small, weedy annual standing between 10 inches and 3 feet tall. The leaves are thin, light green, and ovoid with serrated margins. They often turn reddish-brown in response to cold stress. The female flowers have 3 distinctive red styles that are long and threadlike.

Distribution: Acalypha boasts over 250 species throughout both hemispheres, but these plants are primarily limited to the tropics. From 2,400-7,500 feet, Acalypha neomexicana is found from central Arizona to New Mexico. It frequents disturbed sites such as ditches, roadsides, and over grazed rangelands. Occasionally, it can be found in more pristine areas like canyons sides and shaded rocky slopes. Look for A. lindheimeri throughout the mid-elevation mountains of southeastern Arizona, east to New Mexico and Texas. It can be found in drainage areas and tucked in among boulders.

Chemistry: the genus contains anthraquinones, cyanogenic glycosides, tannins, and other polyphenols

Medicinal Uses: Copperleaf is best used topically to speed resolution of slowly healing wounds and ulcers. It is particularly beneficial to skin afflictions that linger through the involved tissues' lack of innate vitality. Where it is applied topically, Copperleaf stimulates phagocytosis, pro-inflammatory mediators, and general oxidation, literally delivering more biological activity to the area. There is some speculation that Copperleaf is a body-wide immune stimulant. If true, this would clarify why the plant has traditionally been used for such a wide variety of complaints. Copperleaf also has laxative and expectorant qualities ascribed to it.

Indications:
♦   Poorly healing wounds and ulcers (external)

Collection: When collecting Acalypha neomexicana, pull up the entire plant. While in flower prune the last 1-2 feet of branch ends from A. lindheimeri. Dry normally.

Dosage:
♦   Oil/salve/poultice: use as needed

Cautions: Although largely non-toxic, taken internally Copperleaf does have a stimulating effect on the uterus, so it is not recommended during pregnancy. Individuals with G6PD (glucose-6-phosphate-dehydrogenase deficiency) are advised not to orally use Copperleaf. The plant has been shown to cause intravascular hemolysis in these individuals.

COTTONWOOD

Salicaceae – Willow family

Populus fremontii
Fremont cottonwood, Alamo

Description: At maturity, Cottonwood is a large tree, one of the largest in its habitat. It has a broad crown that can reach upwards of 80-90 feet, though usually it is 50-75 feet tall; a 2-4 foot thick trunk is common. The trunk bark is grayish-brown and deeply furrowed. The younger limbs have a thin, grayish-white outer bark coating. The sticky-resinous leaf buds form into leathery and thick leaves; they are deltoid and taper to a terminal point.

Like all other Willow family plants, Cottonwood is dioecious. Each tree is either male or female. The flowers of both sexes form in catkins; the "cotton" of Cottonwood is from the fibrous tufts that surround the mature fruits. In the spring the cottony-seed containing fuzz is carried easily by the wind. Cottonwoods are very fast-growing and in only several decades, are able to reach monstrous proportions. This tree reaches the upper limit of its lifespan at about 100 years.

Cottonwoods are not known for their strength; the light and brittle wood makes for relatively weak branches. In strong winds these trees are notorious for dropping large branches, sometimes at the great inconvenience of campers sheltering under them. Similarly to Aspen, another Populus, in the breeze the leaf patter is disarming and brings to mind times that are serene and peaceful.

Distribution: Cottonwood can be found along streamsides and washes where there is reliable underground water. From 6,500 feet and below the tree is found throughout the Sonoran and Mojave Deserts and generally from Trans-Pecos Texas, the southern half of New Mexico, through to Arizona, central Nevada, southwestern Utah, and central-southern California.

Chemistry: phenolic glycosides: isoferulic acid, ferulic acid, caffeic acid, prenylferulate, prenylcaffeate, pinocembrin, pinostrobin, pinobanksin, chrysin, benzyl-(e)-caffeate, galangin, isosakuranetin, phenylethyl-(e)-caffeate, kaempferol, salicin, salicortin, salireposide, populin, temuloidin, and tremulacin

Medicinal Uses: Although phenolic glycoside content differs slightly from Aspen (Populus tremuloides) and Balsam Poplar (Populus balsamifera),

Cottonwood's uses are very similar. The bark tea is a reliable, broadly acting antiinflammatory agent. Internally use it in sedating the pain of rheumatic conditions. Whether the pain is from an acute sport's injury or long-standing arthritis Cottonwood's cyclooxygenase inhibition will prove relieving. If feverish, the plant lowers body temperature without potentially elevating it first, unlike Elder or many Mint family plants. The bark tea taken before meals is a useful gastric stimulant; its tonic activity is mainly imparted through its bitterness.

Like many Willow family plants, Cottonwood is a urinary tract medicine. The bark tea is mildly diuretic and is indicated in chronic disturbances of the area. Use in long standing kidney inflammation and prostate hypertrophy. Externally the poultice, liniment, salve, or oil made with the leaves and/or leaf buds have use in curbing headache pain, or the inflammation and swelling from contusions, sprains, arthritic joints, and the like. The salve or oil is soothing to burns and scrapes; it will also retard infection due to its antimicrobial activity.

Indications:
◆ Rheumatic conditions/injuries (internal and external)
◆ Fever
◆ Indigestion
◆ Nephritis/prostate enlargement
◆ Burns (external)

Collection: In the spring, when new leaf buds are starting to develop find a secondary branch with light, non-fissured, smooth bark. With a saw cut the branch from the larger one it is connected to, or from the trunk. Clip all of the small branchlets less than a finger-width from the collected branch and discard. With a knife, peel off the bark starting from the cut end. Once started the bark strips easily. Dry the bark in the open, out of direct sunlight.

Preparations and Dosage:
◆ Bark decoction: 4 ounces 3 times daily, externally as needed
◆ External applications of leaf/leaf bud: as needed

Cautions: Use with prudence if taking anti-coagulant pharmaceutics. The chance of Cottonwood triggering reye's syndrome in feverish children is remote, but it is best to err on the side of caution and not use Cottonwood internally is these situations.

CREOSOTE BUSH   *Zygophyllaceae* – Caltrop family

Larrea tridentata (Larrea divaricata var. tridentata, Covillea tridentata)
Chaparral, Greasewood, Little stinker, Hediondilla, Gobernadora

Description: At maturity, Creosote bush is a large shrub, approximately 8-10 feet high by the same dimension wide. The stems are flexible, ash-colored and rise vertically, or nearly so, from the ground. When growing on desert flats it has a distinctive funnel-like appearance with the top section of the plant having the widest radius. Most of the leaves are collected in groupings among the upper branches. The leaflets are fused in pairs and resemble a "packman". The younger leaves are particularly resinous and shiny; with age, their luster diminishes. The yellow petals of the flower have a particular way of twisting perpendicularly to the reproductive center, making the arrangement fan-like. When mature the small fuzzy seed capsules separate into individual wedges, called mericarps.

Beyond normal seed germination, Creosote bush has a relatively unique way of reproducing. The plant is very adept at cloning itself. If you imagine the root crown of Creosote bush as a circle, the clones are created on the circumference, increasing the root crown's diameter. After a time the center roots die of old age, leaving numerous, physically independent, genetically identical clones spread out in a localized area. Eventually as this process continues plants spread outward like ripples in water created from a dropped stone. Some extremely old plants have been dated in southern California to be approximately 11,700 years old. The age of these ancient plants was determined by calculating the known outward growth rates with the furthest distance genetically identical clones were apart from each other.

The aromatics given off by the plant fill the air after a good rain. The wonderful smell is purifying to the spirit and has the ability to cut through the deepest states of emotional self-absorption.

Distribution: Creosote bush can be found throughout the Sonoran, Mojave, and Chihuahuan Deserts. Huge expanses are found in valley bottoms and basins. It more sparsely occupies slopes and rocky hillsides.

Chemistry: lignans: nordihydroguaiaretic acid, dihydroguaiaretic acid, isoguaiaiacin, and norisoguaiacin; flavonoids: apigenin, gossypetin, herbacetin, kaempferol, luteolin, morin, myricetin, and quercetin; saponins: larreagenin a, larreic acid, and erthyrodiol; monoterpenes: α-pinene, limonene, camphene, linalool, borneol, camphor, and bornylacetate; sesquiterpenes: α-curcumene, calamine, β-santalene, edulane, α-bergamontene, cuparene, β-eudesmol, farnesol, and α-agarofuran

Medicinal Uses: If there is one plant that is the medicinal hallmark of the Southwestern Deserts, it is Creosote bush. The plant has such a broad application of use, particularly when combining traditional perspectives from White, American Indian, and Mexican usage, together with science-based evidence, it is no wonder that it is considered a panacea. Looking at Creosote bush's main spheres of influence, that of a unique antiinflammatory, antioxidant, and antimicrobial agent, we are more able to define and understand the plant's therapeutic use.

Creosote bush is sedating to pro-inflammatory mediators. Leukotriene and leukocyte activity, histamine and prostaglandin release are all diminished; this makes Creosote bush useful in lessening rheumatoid arthritis pain and soreness. Used internally with other herbs, such as Yucca, and soaking in a bath made with the plant, is of great value in the above problem. Likewise, in autoimmune initiated asthmatic conditions the plant reduces stuffiness of the bronchial airway through reducing the "heat" of the autoimmune process. For other systemic autoimmune hypersensitivities, Creosote bush may be quite useful, as it is also profoundly antioxidant in nature. Topically Creosote bush has been used with success in resolving psoriasis and eczema, particularly in combination with deeper liver therapies and removing dietary and environmental allergens.

Creosote bush is distinctly inhibiting to several prominent viruses that are troubling in these times of social excesses. HPV (Human papillomavirus), the cause of genital warts and cervical dysplasia, is sensitive to Creosote bush's NDGA content as is Herpes simplex virus types I and II. A douche of Creosote bush tea applied twice daily or a suppository applied before bed is a useful approach for either virus affecting vaginal and/or cervical tissues. Otherwise, topical use of the oil or salve is efficacious. Cold sores respond very well to external salve application.

Studies are not consistent in regard to the plant's antimicrobial/antifungal activity but observable results have been positive, particularly topical application of Creosote bush to infected cuts and skin punctures. The salve is also a "must-have" when living in venomous spider/cone-nose insect territories. Continually applied Creosote bush tends to be remarkable in reducing the deleterious effects of these varmints.

Although internal use of Creosote bush as a cancer therapy is controversial at best, external preparations are useful in resolving a particular form of premalignant squamous cell carcinoma, called actinic keratosis. These reddened and sometimes scaly patches arise on sun-damaged skin. A topical pharmaceutical preparation of NDGA, called Actinex, was used in the treatment of the condition before being removed from the market because of skin hypersensitivity issues. As by dry weight Creosote bush contains 2-10% of NDGA, whole herb preparations are adequate and chances of adverse skin responses are limited.

Indications:
♦ Rheumatoid arthritis (internal and external)
♦ Asthma
♦ Psoriasis/eczema (external)
♦ HPV/HSV, type I and II (external)
♦ Cuts/abrasions (external)
♦ Venomous and non-venomous insect bites (external)
♦ Actinic keratosis (external)

Collection: Collect when new leaf growth is apparent. Using your thumb and forefinger strip the leaves that form in clumps towards the outer-most branch ends. The leaves are easily pulled from their branches; if the flowers and seeds are collected this also is fine. The resin that builds up on your hands does not come off even with the most vigorous scrubbing. Applying a high proof alcohol will help in removal.

Preparations and Dosage:
♦ DPT (75% alcohol): 20-40 drops 3 times daily
♦ Leaf infusion: traditional or cold infusion; 2-4 ounces 3 times daily
    (1 teaspoon of herb to 1 cup of water)
♦ Salve/oil/bath: as needed
♦ Douche: 2 times daily

Cautions: Do not use Creosote bush while pregnant or nursing. Use of the plant is also not recommended if there is existing liver impairment or inflammation. It is also not recommended to use Creosote bush with other drug therapies that may affect the liver, be they over-the-counter or prescription.

There were a number of cases, particularly in the early nineties where Creosote bush was involved to some degree in triggering liver inflammation. Most cases were self-resolving after discontinuing Creosote bush. The two individuals who required liver transplants took the plant for over a year and either drank regularly an undisclosed amount of alcohol or took a cocktail of pharmaceutical and over-the-counter drugs. So in summation, in healthy individuals small to moderate amounts of Creosote bush used periodically is indeed therapeutic if used for the right reasons. Nevertheless, when used zealously with abandon, as a cure-all, for long periods, Creosote bush can be problematic. There are no cautions for the plant's external use.

CROWNBEARD   *Compositae* – Sunflower family

Verbesina encelioides
Anil de muerto

Description: Crownbeard is an herbaceous annual several feet in height. Its grayish-green triangular leaves alternate along slender stems. The small sunflower-like flowers are yellow; each disk petal is 3-notched at its end. Being an aggressive seeder, it is very adept at self-propagation. One distinctive characteristic of Crownbeard is its odor. When the plant is brushed against or when down wind from a stand it exudes a distinctive smell; it is both difficult to describe and unique, but some say it is like rotting meat.

Distribution: Crownbeard enjoys a large range throughout the west. Look to disturbed roadsides, ground around embankments, culverts, and low-lying ditches. If luck is on your side occasionally it can be found in relatively pristine areas, often under Mesquites or on wash banks. In urban areas look to the undeveloped city block with low-lying land; the yellow that catches your eye in the summer is probably the plant.

Chemistry: triterpenes: amyrin, taraxastanone and taraxasterol; flavonoids: quercetin and hyperoside; steroidal glycosides: campesterol, daucosterol, and β-sitosterol

Medicinal Uses: Crownbeard is used externally to reduce inflammation from a variety of causes. It works well to diminish swelling from contusions, bruises, insect bites and stings, burns, and other acute injuries. Alone or combined with St. Johns wort it is well suited for topical application on chicken pox and shingles outbreaks and on herpes cold sores. Rashes from allergic reactions are quieted; also, tissues more quickly heal from cuts and incisions. In combination with Tobacco or Datura, it is efficacious in reducing hemorrhoid flare-ups. Traditional Mexican use dictates the plant's application in gastritis and ulcerative conditions of the stomach. Crownbeard does in fact have promise here through its inflammatory mediating effects on troubled mucosa.

Indications:
- Acute injuries with topical redness (external)
- Shingles/HSV, type I/chicken pox (external)
- Hemorrhoids (external)
- Gastritis
- Gastric ulcer

Collection: Collect the upper half when the plant is in flower; in the southwest this will be after the plant has responded to summer rains. Dry loosely arranged in paper bags or on a cardboard flat. When harvesting the plant be mindful of various insects that may be making a home on it. A number of years ago after laying the plant out to dry, hundreds of unnoticed small inchworms left the plants in mass searching for a way out of the house.

Preparations and Dosage:
- Herb infusion: 2-4 ounces 2-3 times daily
- External applications: as needed

Cautions: There are no problems for external use. Internally in excessive amounts, Crownbeard may slow respiration and decreases blood pressure. Out of principle of not mixing chemically complex herbs and pregnancy, it is not recommended here or while nursing. Use the plant internally two weeks at a time, and then rotate to another plant.

CUDWEED   *Compositae* – Sunflower family

Gnaphalium leucocephalum
Lemon cudweed, Everlasting, Gordolobo, Manzanilla del rio, Lampaquate

Description: In the southwest Cudweed is one of the first plants to show new leaf growth in late winter. The wooly, grayish-green, lance shaped leaves form tidy mounds under the pervious years' dried flower stalks. At this stage, they look like strange, sand-loving sea anemones. The older perennials can send up 30-40, 1-2 foot high stems upon which in the late spring, small, white papery flowers appear. The inflorescence's look to be roundish buttons; there are numerous bracts surrounding the reproductive flower parts at the center. As the flowers age the bracts radiate outward giving the inflorescence a disk-like appearance. The entire plant is sticky to the touch; it smells of a cross between Lemon verbena and freshly crushed pine needles.

Distribution: Cudweed can be found from 2,000-5,000 feet in and around sandy gullies and wash bottoms where water flows seasonally; it ranges from southern Arizona to southern California.

Chemistry: a similarly used Cudweed, Gnaphalium oxyphyllum, contains diterpenoids, flavonoids, acetylenic compounds, and carotenoids

Medicinal Uses: Cudweed lends itself well to initiatory stages of bronchitis where there is a dry and painful cough. The tea is useful in dislodging impacted mucus that is difficult to expectorate. Its mild diaphoretic properties are excellent in dry feverish states where the body is hot and flushed. Lending credence to Cudweed's beneficial effect on the pneumal environment is its genus-wide, mild antimicrobial properties; a number of Cudweed species have been found to inhibit several Staphylococcus and Streptococcus varieties making its application to bacterial associated bronchitis indicated.
    Most other species of Gnaphalium, particularly the aromatic varieties, can be used as well medicinally. The array of varying species in the west enables these plants a wider use. The genuses Antennaria and Anaphalis are closely

related to Gnaphalium and are likewise used similarly, although they are less expectorating and stimulating in nature.

Indications:
- Cough, dry and painful
- Bronchitis with difficult expectoration
- Bronchitis with dry fever

Collection: From early to mid-summer collect the herb just before flowering. Dry either loosely or in bundles. It is a wonderful plant to collect – paper bags, hands, and pruners all become lemon scented. Pruner blades will sometimes stick together from the buildup of lemon waxy-aromatics – oh the hardships!

Preparations and Dosage:
- Herb infusion: 4-8 ounces 3-4 times daily

Cautions: It is best not to purchase Gnaphalium, or as it is locally known in the southwest and northern Mexico, Gordolobo, in commerce. The confusion starts firstly in that Gordolobo is also a common name for Mullein (Verbascum thapsus) in the area, which is not necessarily a major problem for the uses of both plants are somewhat similar. The more important issue is Gnaphalium's occasional adulteration with Senecio longilobus, a rather toxic plant containing pyrrolizidine alkaloids. In Mexico where the bulk of Gnaphalium is collected, it is occasionally mistaken for this look-alike Senecio. This mix-up was responsible for the tragic death of a 6-month year-old baby in Tucson during the late 70's. Cudweed on the other hand is completely non-toxic and can be used freely.

CYPRESS

Cupressaceae – Cypress family

Cupressus arizonica
Arizona cypress

Cupressus sempervirens
Italian cypress

Description: As with many cone-bearing plants, Arizona cypress is a stately tree. At maturity, its pyramidal crown stands between 50-90 feet tall. Like Alligator juniper, the outer brownish-gray bark is fissured in a checkerboard pattern, but can also be thin, fibrous, and vertically layered. In the case of Cupressus arizonica var. glabra the outer branch and tree bark typically sheds leaving a smooth, brownish-red exposed under-layer. Arizona cypress' leaves are small and scale-like. Collectively the branchlet groupings are fan-like. Although not visible all of the time, each leaf has a small, central pitch-secreting gland that appears as a small white dot. The small pollen bearing cones form at branch ends. At full development, the larger seed bearing cones dwarf them. They are normally between ½-1 inch across, round and formed of 6-8 flattened scales. At maturity, the surrounding cone scales open and extend, releasing the seeds.

In its native environment Italian cypress is a large tree reaching 75-100 feet in height. Planted as an ornamental it is usually smaller. The commonly found variety cultivated in the west is conical to columnar shaped. The bark is smooth and gray when young, with age it becomes vertically furrowed. Each scale-like leaf, like Arizona cypress, has a small resin gland on one side. The cones are brownish-gray and are about an inch across.

Distribution: From 3,000-6,000 feet Arizona cypress is found from central-eastern Arizona, southwestern New Mexico, to Big Bend National Park in Texas. Look for the tree in mid-elevation canyons and along streamsides. It particularly gravitates to northern facing exposures. Typical plants found in proximity are Manzanita and Canyon walnut.

Italian cypress is native to the Mediterranean area. Because the tree has been cultivated for thousands of years, the original distribution is impossible to determine with accuracy. It is planted as an ornamental throughout warmer parts of the southwest. Large, mature trees can still be found around remnant homesteads, farms, and old churches.

Chemistry: for Cupressus sempervirens: volatile constituents: pinene, fenchene, camphene, myrcene, carene, terpinene, limonene, phellandrene, terpinolene, cymene, cubebene, copaene, caryophyllene, humulene, muurolene, germacrene d, cadinene and calamenene; sesquiterpenes: cedrene, elemene, carvacrol, preizizaene, acoradiene, selinene, acoradine, curcumene, cuparene, calamenene, and cedrol

Medicinal Uses: Externally, Cypress is used as an antiviral. Continually applied it is useful in removing the average "garden variety" of wart (Verruca vulgaris). Genital warts (Condyloma acuminatum) are less predictably resolved, but the essential oil of Cypress is worth trying. In these cases, it is the preferable article because of its strength. Dilute the essential oil with olive oil when applying to sensitive tissue or use suppositories. Fungal and bacterial infections from a wide array of pathogens are sensitive to Cypress. Apply Cypress to poorly healing wounds, festering bedsores, and other slow to heal external afflictions. For those prone to gingivitis and dental plaque formation, a once or twice a day mouthwash with Cypress tea will prove beneficial through its inhibition of plaque-forming enzymes.

A douche or sitz bath made with Cypress leaves is useful in vaginal Candida infections as is the tea applied topically to other areas of the body that are similarly affected. Typical places are around the mouth, under arms, between mid-section rolls of skin, and other moist and dark areas of the body. Scaly and crust-like skin afflictions such as cradle cap (seborrheic dermatitis) and chronically dry eczema respond well to Cypress.

Internally, Cypress checks negative flora populations in the colon and specifically is useful in diminishing intestinal Candida overgrowth and other colonic flora imbalances characterized by gas and diarrhea with alternating constipation. Various aromatic constituents of Cypress have been shown to inhibit water and food borne pathogens responsible for gastrointestinal tract distresses, such as Giardia lamblia, Salmonella spp., and most likely the Ameba group of organisms, notably Entamoeba histolytica. The tea is considered the primary preparation because of the large surface area it covers as it descends along the gastrointestinal tract.

Cypress is clearly immune stimulating to surfaces with which it comes into contact. The plant initiates innate immune activity, but also to some degree, acquired immunity, particularly T-cell activity. This effect of Cypress has its greatest influence on the lungs and urinary tract. In chronic cases of bronchitis where expectoration is copious, mucus is green or yellow and the lungs feel weakened Cypress helps to resolve the situation. Resident macrophages or dust cells within the alveoli are stimulated and boost the lungs infection-fighting prowess. The plant's aromatics, which are excreted through the lungs, serve also to inoculate the area with antimicrobial constituents. Weakened, lingering coughs tend to resolve. The inhaled steam from the infused leaf tea, or diffused essential oil can be used to similarly effect the bronchial environment. In addition, it is a simple way to facilitate resolution of a sinus infection, particularly if it has been long standing. Chronically sore throats and even Strep throat are additionally benefited by Cypress steam inhalations.

The urinary tract is benefited as well. Acting as a urinary tract antiseptic and localized immune stimulant, lower urinary tract infections, particularly involving Escherichia coli are resolved. If infection is dependent upon urinary tract weakness or there is a constitutional laxity of the area, it is often strengthened by Cypress. Dribbling of urine and partial incontinence, especially upon physical exertion, coughing, or laughing, are diminished as are the same problems in older men dependent upon chronic prostatitis. Small doses of the tincture, 5-10 drops before bed, often lessens chronic bed-wetting in children.

Cypress has been used with success in treating valley fever, or coccidioidomycosis, caused by the soil mold Coccidioides immitis, commonly found in alkaline soils throughout the hot and dry American southwest. It is responsible for flu-like symptoms of fatigue, fever, headaches, aches and pains, and cough. Susceptibility is largely dependent upon the state of the immune system, overall vitality, and racial/genetic disposition. Cypress is best used as an emmenagogue when menses is slowed from uterine laxity, chronic illness, or relocation to a colder living area.

Indications:
- Warts, common and genital (external)
- Wounds/bedsores/slow to heal tissues (external)
- Gingivitis (mouthwash)
- Infections, fungal and bacterial (external)
- Candida infections (internal and external)
- Dermatitis, dry and scabby (external)
- Intestinal flora imbalances with diarrhea, constipation, and flatulence
- Food poisoning/ameba and Giardia infections
- Bronchitis with copious phlegm and weak cough

- Strep throat/general sore throat
- Urinary incontinence/bed wetting from lack of bladder tone
- Cystitis/urethritis/prostatitis/as an antiseptic/weakened and lax urinary tract tissues
- Valley fever

Collection: In the spring when new growth is noticeable, collect entire fan-like leaf sprays by breaking them off at larger branch junctures. Lay out, well spaced to ensure proper drying.

Preparations and Dosage:
- FPT: 20-40 drops 3 times daily
- Leaf infusion: 4-6 ounces 3 times daily
- Inhaled steam from the infusion or essential oil: 5 minutes 3 times daily
- Oil/salve/wash/poultice: as needed

Cautions: Do not use during pregnancy or while nursing. Excessive doses of internal and steam derived preparations can irritate the lungs, upper respiratory tract tissues, and kidneys. Italian Cypress has the tendency to pick up heavy metals in its bark. The leaves may or may not exhibit the same tendency, but since no plant should be collected next to industrial sites or roadways, this should not be a problem.

DANDELION   *Compositae* – Sunflower family

Taraxacum officinale (Leontodon taraxacum)
Chicoria, Consuelda

Description: Dandelion is a small perennial arising from a single or branched taproot. Both the leaves and flowers originate from the plant's root crown. The plant completely lacks branches or stems. The dark green leaves are between 2-12 inches long and are deeply lobed. The golden yellow flower heads arise on hollow flower stems, which can be several inches to 1-2 feet long. The puff-like seed clusters are wind or breath dispersed. Each achene is attached to a parachute-like grouping of silky hairs making dispersal easy. If damaged, the entire plant exudes a milky sap. Dandelion in low elevation, arid locales tends to be diminutive in size and weaker in strength compared to its high mountain and cold country relatives.

Distribution: Dandelion is found throughout most of the country. This European native is extremely robust and versatile, making the best of what it is given. Lawns, gardens, grassy parks, and roadsides are common places for the plant.

Chemistry: sesquiterpene lactones: eudesmanolides, germacranolides, and guaianolides; phenylpropanoids; phenolic acids: caffeic acid and chlorogenic acid; flavonoids: apigenin, luteolin, and chrysoeriol; coumarins: scopoletin and aesculetin, cinnamic acid esters (monocaffeyltartaric acid, chlorogenic acid, and chicoric acid) and hydroxycinnamic acid; triterpenes; β-amyrin, taraxol, and taraxerol; carotenoids: lutein; phytosterols: sitosterol, stigmasterol, and taraxasterol; polysaccharide: inulin

Medicinal Uses: Dandelion's use as a gastric and hepatic/biliary stimulant is straightforward. The tea or tincture taken before meals is a reliable bitter tonic. It increases digestive prowess by stimulating an array of gastric secretions. Use the plant if prone to indigestion and combine with Dogweed or Mountain marigold if there is a tendency for bloating. Dandelion is stimulating to bile production by the liver and release by the gallbladder, and likewise small intestinal fat digestion is augmented. The plant tends to be more cooling to the liver than other hepatic stimulants such as Desert barberry, so its use in liver inflammations, like hepatitis C, is better suited. In fact alone or combined with Milk thistle, Dandelion reduces liver sensitivity, upper body tightness, and itchy eyes and skin associated with subacute liver inflammation. Moreover, a cup of roasted or plain Dandelion root tea in the morning before breakfast is an effective way of thinning bile so gallstones tend not to develop. Small amounts of the tea over a longer period will diminish established gallstones from overly concentrated bile.

Dandelion, particularly the leaf, is diuretic. It is indicated in resolving uric acid kidney stones and acts systemically in eliminating uric acid deposits responsible for gout. Dandelion roots have substantial inulin content, a complex carbohydrate that enters the colon intact due to the body's inability to digest it. In the colon, inulin promotes beneficial flora growth, particularly of bifidobacteria. This in turn stabilizes the large intestinal environment, limiting pathogenic bacteria and their destructive by-products. Use Dandelion in the nefarious "leaky gut syndrome" – a title meant to describe a symptom picture of skin allergies, joint inflammation, fatigue, and colon instability dependent upon proliferation of harmful colon bacteria, their by-products, and heightened leukocyte activity. For this purpose, combine Dandelion with Yucca. The combination tends to stabilize beneficial flora levels, while binding harmful endotoxins.

Indications:
♦   Indigestion
♦   Liver/biliary congestion
♦   Poor fat digestion
♦   Uric acid kidney stones/gout
♦   Poor intestinal health

Collection: Gather Dandelion leaf when verdant and hydrated during the spring and summer. The roots of the plant can be dug all year, but are strongest during colder seasons, particularly in the fall when they can contain 40% inulin. Dry the leaves normally. Split the taproots length-wise before drying.

Preparations: The root powder in capsules is the best way to receive the plant's inulin content.

Dosage:
♦   Leaf infusion/root decoction: 4-8 ounces 3 times daily
♦   FPT/DPT (50% alcohol): 60-90 drops 3 times daily
♦   Fluidextract (root): 20-40 drops 3 times daily
♦   '00' capsules (root): 2-3, 3 times daily

Cautions: Do not use if there is a biliary blockage.

Other Uses: Although slightly bitter, the young leaves are used as a potherb. Add them to salads, other cooked greens, and the like.

Writing about Dandelion and its virtues Doctor Geo F. Collier stated in an 1843 issue of The Lancet: "The great objection to its use will be that it costs nothing, and may be made by everyone, without pharmaceutical mystery or expense." (Some things just never change)

DATURA

Solanaceae – Nightshade family

Datura meteloides (Datura wrightii, D. innoxia)
Sacred Datura, Toloache

Datura discolor
Desert thornapple

Datura stramonium
Jimsonweed, Jamestown weed

Description: Datura meteloides is a large, herbaceous, 2-3 foot high perennial. It tends to be mound-like in growth and has large, grayish-green leaves. They are ovoid in shape, can be toothed and deeply lobed, and are narrowed at the tip and wider at the base. They are aligned alternately along the many-branched stems. The flowers are folded into compact swirls before they fully form. After unfurling the large funnel-form flowers are white and sometimes suffused with violet. They originate from forks in the upper branch stems. Each flower does not last long; they open in the evening and typically wither by the middle of the next day. The green circular seedpods droop downward (as opposed to D. stramonium's, which remain upright) and are covered with coarse, slender spikes. After drying the brown pods contain numerous, compact, small kidney shaped seeds that are light brown. Brought to my attention by Y.C., an acquaintance, the whole plant smells peanut-like.

Datura discolor is a smaller, 1-2 foot high annual with grayish-green, several inch long, ovate leaves. The flowers, which emerge from a 2-3 inch long calyx, are trumpet-like. The floral tube is constricted, opening widely at the very end. The corolla is white, tinged with violet, and is 10-toothed. The spiny, drooping seedpods contain numerous black seeds. D. stramonium is a leggy annual sometimes reaching 5 feet in height. Its coarsely lobed-toothed leaves are dark green and prominently veined. Depending on variety D. stramonium's trumpet shaped flowers are 3-5 inches long and are either white or purplish. The upright seedpods are situated between the upper stem branches. The seeds are dark brown to black at maturity.

Distribution: Datura meteloides is widely distributed throughout the southwest. It can be found from central California, east to Colorado and Texas, and south through Arizona and New Mexico. The plant frequents numerous vegetative zones: Creosote Bush and Coastal California Sage Scrub, and mid-elevation Grasslands, among other areas. From sea level to nearly 6,500 feet look for the plant along slopes, washes, and other drainage areas. D. meteloides is fond of disturbed soils – roadsides, the sides of washes, and over grazed rangelands are some of its favorites.

Datura discolor is limited to elevations below 2,000 feet, but on occasion it has been reported up to 4,000 feet. The plant is found from southeastern California to southern Arizona. Disturbed soils, washes, and other drainage areas are places where the plant is found. D. stramonium, native to Tropical America or North America (no one is sure), is sporadic in distribution. Look for it in vacant lots and waste areas throughout the country.

Chemistry: tropane alkaloids for Datura discolor, very similar for D. meteloides: hyoscine (scopolamine), apohyoscine, norhyoscine, hyoscyamine, meteloidine, tropine, atropine, littorine, and cuscohygrine; flavonoids: quercetin and kaempferol

Medicinal Uses: Datura is one of the strongest analgesic herbs we employ. Its influences are drug-like. The leaf poultice, oil, or liniment will give symptomatic relief to swollen and painful sports injuries, contusions, sprains, and the like. The freshly pureed leaf, alone or mixed with Prickly pear or Aloe leaf pulp, is soothing and will relieve pain from burns. Datura's broad antimicrobial activity keeps infection from setting in damaged, susceptible tissues. Datura oil applied to hemorrhoids reduces swelling and associated discomfort. A liniment soaked cloth applied to a throbbing headache is pain relieving. The same external preparations are applied over the lower abdomen for menstrual and intestinal cramps. It is also of use in diminishing back or leg muscle spasms from over work, injury, or stress.

The dried foliage of Datura is crushed and rolled to make a cigarette, packed into a pipe, or simply lit on a small tray. Several inhalations of the smoke are taken for the bronchial constriction of asthma or severe allergies from pollen or insect stings. It by no means is safer than regular medications, but it works in a pinch when the latter are not available. Datura exerts an anticholinergic effect on bronchial passageways, opening the area so air can be more fully inhaled and exhaled.

Indications:
♦   Acute injuries, unbroken skin (external)

- Burns (external)
- Hemorrhoids (external)
- Menstrual/intestinal cramps (external)
- Muscle spasm (external)
- Bronchial constriction (smoke)

Collection and Preparations: The entire plant is medically active, although the leaves and/or seed capsules are the most practical part to collect. Dry the leaves and seed capsules for storage or tincture fresh for the liniment.

Dosage:
- Liniment: topically 3-4 times daily
- Oil/salve/wash: topically 3-4 times daily
- Smoke: several inhalations 2-3 times daily in acute situations

Cautions: Apart from smoking small amounts, Datura should not be used orally. Internally, in very small amounts, the plant does have other therapeutic uses, although it is best to leave those to advanced practitioners. Ingested the plant is toxic and can lead to a number of nervous system derangements, temporary or permanent blindness not being the least of them. Do not use if pregnant or nursing. Prolonged external application can affect the central nervous system. Remember, exposed surface area plus duration equals dosage. Stop external application, particularly for headache pain, if dizziness and altered vision are sensed.

DEERWEED

Compositae – Sunflower family

Porophyllum gracile (*Porophyllum junciforme, P. putidum*)
Yerba del venado

Porophyllum macrocephalum
Odora

Description: Porophyllum gracile is a small, many-branched perennial, not more than 2 feet tall by the same wide. Except for a few linear leaves, the slender branches are practically leafless. In the spring P. gracile's bluish-green coloration distinguishes it from surrounding plants. The inconspicuous flowers are purplish-white; they are supported on ½-¾ inch long involucres. New stem growth, leaves, and flowers are strongly aromatic.

Porophyllum macrocephalum is a 1-2 foot tall annual with ovoid, mostly opposite, thickened leaves. Like P. gracile, the involucres are also thickened, and on them rest inconspicuous, purplish-white flower heads. When crushed the whole plant is aromatic; the odor is pungent and not at all unpleasant.

Distribution: Porophyllum gracile populates hillsides and basins of the Chihuahuan, Mojave, and Sonoran Deserts. From 4,000 feet and below P. gracile is found throughout southern Nevada, southern California, and Arizona. P. macrocephalum is essentially a southern Arizona plant. South from the Peloncillo and Baboquivari Mountains it is found between 3,500-5,000 feet on rocky slopes, hillsides, and canyons.

Chemistry: acetylenic thiophenes; monoterpenes: α-pinene, sabinene, and myrcene; sesquiterpene: β-cubebene; fatty acid derivatives: 7-tetradecene, cis-4-decenal, pentadecanal, and heptadecanal

Medicinal Uses: Use Deerweed when in need of a simple gastric carminative. When the stomach feels full and distended from improper dietary choices several sprigs of the fresh plant or a little of the fresh plant tincture will relieve the distress. Eating several leaves or flowers has the uncanny ability of making anyone with trapped stomach air, burp. For colicky babies it can be thought of as an equivalent to Catnip, working well to relieve trapped gas and spasm.

Indications:
◆ Dyspepsia with bloating and nausea
◆ Colic

Collection: In the spring or summer when new growth is apparent, collect the top several inches of fresh branches from the plant. Leave older, woody sections as they have little value, which is evidenced by their lack of scent.

Preparations: Individuals who live close to Deerweed will benefit most from the plant, as eating a small handful of the fresh herb is by far the most efficacious way of receiving its benefits. The fresh plant tincture is second in serviceability. After drying the plant, the scent diminishes. The herb infusion is less effective than the fresh plant or the fresh plant tincture.

Dosage:
◆ Fresh leaves and flowers: eaten as needed
◆ FPT: 30-60 drops 3 times daily
◆ Leaf infusion: 4-8 ounces 3 times daily

Cautions: None known.

DESERT ANEMONE   *Ranunculaceae* – Buttercup family

Anemone tuberosa
Desert windflower

Description: Desert anemone is a small, herbaceous perennial. Thin stems arise 1-2 feet from the plant's tuberous roots. The divided, semi-succulent leaves are few, mostly originating from the base and mid-stem. The 1½-inch diameter flowers are positioned at stem ends and are composed of approximately 10 modified sepals, appearing as petals. The sepals are often white but can also have pink or purplish twinges. The seeds are wooly and form in dense, cylindrical heads. Throughout much of Desert Anemone's western expanse, the plant is dependent upon winter-spring rains to sprout above ground. In dry years, it is common for the plant to forgo rising from its tuberous roots.

Distribution: From 2,500-5,000 feet Desert anemone is found on slopes and hillsides crowded among rocks and boulders and occasionally under shrubs and trees. The plant is found from the southern California Desert to southern Nevada and Utah, through much of Arizona, to New Mexico.

Chemistry: lactones: anemonin and protoanemonin; triterpenoid glycosides; flavonoids

Medicinal Uses: The understanding of Desert anemone comes to us largely from the associated use of Anemone patens or Pulsatilla by nineteen and twentieth century Eclectic and Homeopathic physicians. For all practical purposes, Desert anemone is just as useful. The plant is both an emotional and physical medicine. Use small doses of the fresh plant tincture in episodes of fear, gloom, and depression. The plant works well if there is also restlessness, insomnia, and nervous system debility from substance abuse, laziness, or too much cerebral work. Desert anemone has the ability of lifting the spirits and making needed rest possible. It is of particular use to individuals who are thin, cold-bodied, and tend to have reactive skin allergies.

Desert anemone is not to be underestimated in calming premenstrual emotional yo-yos and first or second day period cramps. In addition, slowed menses tends to be stimulated slightly, particularly if there are accompanying feelings of chilliness of the pelvic area and lower back. Ovarian pain during ovulation or otherwise is sedated by Desert anemone. For men, the plant proves relieving to epididymitis, idiosyncratic orchitis, and varicoceles. In fact, through its restorative influence on venous circulation, relief is provided to most chronic inflammations of the genital/urinary systems, if dependant upon debility. Use it also if there is decreased libido and lack of sexual interest from stress, overwork, and nervousness.

Like Clematis, Desert anemone is used as a migraine abortive. Because it is vasodilating it is best applied when visual disturbances and the classic migraine aura is noticeable. 5-10 drops directly on the tongue can stop the progression almost immediately, although if in the advanced pain of a migraine Desert anemone may worsen the episode.

In small amounts, Desert anemone is a gastric stimulant; it provides more blood to the stomach walls through its dilatory effect. For indigestion and digestive atony combine the plant with bitters and take before meals, particularly if the emotional picture fits as described previously.

The plant reduces cerebral spinal fluid and intraocular pressure; use in mild cases of glaucoma. An eyewash made with the fresh plant tincture is of value in chronic conjunctivitis, ocular irritation, and styes. Topically, Desert anemone, like Clematis, is rubefacient. It will cause vasodilation, bringing more blood to surface tissues in a matter of minutes. Apply a fresh plant poultice to chronic arthritic conditions. Remove the poultice at the first sign of redness.

Indications:
- Depression, gloominess
- Genital-urinary system debility
- Decreased libido
- Dysmenorrhea/amenorrhea
- Migraines, beginning stages
- Indigestion
- Glaucoma/conjunctivitis/styes (internal and eyewash)
- Arthritis, as a counter-irritant (external)

Collection: Gather the foliage – leaves, flowers, and stems – in early spring. Chew a small piece of leaf to better understand the plant's medicinal effect. There is no need to dig the tubers since the above ground portion is medicinally potent.

Preparations: Tincture fresh. Desert anemone's potency tends to degrade quickly. It is best to make a fresh batch of tincture every year or two. Drying the plant greatly diminishes its potency. For an eyewash mix 10 drops of fresh plant tincture in 2 ounces of isotonic water; make fresh daily.

Dosage:
- FPT: 3-10 drops 3-4 times daily
- Fresh poultice: apply as needed
- Eyewash: 3-4 times daily

Cautions: For robust people with strong circulation Desert anemone can be emotionally unsettling. Too much of the plant will cause gastric irritation and diarrhea. Do not use in any condition that is hot, fiery, and acute. In addition, like most other Buttercup family plants do not use Desert anemone during pregnancy due to its dilatory effects on uterine vasculature.

DESERT BARBERRY   *Berberidaceae* – Barberry family

Mahonia fremontii (Berberis fremontii)
Fremont barberry, Holly-grape

Mahonia haematocarpa (Berberis haematocarpa)
Red barberry

Mahonia trifoliata (Berberis trifoliata)
Algerita

Mahonia nevinii (Berberis nevinii)
Nevin's barberry

Description: The species profiled here are large, spiny-leaved shrubs with 6-petaled yellow flowers, mostly juicy fruits, and deeply yellow inner roots. Mahonia fremontii is often a large shrub, occasionally reaching 12-15 feet in height. The stiff bluish-green leaves have 3-7 pinnately arranged, spined leaflets. The developing fruits are yellow or sometimes red; at maturity they are bluish-black. M. haematocarpa is a large many-branched shrub obtaining 12 feet in height. Each leaf is comprised of 3-7 lanceolate leaflets with one terminating the group. Its typical Barberry flowers are 6-petaled. At maturity, the berries are pea-sized, red, and juicy. M. trifoliata reaches 10 feet in height. This dense shrub has stiff, grayish-blue, spined leaves that are composed of 3 leaflets. After flowering, red, tart, and juicy fruits develop. M. nevinii is also a large rounded shrub. Although not as stiff as the others, the holly-like leaves are comprised of 3-5 spiny, lanceolate leaflets. The yellow flowers form in loose racemes. The fruits are yellowish-red to red and are succulent.

Distribution: Mahonia fremontii is found between 4,000-7,000 feet, mostly throughout Desert Grasslands and Juniper-Pinyon Woodlands; occasionally it is found lower in elevation in isolated pockets in southern California. From these holdouts in California the plant is found east through southern Nevada, central-northern Arizona, Utah, Mesa and Delta Counties in Colorado, to the Sandia Mountains of New Mexico. From 3,000-7,500 M. haematocarpa ranges from Arizona where the bulk of the plant practically cuts a diagonal swath across the state just below the Mogollon Rim. It is also abundant throughout southeastern Arizona; from there the plant is distributed east to

{ 78 }

central-south New Mexico and finally to Trans-Pecos Texas. The plant is commonly found in Desert Grasslands and in Oak Woodlands.

Mahonia trifoliata's most expansive range is along the Pecos River Basin in New Mexico and south and east through most of western Texas. The plant is prominent on hillsides and slopes overlooking drainages. Below 2,000 feet in southern California M. nevinii is found in Coastal Sage and Chaparral Scrub habitats. Look for the plant in arid sandy valleys.

Chemistry: (for Mahonia repens; other species are similar) isoquinoline alkaloids: oxyacanthine, berberine, columbamine, corydine, isocorydine, glaucine, jatrorrhizine, magnoflorine, obaberine, obamegine, palmatine, thaliporphine, and thalrugosine; lignan: syringaresinol

Medicinal Uses: Desert barberry is inhibiting to a wide array of pathogens. The plant is broadly antibacterial and fungicidal. Topically the salve or oil applied to infected cuts or wounds, as well as to various skin and nail fungi, will prove beneficial. Internally the root tea or tincture is used as a systemic support for the same issues. Its use is also indicated in bacterial or mold induced sinus infections and for sore/strep throat. From its berberine content, Desert barberry is directly inhibiting to pathogenic gastrointestinal microbes and their harmful endotoxins. Take the plant if suffering from food poisoning, Giardia infection, amebiasis, and other GI tract parasitic/microbial infections. It combines well with Western mugwort.

As a functional bitter tonic, the tea or tincture is of use in indigestion. Although not as direct in its effect here as Gentian or Swertia, Desert barberry stimulates hydrochloric acid, pepsinogen, bile, and succus entericus secretion facilitating food breakdown in the stomach and small intestine – some even may experience a laxative effect through the plant's stimulation of these digestive secretions. Like its close relative Oregon grape, the plant has an interesting effect on the skin and liver. On both areas, although through diverging mechanisms, it diminishes inflammatory excesses. Applied externally the oil or salve slows excessive cellular proliferation, turnover and lipid peroxidation making it valuable in treating psoriasis. Internally the plant's effect on the liver is cooling and protective. It has been shown to normalize liver enzyme elevations, as well as other inflammatory markers associated with hepatitis and liver toxicity from environmental/dietary causes. It is hepaprotective possibly through its influence on the liver's cytochrome P450 pathway. Traditionally Desert barberry was used for "bad blood" and like Oregon grape (Mahonia aquifolium) and European Barberry (Berberis vulgaris) it is considered a classic alterative along with plants like Golden smoke, Stillingia, and Echinacea. It is highly indicated in conditions where the skin is dry, red, and heals poorly, or for what were once called scrofulous conditions.

Moreover, Desert barberry is broadly antiinflammatory and is well used internally in febrile states; it tends to clear pyrogenic compounds within the body. Broadly speaking the tea also has use in inflammatory conditions such as chronic allergies, psoriatic arthritis, lupus, and a range of others.

Indications:
♦ Bacterial, fungal infections (internal and external)
♦ Sinusitis/strep throat (internal and gargle)
♦ Food poisoning/giardiasis/amebiasis
♦ Indigestion with insufficient protein/fat digestion
♦ Psoriasis (internal and external)
♦ Hepatic inflammation, sluggishness
♦ Fever/autoimmune inflammation

Collection: Leave the trowel and pruners behind; bring a man's tools – a shovel and a pick. Collectors are advised to wear a long sleeved shirt and pants to provide protection from the sharply spined leaves. On larger plants, secondary rhizomes that are closer to the ground's surface are collected; leave the main taproots, at least on older plants. The entire taproot can be collected from smaller plants that have several stems rising from its root crown. It is a hard plant to dig in compacted soils, but worth it. Although not as high in berberine content, the leaves can be collected for oils and salves.

Preparations: Cut the roots into ¼-½ inch sections before drying, otherwise, like Red root, unless you own an industrial wood chipper they will be worthless. Because the roots are woody and lack substantial water content, unlike Oregon grape, the tea and dry plant tincture are the best preparations.

Dosage:
♦ Root decoction/cold infusion:2-4 ounces 3 times daily
♦ DPT (50% alcohol): 20-60 drops 3 times daily

Cautions: Berberine can cause hemolysis in babies with G6PD (glucose-6-phosphate-dehydrogenase) deficiency. Like other cholagogues do not use if there is a biliary blockage.

Other Uses: The fruits of Desert barberry can be used for jams and jellies, or can be eaten alone.

DESERT COTTON   *Malvacea* – Mallow family

Gossypium thurberi
Wild cotton

Description: As a many branched, moderately sized shrub, Desert cotton can reach heights of 12 feet, but usually 3-5 feet is normal. Its petioled leaves are palmately 3-5 parted; each lobe is pointed. The large, showy, white flowers are occasionally crimson spotted; they exist in groups of 2-3, are 5-petaled, and 2-3 inches across. The seed capsules are round and 3-parted. Look closely for the small cotton fibers after the seed capsules split open from age.

Distribution: In the United States Desert cotton is limited in distribution to central and southeastern Arizona. Look for the plant along washes, streamsides, and canyon bottoms – at higher elevations, look to draws, among foothills, and rocky slopes. Although limited in range it is a fast-growing, successful plant; it sprouts easily and is not difficult to propagate.

Chemistry: phenolic acids, condensed tannins and the sesquiterpene: gossypol

Medicinal Uses: Desert cotton is primarily an emmenagogue. Use the fresh plant tincture (the most active preparation) when menses is slow to start and there is pelvic and lower back pain. In larger doses, the plant may even cause mid-cycle spotting. Alone or in combination with other herbs that address constitutional imbalances Desert cotton is of help in resolving uterine and breast fibroids. In combination with Wild peony or Hopbush, it is well suited in diminishing first and second day period cramps. Modern day use of Desert cotton primarily originates from Eclectic practitioners, traditional Mexican use, and the associated use of Gossypium spp. by slaves throughout cottonlands in the southeast.

In recent years, light has been shed upon gossypol's physiological effects. The compound is largely present in the seed and in smaller amounts throughout the whole plant. Initially discovered in China where the poor in times of scarcity eat cottonseed meal cakes, the plant disrupts fertility in men. In at least one study funded by the World Health Organization it was determined that proper sperm formation in the testes was inhibited. Apparently, spermatogenesis is negatively affected by gossypol's disruptive effect on the testes' sertoli cells. In a small percentage of men taking the isolated compound fertility was impaired permanently. In conclusion, men are ill advised to use Desert cotton.

Indications:
♦ Menses slow to start with back and pelvic pain
♦ Breast and uterine fibroids

Collection: In the spring when Desert cotton is beginning to leaf out dig the slender, woody taproots; on older plants, they are occasionally forked.

Preparations: Clip the fresh roots into small ¼-½ inch sections and tincture. High-grade Desert cotton by only tincturing the thin layer of outer root bark. Although this is time consuming a much stronger medicine will be gained.

Dosage:
♦ FPT: 20-40 drops 3 times daily

Cautions: Do not use while pregnant or nursing. As stated previously, men should not use Desert cotton, and should avoid food containing cottonseed oil, if wanting to keep sperm intact and healthy.

DESERT LAVENDER   *Labiatae* – Mint family

Hyptis emoryi
Bee sage

Description: As a member of the Mint family, Desert lavender has the typical square stem-opposite leaf setup. The leaves and young stems are covered with a wooly pubescence. The flowers are purplish-blue and are arranged in clusters among the upper leaves or in terminal spikes. Desert lavender is a medium to large sized shrub that when flowering attracts a whole assortment of pollinators, particularly bees. When the plant is in full bloom the lavender scent is heady.

Distribution: From 4,000 feet and below Desert lavender is found from southern parts of the California Desert, north to southern Nevada, and east throughout much of southwestern Arizona and southern New Mexico. At lower elevations Desert lavender is commonly found along washes on alluvial fans. Where it is slightly colder at higher elevations, the plant prefers rock and boulder strewn foothills where it receives extra sustaining warmth. The rocks warmed by the sun during the day act as atmospheric heating blankets enabling Desert lavender and other warmth loving plants such as Brittlebush to thrive.

Chemistry: general essential oil content for the genus: α-pinene, β-pinene, thymol, and rosmarinic acid; lignans; flavonoids

Medicinal Uses: Desert lavender is a sedative of mild strength. Like Verbena, a distant cousin, its sedation on the central nervous system makes usage appropriate in times of emotional stress and anxiety. It is particularly useful as a sudorific in febrile states when the skin is hot and dry and the mind and body are tired and restless. A cup or two of the hot tea is a sure way to break a mild to moderate fever.

Topical application of Desert lavender makes an excellent injury dressing. Many Mint family plants contain aromatic oils that are antimicrobial and anti-inflammatory. Desert lavender is no exception to this. These properties lend themselves well in limiting bacterial growth, capillary bed inflammation, and subsequent leakage. A salve or poultice applied to burns, contusions, cuts, and other injuries speeds healing. For Candida flare-ups, the leaf infusion applied as a wash to involved tissues will help speed resolution. Sitting in a warm sitz bath of tea for 15-20 minutes is one of the better methods of directly limiting Candida growth affecting vaginal and urethral tissues.

For inflammatory conditions of the stomach such as gastritis and peptic ulcer Desert lavender has the distinct effect of not only reducing inflammation (through several mechanisms, but notably by inhibiting pro-inflammatory prostaglandin synthesis) but also of reducing hyper-secretions of the stomach. Hydrochloric acid secretion is lowered with internal usage of the plant making these overly acidic, hyper-secretory conditions more apt to heal.

Indications:
- Anxiety/tension/sleeplessness
- Fever, dry, moderate temperature
- Gastritis/peptic ulcer
- Burns/cuts/scrapes (external)
- Candida infections (external)

Collection: Gather the plant in the spring or summer when growth is new. Crush a leaf – it should be hydrated and lavender scented. Collect the leaves and flowers since these parts have the greatest concentration of medicinal aromatics.

Preparations and Dosage:
- Leaf infusion: 4-8 ounces 2-3 times daily
- FPT/DPT (60% alcohol): 30-60 drops 2-3 times daily

Cautions: It is unwise to use during pregnancy due to Desert lavender's array of uterine stimulating aromatics.

DESERT MILKWEED

Asclepiadaceae – Milkweed family

Asclepias subulata
Rush milkweed, Leafless milkweed

Description: Desert milkweed is a large, 4-6 foot tall, clump-forming perennial. Its greenish-white stems are rush-like, slender, and form in numerous clusters that rise up from a central root crown. Its leaves, which are small and thread-like, are ½-1 inch long and usually fall away quickly in response to drought or cold temperatures. The light yellow flowers form in umbels at the branch ends and have a typical milkweed structure: 5 united sepals and 5 petals, which generally appear dumb-bell like. The seedpods are 2-3 inches long by a ½-inch wide and upon opening release densely tufted seeds to the wind. When any part of the fresh plant is broken, a white-milky sap exudes from the wound. The form of Desert milkweed's roots change in relationship to the types of soil it is found in. The plant, in fine, sandy soils often has one main taproot reaching depths of 3-4 feet. Roots with secondary rhizomes that are more tortuous occur in soils that are composed of gravel and larger sediments.

Distribution: From nearly sea level to 2,500 feet Asclepias subulata is found from Clark County, Nevada, south along the Colorado and Gila River Basins in Arizona, to lower portions of the California Deserts. The plant is commonly found next to washes, sandy and gravely plains, and on dry, rocky slopes. Desert milkweed is cold sensitive, a factor that limits its range in more northerly locations.

Chemistry: at least three cardenolide-type cardiac glycosides; lignan: lariciresinol

Medicinal Uses: The medicinal qualities of all Milkweeds tend to have more similarities than differences. They largely differ in the extent to which they stimulate the heart. Desert milkweed and other closely related species that are chemically or structurally similar, such as Asclepias erosa, A. albicans, and A. linaria, are known to have high cardiac glycoside contents. Desert milkweed will affect the heart more profoundly than other commonly used Milkweeds, i.e. Pleurisy root (A. tuberosa) and Antelope horns. Think of this plant as Antelope horns plus more "heart". Unlike Antelope horns, the plant does not have a coherent history of traditional use, or at least one that has been recorded or revealed. The plant's lung and skin affecting attributes are predictable, its effects on the heart, uterus, and intestines less so. For a general overview of medicinal uses and indications, see Antelope horns.

Collection: Gather the roots in the fall or winter. Sandy soils will make digging easier, but that luxury is not always available. Pick a large, robust plant. Dig a hole to one side of it, 1 foot or so out and 1-2 feet deep. Slowly work in to the main root mass; as you do collect any secondary rhizomes you encounter. When the main root mass is reached take a pound or two while being as gentle as possible as not to disturb the entire root complex.

The latex of Desert milkweed can be harvested by chopping ½-inch sections of the stems off starting at the top of the plant. After several minutes, the latex will harden. Scrape it off with a razor blade or knife; chop another piece off from the same branch ½-inch lower, repeat. Like harvesting Wild lettuce latex, the process is time consuming, but all good things come with time and hard work. For the plant's sake do not denude all of its stems, leave at least half for flower growth and reproduction. After drying to a glue-like consistency, the latex can be tinctured or rolled into pellets and swallowed.

Preparations: Clean the roots well of any debris and embedded stones. Chop them into ¼-½ inch pieces. Dry, then store. After a year, the root oils tend to oxidize. Use within this time.

Dosage:
- DPT: (50% alcohol) 5-20 drops 3 times daily
- Fluidextract: 5-10 drops 3 times daily
- Latex tincture: (50% alcohol) 5-20 drops 3 times daily
- Latex pellets or '00' capsules: 1-2, 3 times daily

Cautions: Same as Antelope horns, but place more awareness on heart interactions.

DESERT OREGANO
Verbenaceae – Vervain family

Aloysia wrightii (*Lippia wrightii*)
Beebush, Vara dulce, Altamisa, Oreganillo

Description: Desert oregano is a small, rounded sub-shrub, often growing next to or under larger shrubs and trees. The younger stems of the plant are ridged, the older growth lesser so. Desert oregano's leaves are small, oval, oppositely arranged, and delicately perched beneath tiny, whitish flower spikes. Bees are quite fond of the plant during the spring and summer when it is in flower. The scent of Desert oregano after brushing up against it or crushing a few leaves between the fingers is friendly and disarming. Actually, the plant smells much closer to a cross between Lavender and Lemon verbena – certainly not Oregano with its cutting pungency.

Distribution: From isolated outposts in southern California it ranges southeast through Arizona, southern New Mexico, and southern Texas. It is typically seen growing on hillsides, rocky slopes, and on the edges of drainage areas between 1,200-6,000 feet.

Chemistry: α-pinene, sabinene, limonene, cineole, linalol, β-caryophyllene, neral, α-terpinyl acetate, geranial, citronellol, nerol, geraniol, caryophyllene oxide, cisnerolidol, and spathulenol
    This is an essential oil listing for Aloysia triphylla or Lemon verbena. Desert Oregano contains similar compounds, but owing to its bitterness and other differences, some variation is to be expected.

Medicinal Uses: The tincture or the tea taken before meals is a functional, aromatic bitter. Through reflex, in response to bitterness, digestive secretions (particularly pepsinogen and hydrochloric acid) are stimulated. Blood flow is shifted to the stomach walls by the dilating nature of the plant's aromatics. Take Desert oregano when there is indigestion after a meal. If a recently eaten meal feels immovable and the stomach is bloated Desert oregano is warranted.

Indications:
♦   Indigestion with bloating

Collection: If the foliage smells strongly Lavender-like, it will make good medicine. Gently strip the leaves and flowers from the upper branches. Dry the herbage for tea or use fresh.

Preparations and Dosage:
♦ Leaf infusion: 4-8 ounces 3-4 times daily
♦ FPT/DPT (50% alcohol): 30-60 drops 3-4 times daily

Cautions: Do not use during pregnancy due the plant's potential of stimulating uterine vasculature.

DESERT RHUBARB   *Polygonaceae* – Buckwheat family

Rumex hymenosepalus
Wild rhubarb, Tanner's dock, Canaigre

Description: In early spring, Desert rhubarb is one of the first plants to challenge the surrounding straw colored land by sending up small clusters of leaves from beneath the ground. The leaf tips, which are seen first, quickly progress into large, smooth, wavy-margined, deeply green leaves. At maturity these lower basal leaves are generally 1-2 feet long by 2-4 inches wide. They progressively become smaller and less abundant along the rising flower stalks. The flower clusters are similar to other Docks and are borne on central fleshy stalks. After maturing, the seeds become reddish, waiting in large clusters to be released by the wind. The whole plant is rather succulent and is able to withstand drought through numerous underground tubers, thus providing the upper portion with necessary water and nutrients in times of scarcity.

Distribution: Desert rhubarb can be found from western Texas to stretches of the Mohave Desert in California, south from Wyoming, Utah, and Colorado, to Arizona and New Mexico. Look for the plant from 6,000 feet and lower in sandy and moist soils. Washes, fields, and roadsides are some of its favorite abodes.

Chemistry: condensed and hydrolyzable tannins; chrysophanol, emodin, and physcion

Medicinal Uses: Desert rhubarb is used topically for its astringency. External preparations are tightening to surface tissues and will lessen skin irritation and redness from burns, rashes, and scrapes. The plant, being moderately hemostatic is applied well to superficial cuts in order to staunch bleeding. Although symptomatic in effect, it can be almost miraculous in limiting the spread of stress or chemical sensitivity induced rashes, probably through its inflammatory-prostaglandin mediating properties. In these cases, use the juice liberally as a paint. In addition, the juice as a mouthwash or gargle is soothing and astringing to mouth sores, bleeding gums, and sore throats.

Indications:
♦ Cuts/abrasions/burns (external)
♦ Rashes (external)
♦ Sore throats/mouth sores (gargle)

Collection: During the late winter or early spring when Desert rhubarb's leaves are just starting to show themselves, with a trowel, dig to a depth of about 1 foot, 6-10 inches beyond the outer leaves. Slowly work in to the central area underneath the plant. Depending on the softness of the soil, this can sometimes be done with hands alone. Along the way tubers of varying sizes will be found, some will be younger, pale, and flesh-colored, others will be darker, having a rust-brown coloration; also, some will be dried out, remnant tubers of the year before. Collect no more than half the tubers one plant has of both light and dark types. Next year, although diminished in strength the plant will again grow and flourish.

Preparations: The roots can be used in several different ways. To dry, thinly slice the tubers, and then lay out well spaced.

The following description describes how best to make Desert rhubarb root juice, which in many ways is the superior preparation. This method is an adaptation of a technique used by Peter Bigfoot: Wash and clean the roots well, as running small pebbles through a juicer is never a good idea. Dice the fresh tubers in ¼-inch pieces. Slowly in small handfuls juice the entire root; periodic cleaning of the metal juicer screen may be necessary as you progress, as the root fibers tend to collect there. Overall, this is a difficult root to juice and will challenge the best of juicers, but the result is worth it.

Pour the juice in a glass container; a mason jar works well. Place the covered Desert rhubarb juice in an area where it is easily observed but will not be disturbed. After several hours, the juice will form two layers. There will be a top layer, deeply rust brown, most likely tannic acid in solution and a bottom layer – mostly remnant pulp and bound tannins. After the two layers have separated fully, ladle off the top tannin layer and preserve it with 20% grain alcohol (4 parts juice to 1 part undiluted grain alcohol). Discard the remaining yellowish-orange pulp. The tannin solution does not need to be refrigerated.

Dosage:

♦ Tannin juice/root powder/root decoction: externally as needed

Cautions: Externally, none known.

Other Uses: Some ethnobotanical literature cites Desert rhubarb tubers being used for food. Since they are so high in tannins, realistically this may be possible only after a ½-dozen changes of water, which itself is a highly valued and often scarce substance in most arid places where Desert rhubarb grows. If eaten fresh, directly from the ground Desert rhubarb's high concentration of root tannins are so deranging to sensitive mucosal layers, which the mouth and gut are primarily lined with, even if an individual was starving, it would hurt more than help.

The fleshy flower stalks and leaf petioles can be eaten more liberally raw and also are used as a substitute for "true" Rhubarb. Carolyn Niethammer, in her book American Indian Food and Lore has a tasty recipe for Desert rhubarb pie. The young and tender leaves can be boiled through a couple of changes of water to remove the bitterness then eaten alone or with other greens.

DESERT WILLOW

Bignoniacea – Bignonia family

Chilopsis linearis
Mimbre, Sauce

Description: Desert willow, being totally unrelated to true Willow (Salix spp.), is a small deciduous tree with linear leaves arranged alternately along its branches. The tree's conspicuous funnel-like white, pink to purple flowers are difficult to miss, both visually and because of their strong fragrance. Like Trumpet flower, the narrow and elongated seedpods hold numerous seeds that take to the air by way of their winged outer coating.

Distribution: Desert willow needs ample water supply to thrive, making it is a reliable indicator of permanent underground water. Most often the tree can be seen growing along washes, gullies, and other drainage areas. The tree is found from southwestern California, north to Kansas, where it has been added recently to the state's flora, south through Oklahoma and Texas.

Chemistry: unknown, besides typical cyanin flavonoids in the flower

Medicinal Uses: A simple leaf infusion of Desert willow applied externally, like other Bignonia family plants, is antifungal. It is useful in treating various skin and nail funguses; it is also effective against Candida infections. A douche or sitz bath of warm Desert willow tea is an excellent localized application for vaginal Candida overgrowths from antibiotics or steroid use. The tea internally can be systemically useful in the above-mentioned issues.

Desert willow has promise in treating valley fever or coccidioidomycosis. The responsible organism, Coccidioides immitis, is a soil mold common in the arid American Southwest. Exposure in susceptible individuals is usually self-resolving but can manifest fever, malaise, cough, and skin rashes among other symptoms. In immune compromised and dark skinned individuals, deeper pulmonary and systemic infections are more apt to result. Allopathic intervention is warranted in these advanced cases. Desert willow in combination with pulmonary inoculating herbs such as Ligusticum or Lomatium is of use in mild or moderate cases of exposure.

Indications:
♦ Candida albicans and other fungal infections (internal and external)

Collection: In late spring to early summer when Desert willow is in bloom collect the last 8-12 inches of branch ends, as these will have the newest leaves and developing flowers. The bark can be collected, as it is also medicinally active (this only being necessary in colder times of year when the leaves are absent).

Preparations and Dosage:
- FPT/DPT (50% alcohol): 30-60 drops 3 times daily
- Leaf infusion/bark decoction: 4-6 ounces 2-3 times daily
- Douche/sitz bath/wash: 2-3 times daily

Cautions: None known.

Other Uses: Being a fast grower, rather adaptable to various planted conditions and ascetically appealing, particularly when in flower, Desert willow is often cultivated as an ornamental throughout the southwest.

DOGWEED   *Compositae* – Sunflower family

Dyssodia pentachaeta
Golden fleece, Golden dyssodia, Parralena

Dyssodia acerosa
Needle leaf dogweed, Prickleleaf dogweed

Dyssodia papposa
Fetid marigold, Pagué

Description: Dyssodia pentachaeta is a small plant, usually no more than 8-10 inches high. This perennial forms in clumps and has opposite, pinnatifid leaves arranged in 5-7 linear divisions. The yellow flowers are ½-inch across and form on slender stalks above the foliage clumps. When crushed (as with most Dogweeds) the aromatics emit a pleasant scent. D. acerosa is another small perennial. It is woody at its base and stands approximately 1 foot tall. The dark green linear leaves are attached to the main stems either oppositely or alternately. Small circular glands are noticeable on the leaf surfaces. The yellow flowers are ¾-inch across and form at branch ends. D. papposa is a small 4-16 inch tall annual. Its leaves are 1-2 inches long, pinnatifid, and linearly divided. The flowers are small and tend to be surrounded by inconspicuous rays. All Dogweeds are aromatic. Judge the medicinal potency of individual plants by their pungency.

Distribution: Dyssodia pentachaeta is found from 2,500-5,600 feet sporadically throughout southern California, southern and western Arizona, and parts of New Mexico to Texas. Roadsides are a typical favorite of the plant. Otherwise, it is found in washes and on dry slopes and hillsides. D. acerosa ranges from western Texas to southern and central New Mexico to southeast and central Arizona, and finally throughout the Grand Canyon area. Look for this Dogweed on limestone soils between 3,500-6,000 feet. D. papposa inhabits a wide range of territory: from Illinois to Montana, south to Louisiana and Arizona. Throughout the arid southwest, it is often found in waste places – ditches, fieldsides, etc.

Chemistry: flavonoids, acetylenic thiophenes, and monoterpenes

Medicinal Uses: Dogweed, like closely related Mountain marigold and Deerweed, is used as a tea to settle an upset stomach. It serves as a useful carminative, used in relieving gas pains from poorly digested food dependant upon stress or general debility of the area. A small amount of the tea is likewise good for colicky babies. When the stomach lining is inflamed from an over production of hydrochloric acid, an excess of alcohol or other gastric insults, Dogweed tea is soothing. Try a cup of tea after a meal that has caused bloating and fullness.

Indications:
♦ Gastritis
♦ Indigestion/gas pains/colic

Collection: Prune the upper herbage from the plants at the height of their potency, when they are non-stressed and before or during flowering. Throughout the southwest Dyssodia papposa is collected between late July and August, after it responds to Monsoon rains. The other perennials are collected throughout the spring and summer.

Preparations and Dosage:
♦ Leaf infusion: 4-8 ounces 3 times daily

Cautions: None known.

ELDER   *Caprifoliaceae* – Honeysuckle family

Sambucus mexicana (Sambucus caerulea var. mexicana)
Mexican elder, Flor sauce, Flor de saugua, Saúco

Sambucus glauca
Blue elderberry

Sambucus microbotrys
Red elderberry

Description: Mexican elder is a small tree reaching 15-35 feet in height. Its appearance can be unruly and non-uniform, given the tree's propensity for dropping branches in favor of conserving water – a common survival mechanism seen in desert trees. The branches have an erratic way of growing and can be angled, arched, drooping, or nearly horizontal. Upon maturation, the crown is wide and rounded. The bark is finely fissured and yellowish-brown. The leaves are composed of 3-5 ovoid, thickened leaflets which are smooth above, occasionally hairy beneath and have finely serrated margins; when crushed they are strong-scented. The small cream-colored flowers form in flat-topped clusters 6-8 inches across. The fruits that follow are clustered, a ½-inch across, and are sweet and very edible.

The closely allied Blue elderberry is smaller, at least at higher elevations. The leaves are composed of 3-9 lanceolate leaflets and like Mexican elder has edible fruits. Red elderberry is typically a large shrub with 5-7 thin, coarsely serrated leaflets. Bright red, semi-poisonous berries follow the whitish flower clusters.

Distribution: Mexican elder is found along drainages from 2,000-4,000 feet. It is distributed disjointedly throughout the southwest. Pockets of the tree can be found from coastal mountainous regions of southern California to central-eastern Arizona, Gila River and Rio Grande Drainages in New Mexico, and finally to the Nueces River area of western Texas.

Blueberry elder is common throughout the coastal and inter-mountain west. It is typically a tree found with Douglas fir and other conifers. Red elderberry, a

ELDER

non-native shrub-tree originally from Eurasia, has naturalized extensively throughout the country. In the west, it is found in moist coniferous forests.

Chemistry: for Sambucus canadensis, a closely allied blue-fruited Elder: triterpenes: α-amyrin palmitate, balanophorin and oleanolic acid; flavonoids: cyanidin, cyanin, quercetin, and rutin; monoterpene: morroniside; steroids: campesterol, β-sitosterol and stigmasterol; sambucine

Medicinal Uses: Elder is chiefly diaphoretic, making its application to fevers, particularly if they are low to moderate in temperature, warranted. If the skin is hot and dry Elder will reliably promote sweating. The tea drunk cold is diuretic, especially if there is no elevated temperature. External preparations are distinctly antimicrobial and antifungal. Elder is usefully applied to these situations particularly if the affected tissues are edematous, slow to heal, and tend to ulcerate.

Mexican elder has been found to inhibit Salmonella spp. and Shigella dysenteriae, so its application to gastroenteritis coincides with traditional use for the plant in Guatemala. Elder has some use in lung centered viral conditions particularly if the insult has produced a dry fever. The leaf and flower tea are somewhat similar in effect to the now popular European black elderberry (Sambucus nigra) preparations.

Indications:
- Fevers, dry, low to moderate temperature, with lung centered viruses
- Fluid retention
- Wounds, edematous, ulcerated, slow to heal, with or without bacterial or fungal involvement (external)

Collection: Prune the last foot or so from the flowering branch ends, or collect the flower and leaves separately. The fruit clusters can be collected in bunches and then separated from their respective small stems.

Preparations: The flowers are simple enough to dry; the leaves though can be problematic. If they are not dried quickly they often mildew, turn black and become unusable. Dry quickly in a warm and arid environment or use a dehydrator.

Dosage:

♦   Leaf/flower infusion: 2-4 ounces 3 times daily, though often less of the
    leaf tea is needed as it can be more stimulating

Cautions: American elders all contain varying amounts of sambucine and
cyanogenic compounds. Although individual populations can markedly differ
in concentrations it is best to use flower and leaf preparations, verses the bark
which tends to contain higher amounts of these compounds. Red elder berries
are considered generally toxic and should be avoided. The fruits of Sambucus
racemosa, a native Red elderberry, were rendered safer to eat by various
American Indian tribes by applying heat, through boiling, steaming, or
roasting. Heat has been shown to reduce cyanogenic compounds significantly.
Some sensitive individuals may find the flower and especially leaf
preparations mildly laxative. Like any vasodilating herb, Elder can potentially
increase body temperature very briefly before promoting diaphoresis; be
mindful of this when using it in higher febrile states.

Other Uses: The fruits of blue Elder types, in moderate quantities, are sweet
and edible raw. The fruits are popular in making jams, jellies, and wines.

FILAREE   *Geraniaceae* – Geranium family

Erodium cicutarium
Storksbill, Alfilerillo, Alfilaria

Description: Filaree is a small herbaceous annual, rarely biennial, that
typically has laterally oriented leaves during its first growth phase. Its
spreading basal leaves radiate out to form compact rosettes; the lobed leaflets
form in alternate pairs along the stems. They are hairy and can reach several
inches in length. Later Filaree's growth can be more erect and in ideal
conditions reach 1-1½ feet in height and often twice that stretched along the
ground. The stems are reddish and branched. The small, 5-petaled, purplish-
pink flowers are clustered in small groupings on slender stalks originating
from the leaf axils. Another common name, Storksbill, applies to the massed
pointed fruits. The fruit clusters separate into 5 individual seeds, all having a
tail-like appendage that coils and uncoils in corresponding dry and wet
conditions, thereby assisting the seed's placement in the ground.

Distribution: This non-native, European originator is found throughout the west and much of North America. From practically sea level to 9,000 feet, look for Filaree along roadsides, vacant lots, fallow fields, gardens, and any other area where the earth has been disturbed allowing for the easy seeding of the plant.

Chemistry: flavonoids: quercetin, kaempferol, luteolin, and ellagic acid

Medicinal Uses: Traditionally Filaree is used as a mild astringent in various external and internal conditions. Internally the tea reduces heavy menstruation and is considered soothing to the urinary tract when tissues are inflamed and it hurts to urinate. In addition, the plant is mildly hemostatic to the area, lessening passive hemorrhaging. Because of the mildness of Filaree, it is best not to over estimate the power of the plant. Filaree has a reputation as a reliable diuretic particularly indicated when there is rheumatic pain and associated fluid retention centered around the joints.

Similar to Geranium, Filaree is a soothing gargle for sore throats. In addition, the tea or fresh plant poultice can be applied topically to diminish redness and sensitivity from sunburn, scrapes, and rashes. Used as a sitz bath or douche the plant is soothing to inflamed vaginal and cervical tissues.

Indications:
♦ Heavy menstruation
♦ Urinary tract inflammation/haematuria
♦ Fluid retention with accompanying rheumatism
♦ Sore throat (gargle)
♦ Burns/rashes (external)
♦ Vaginal, cervical inflammation (external)

Collection: When the herbage is still fresh and verdant, pull the entire plant up, root and all. The slender taproot should come up easily especially if the plant is in moist, non-compacted soil. Larger roots may have to be split lengthwise as to insure their proper drying. It is acceptable to mix the herb and root together in storage as they complement each other well; the root's lack of density makes the infusion method fine.

Preparations and Dosage:
♦ Herb/root infusion: 4-8 ounces 3 times daily

♦   Sitz bath/douche: 2-3 times daily

Cautions: Filaree growing in the desert occasionally is a host for Synchytrium papillatum, a fungus that causes the plant to produce a burgundy pigment on its leaves. Do not gather and use infected plants.

Other Uses: The young green leaves are edible and can be added to salads and the like.

FLAT-TOP BUCKWHEAT *Polygonaceae* – Buckwheat family

Eriogonum fasciculatum
California buckwheat

Description: Flat-top buckwheat is a compact, dense sub-shrub growing 2-3 feet wide by the same high. Its initial appearance is often larger since the plant is occasionally found in clump-forming colonies. The main stems are woody and around the plant's circumference, they tend to prostrate themselves along the ground, where some varieties aggressively root at stem nodes. The leaves are bunched in crowded groupings along the stems and point upward. They are linear and are approximately ½-¾ of an inch long, greenish above and lighter underneath. The flowers are white to pink and form in dense flattened clusters at branchlet ends where they appear to hover over the body of the plant.

There are a number of varieties of Eriogonum fasciculatum that overlap in range and appear very similar to one another. For simplicity, the varieties here are described as a whole. Besides the Flat-top buckwheat types, which are uniform in growth, dense and bushy, there are the Skeletonweed morphologies (E. deflexum). They tend to be annuals, but not always, have basal rosettes of petioled leaves that are often kidney shaped. They tend to have 1 or several central, sometimes inflated, leafless or nearly so, vertical stalks on which spreading and tiny inflorescences are borne. Another biotype is that of Desert buckwheat or E. wrightii. These are bushy perennials similar to E. fasciculatum but they lack the stoutness of the latter. New growth tends to be non-uniform and weak-branched. The elliptical leaves are approximately a ½-inch long, downy, and are spread alternately along the stems; the flowers also form in clusters at branch ends.

Distribution: Flat-top buckwheat can be found from Santa Barbara and Monterey Counties, California, east through southern Nevada and western Arizona. Look for the plant on bluffs and cliffs over looking the ocean in southern California, on disturbed soils, the edges of washes and occasionally on desert flats throughout the rest of its range. Overall, the genus contains 200+ species throughout the United Sates; they are particularly abundant across the west.

Chemistry: Buckwheat family array of hydrolyzable and condensed tannins; other flavonoids

Medicinal Uses: All Eriogonums can essentially be used the same way. The bushier perennials, because of their mass and subsequent collectability lend themselves more to therapeutic use. Flat-top buckwheat is a simple remedy for simple complaints. Its mild astringency lends itself well to several applications, these also being common to other plants that have similar constituent make-ups. When it is painful to urinate, and the lower urinary tract is raw and inflamed, possibly from urine pH changes or from the throes of a lower urinary tract infection, Flat-top buckwheat will cool and contract urinary tract tissues enough to diminish the pain and inflammation.

The leaf tea will check diarrhea, be it from dietary or stress reactions. Similarly, the plant has use in diminishing simple intestinal inflammation. Externally the crushed plant applied fresh or the strong infusion used topically is soothing to burns, weepy rashes, and other outbreaks that tend to be moist and red.

Indications:
♦ Lower urinary tract pain and irritation
♦ Diarrhea with intestinal inflammation
♦ Skin inflammations (external)

Collection: In the spring when new leaf growth is apparent, collect Flat-top buckwheat by pruning upper growth from the plant. After drying, garble the leaves and flower from the stems. Discard the stems.

Preparations and Dosage:
♦ Herb infusion: 4-8 ounces 3 times daily

Cautions: Due to the plant's potential vasoconstriction of uterine lining, Flat-top buckwheat is not recommended during pregnancy.

GLOBEMALLOW   *Malvacea* – Mallow family

Sphaeralcea spp.
Desert hollyhock, Desert mallow, Sore eye poppy, Yerba de la negrita

Description: Globemallow is a 1-4 foot high, short-lived, perennial bush, although several species are in fact smaller annuals. These plants are covered with small star-shaped hairs making them fuzzy to the touch. Due to individual species and environmental conditions, the leaves are of varying size and shape, but most are palmately lobed or at least shallowly dentate; when crushed they are mucilaginous. The thickened leaves alternate along the main stems. The flowers form in racemes or panicles; they are 5-petaled and showy. Orange and red are usually the predominate colors but occasionally varieties can be white, lavender, or pink. The seedpod is wheel shaped, composed of 5 or more carpels and surrounded by a persistent calyx. Kidney shaped, pubescent seeds are held within each wedge-shaped carpel. Globemallow is notorious for inter-species crossbreeding, making individual species classification sometimes difficult.

Indian mallow or Abutilon spp. and Hibiscus spp. are other regionally available native plant genera in the Mallow family that can be used in a similar fashion. Depending on species, Indian mallow is a small, deciduous shrub or herbaceous plant. The leaves, like Globemallow, are covered with small hairs and alternate along the stems. They are petioled, entire, or toothed and often cordate, at least towards the base. The 5-petaled flowers are usually yellow or orange, but sometimes according to species, they can be white, pink, or red. The seed capsules are cylindrically shaped and composed of seed containing carpels. H. denudate and H. coulteri are perennial, herbaceous multi-stemmed small plants. H. denudatus's leaves are ovoid or obovate, with prominent teeth. The large lavender flowers are quite a contrast to its light green leaves. H. coulteri's mature leaves are deeply 3-lobed; the lower leaves are lesser so. The plant's large flowers are yellow with a red spot at their base. There are several seeds in each wedge-shaped carpel.

Distribution: Globemallow is abundant throughout the interior west and can be found in a wide array of elevations and climates. Sphaeralcea coccinea, one of the larger distributed species, stretches from Arizona and New Mexico, north to Saskatchewan and Alberta. Other species' ranges are similar, although the densest populations of all species combined occur within the arid southwest. Look to dry hillsides, roadsides, trailsides, and disturbed soils.

Indian mallow is generally a plant of the southwestern Deserts. Southern California, Arizona, New Mexico, and Texas contain the bulk of the plant. It is found from 1,000-5,500 feet on rocky slopes, streamsides, and canyon bottoms. Hibiscus denudatus is found from sea level to 4,000 feet in southeastern California, east through much of southern Arizona, skipping the bulk of New Mexico to southern Texas, west of the Pecos River. A disjointed pocket exists in Clark County, Nevada. H. coulteri is found from 2,000-4,000 feet throughout Arizona's Sonoran Desert and southeast Cochise County to the Big Bend area of Texas.

Chemistry: various polysaccharides (pectin, mucilage, and starch), namely arabinogalactans; tannins: similar to Mallow

Medicinal Uses: Use Globemallow in beginning stages of bronchitis. When the lungs and throat feel hot and irritated and there is an unproductive cough the tea sipped throughout the day will gently diminish the cough reflex through its soothing effect on inflamed bronchial and throat tissues. Globemallow's pharmacological activity provides a slight immunologic boost to the lung environment. Dust cells or macrophages that reside in the alveoli are stimulated by Globemallow's polysaccharide content. These immunologic mucilages - mainly arabinogalactan and other related compounds - serve as the main stimulator to the area. The dust cells reside deep within the lungs, beyond the larger bronchi, in the air sacs. They engulf and eliminate foreign particles that are small enough to become deposited within the alveoli. Globemallow intensifies this process, making our local respiratory environment more resilient and active.

Urethral and bladder irritation respond well to this soothing plant. The surrounding urinary tract tissues are soothed through their contact with the Malvacea constituents, which are eliminated through the urine. Extra benefit will be gained, if in fact there is an infection, from an appropriate urinary tract antibacterial herb such as Manzanita or Juniper.

Externally Globemallow makes an excellent emollient poultice. It is very useful in reducing swellings from injury, bringing abscesses to a head, and getting splinters to slowly gravitate to the skin's surface. Globemallow's immunological stimulation quickens the tissue's natural process of resolution. The body then proceeds to encapsulate spent phagocytes, damaged tissue cells, and other cellular wastes created by this process. This mass is then slowly resolved from the inside or comes to a head on the outside and is released. Copperleaf or Leadwort can be added for an additional stimulating effect.

Indications:
- Bronchitis, with an irritative cough
- Urinary tract irritation
- Abscess/splinters (internal and external)

Collection: Collect Globemallow in the spring after it has been enlivened by winter-spring rains. Its growth will be full and new, as opposed to early summer collection where the leaves are smaller, more condensed, a bit more astringent, but still good medicine. Snip the upper herbage that consists of the stem, flower, and leaf. Dry normally.

Preparations: Globemallow has a pleasantly sweet, slippery, and astringent taste. When making the foliage infusion, strain it well to remove the very small leaf hairs. Use a cloth for best results. If left in the tea they can be irritating to the throat.

To prepare a poultice, slowly stir in enough hot water to dried and powdered Globemallow leaves to achieve a thick, pudding-like consistency. Place this glob in several folds of cheesecloth and then place this on the affected area when it has sufficiently cooled down – but is still warm. Cover with a warm damp towel. Repeat the process as needed.

Dosage:
- Herb infusion: 4-8 ounces 3 times daily
- Poultice: as needed

Cautions: A friend related a story to me once about Globemallow. He and several buddies were driving a truck with the windows down on a dirt road with Globemallow on both sides. As they traveled, the side mirrors slapped the 4-5 foot high plants creating a fine cloud of leaf hair in the cab. After several minutes of this their eyes were red from the contact irritation of the fine leaf hairs…Sore eye poppy. Also, when children rub their eyes after playing with the plant the same can result.

GOLDEN SMOKE

Papaveraceae – Poppy family

Corydalis aurea
Scrambled eggs

Description: Golden smoke is a small, weak-stemmed biannual or short-lived perennial. The plant is bluish-green, glaucous, and between 4-16 inches tall. Its distinctive yellow, spurred flowers tend to form in racemes at the branch ends. These little clump-forming plants have deeply lobed leaves that appear feather-like. The resulting seedpods are elongated, slightly curved, and scimitar-like; they are approximately 1 inch long and contain numerous small black seeds.

Distribution: Although the plant is sporadic in local distribution, it is a common plant throughout much of the west and can be found at most elevations. Look for Golden smoke along streamsides, in washes, and other drainage areas beneath overgrowth. It also frequents disturbed areas and is occasionally seen along road and trailsides. It is one of the first plants to bloom in the spring in arid, lower elevation areas.

Chemistry: berberine, bulbocapnine, corpaverine, corybulbine, protopine, sanguinarine, and other isoquinoline alkaloids

Medicinal Uses: Golden smoke is a sedative of moderate strength. It is particularly useful when nervous system distress manifests as muscular twitching, tics, and mild seizure activity. Use Golden smoke when these excessive discharges are accompanied by pain. Chronic skin conditions that are of a low-grade, allergic nature respond positively to Golden smoke. The plant seems to be particularly suited to thin individuals whose skin and nervous systems are hypersensitive. If prone to lymph node enlargements, general lymph sluggishness, and blood dyscrasias then Golden smoke will prove corrective.

Golden smoke positively influences digestion and is used when the tongue is chronically coated, the stomach easily becomes distended, and there is a general sluggishness of upper digestive process. Think of Golden smoke as a combination of Desert barberry, California poppy, and Red root (Ceanothus spp.); it is a complex plant worthy of revitalization in modern-day herbal use.

As an alterative or sedative, Golden smoke is best used in combination with other herbs.

Indications:
♦ Lymph node enlargements
♦ Poorly healing tissue with tendency towards ulceration
♦ Atonic gastric digestion
♦ Chronic skin conditions from allergy or autoimmune disturbances
♦ Nervous system irritability/mild seizure activity/muscular tremors/tics

Collection: Collect the whole plant when flowering in early spring.

Preparations and Dosage:
♦ FPT/DPT (50% alcohol): 10-30 drops 3 times daily
♦ Leaf infusion: 2-4 ounces 3 times daily

Cautions: Pharmacologically Golden smoke is a complex plant. It has been shown to inhibit platelet aggregation, so is not recommended if taking medications that effect blood viscosity. If used alone, keep Golden smoke use to short term (2-3 weeks) or longer at lower doses in combination with other herbs. Do not use Golden smoke during pregnancy or while nursing.

GREENTHREAD

Compositae – Sunflower family

Thelesperma megapotamicum
Navajo tea, Hopi tea, Cota

Description: Greenthread is a deep-rooted perennial. The plant usually stands 2-3 feet tall and has numerous long and narrow stems, which are smooth, bluish-green, and glaucous. The leaves, of similar characteristic, are opposite and either entire or divided into 1 or 2 linear divisions. The nodding yellow flower heads sit atop long peduncles; they seem too large to be properly supported by the thin stem. The flowers fade to tannish-brown with age. Other species of Thelesperma are similarly formed. T. subnudum is a smaller plant also with large yellow flower heads. T. longipes' flowers are smaller; its delicate leaves are prominently divided.

Distribution: Greenthread has a large distribution throughout the interior west. From Nebraska and Wyoming, the plant is found south through most of the plains states, to Arizona, New Mexico, and Texas. From 4,000-8,000 feet look to open woodlands, grassy flats, mesa tops, on the edges of gullies, and along secondary roads.

Chemistry: not known

Medicinal Uses: The Hopi, Navajo, and Hispanic New Mexicans have used the plant as a beverage tea. It is drunk simply for the taste. The tea is non-bitter, pleasant tasting, and sweetens well with a little honey or sugar. Greenthread tends to be mildly diuretic.

Collection: Gather Greenthread while it is in flower for easier identification. Snip the above ground foliage and bundle loosely or dry normally.

Preparations and Dosage:
♦ Herb infusion: as desired

Cautions: None known.

Other Uses: The foliage and roots have been used as a traditional dye; they provide a yellow, brownish-orange coloration.

HOPBUSH

Sapindaceae – Soapberry family

Dodonaea viscosa (Dodonaea viscosa var. angustifolia, D. viscosa var. linearis, D. arizonica)
Switch sorrel, Jarilla

Description: Hopbush is a perennial shrub, usually 4-8 feet tall. The leaves are evergreen, several inches long, much less wide, and generally lanced shaped. If crushed the foliage is sticky, afforded by an evenly distributed coat of resin. The male and female flowers are insignificant and are dwarfed by the 3-4 winged, yellowish-green, occasionally pink tinged fruits. Although they do not really resemble true Hops flowers (Humulus), the coloration is similar and they are relatively papery. The winged fruit clusters are noticeable during mid-spring and are showy.

Distribution: Hopbush is primarily found in central-southern Arizona and parts of Florida. Various species are found throughout much of the tropical and subtropical world; it is a far-reaching genus that is even dominant in parts of Australia. Look for Hopbush from 2,000-4,000 feet among rocky hillsides and boulder strewn slopes. The bush is one of the first to begin repopulation of burned and disturbed land in upper desert areas.

Chemistry: diterpenoids: dodonic acid and hautriwaic acid; flavonoids: pinocembrin, viscosol, santin, and penduletin; dodonones: methyldodonate and dodonolide; saponins: dodonosides a and b

Medicinal Uses: Traditionally Hopbush is used by cultures unrelated to each other, some even existing on opposite ends of the planet. The alignment of American Indian, Mexican, and South African use is striking. The plant is used extensively in sedating smooth muscle contractions; Hopbush is useful in limiting spasmodic diarrhea and stomach cramps. It quells the body's exaggerated reaction to these types of gut centered stresses, be they viral initiated or otherwise. Also, on a purely symptomatic level Hopbush is used in diminishing uterine cramps.

Gallbladder colic, whether from gallstone formation or an adverse response to dietary fat, is lessened. All of these areas – upper and lower gastrointestinal tract, gallbladder and uterus – can be further affected by an externally applied poultice of fresh leaves or a paste made of the moistened leaf powder. It has been suggested that Hopbush exerts this spasmolytic effect by interfering with calcium uptake in smooth muscle cells subsequently inhibiting contraction.

Externally Hopbush applied as a wash or poultice is soothing to any number of rashes and inflammations. The plant is mildly antimicrobial and has been found to inhibit numerous pathogens, namely Escherichia coli, Staphylococcus aureus, and Candida albicans. For lessening Candida flare-ups use a topically applied tea, sitz bath, soak, or douche.

It is interesting to note that Dodonaea growing in different parts of the world shows differences in antimicrobial activity on the same pathogens. As with most plants, environmental conditions greatly influence their internal chemistries, even plants of the same species.

Indications:
♦ GI tract cramps with or without associated diarrhea
♦ Bilious colic
♦ Uterine cramps (internal and external)
♦ Rashes and inflammations, allergy and/or mechanically induced (external)
♦ Skin infections (external)
♦ Candida outbreaks (external)

Collection: From spring through summer, collect Hopbush leaves when they are green and sticky. Dry normally for tea.

Preparations and Dosage:
♦ Leaf infusion: 4 ounces 3 times daily
♦ FPT/DPT (60% alcohol): 30-60 drops 3 times daily
♦ Externally used infusion/fomentation/poultice/oil/salve: apply as needed
♦ Sitz bath/douche: 2-3 times daily

Cautions: It is not wise to use during pregnancy due to the plants effect on uterine musculature.

HOREHOUND

Labiatae – Mint family

Marrubium vulgare
White horehound, Marrubio, Mastranzo, Concha

Description: Horehound is a short-lived perennial. It is 1-2½ feet tall and generally erect and bushy. The classic mint characteristics of opposite leaves and square stems are apparent. Horehound's stems are distinguishable from other related plants in that, particularly towards the base, they are covered with dense, woolly-white fuzz. The leaves are toothed, rounded, green above, and lighter beneath. Where the leaves join the stems, the small, white tubular flowers form in dense clustered whorls. The flower calyxes are toothed and after drying as a group, are bur-like. The seeds are small, egg-shaped, and brown.

Distribution: Horehound is an opportunistic non-native, originally from Europe. It is found in great abundance throughout the west at most elevations. It frequents places of disturbed soils such as roadsides, trailsides, and drainage areas. Just as Prickly poppy's abundance seems to be indicative of cattle activity, Horehound indicates horse movement. Find an old stable or horse trail and surely there will be Horehound close by.

Chemistry: flavonoids: luteolin, apigenin, and vitexin; labdane; diterpenoid: marrubiin; phenylpropanoid esters: (e)-caffeoyl-l-malic acid, acteoside, forsythoside b, arenarioside, and ballotetroside

Medicinal Uses: Horehound is truly a multi-faceted plant. Because it affects several organ systems, it is a prosaic tool worthy of understanding. Use it as a stimulating expectorant. It tends to break up impacted bronchial mucus by its invigorating effect on the area. Bronchial secretion is enhanced; mucus is thinned and therefore easier to expectorate. Horehound also has a time-honored reputation in constricted lung conditions. Its decongesting effect is noticeable in humid asthma with associated phlegm. The plant's cyclooxygenase inhibition may play a role in its therapeutic effect here. As a remedy for hoarseness and coughs, the syrup particularly allays throat and bronchial irritation.

The room temperature tea or tincture taken before meals is used to stimulate an array of gastric, hepatic, and small intestinal secretions. The plant enlivens these areas and is useful in dyspepsia with poor protein and fat digestion. Moreover, Horehound is stimulating to appetite, often turning indifference to food into moderate hunger. The tea drunk hot is diaphoretic and is appropriately used when there is a low to moderate fever with dry skin. Drunk cool the tea is mildly diuretic and can be helpful in eliminating fluid retention from non-organic causes.

Indications:
- Bronchitis with a productive or non-productive cough
- Asthma with copious phlegm
- Indigestion/lack of appetite
- Fluid retention

Collection: In the spring, collect the upper half of the plant. Strip the leaves and flower clusters from the stem; discard the stems, as they are medicinally ineffective.

Preparations and Dosage:
- Leaf infusion: 4-6 ounces 3 times daily
- FPT/DPT (50% alcohol): 30-60 drops 3 times daily
- Syrup: 1 tablespoon 3-4 times daily

Cautions: Idiosyncratically, Horehound can cause short-term hypoglycemic episodes and in large quantities may slightly elevate blood pressure.

HORSETAIL

Equisetaceae – Horsetail family

Equisetum arvense
Common horsetail, Canutillo

Equisetum laevigatum
Smooth scouring rush, Cola de caballo

Equisetum hiemale
Scouring rush, Cola de caballo, Canutillo de llano, Caballo

Description: Equisetum arvense, like other Horsetail species, has underground spreading rhizomes. This perennial has two functionally different stems. Spore-filled cones top the fertile stems, which arise in early spring. They are flesh-colored and 6 inches to 1 foot tall. The infertile stems develop shortly after; they have numerous whorls of small jointed branchlets radiating from the main stem. Overall, they have the appearance of upturned cylindrical feather dusters.

Both Equisetum laevigatum and E. hiemale are scouring rush biotypes. They are rather similar in appearance. These perennial plants also arise from spreading rhizomes. The wand-like stems are hollow and jointed. The fertile stems are distinct in appearance in that they also have a small cylinder-like cone terminating the end of the stem. Given its prominent silica formed ridges E. hiemale's stems are rougher than E. laevigaum's.

Distribution: All Equisetum species profiled here are found throughout most of the United States and much of Canada. They are commonly encountered along streams, moist soils, and drainage areas. Throughout the arid southwest, they are typically mid to high elevation plants.

Chemistry: flavonoids: chlorogenic acid, kaempferol, dihydrokaempferol, hydroxycinnamic acid, equisetumpyrone, quercetin, protogenkwanin, gossypetin, luteolin, apigenin, protoapigenin, genkwanin, and naringenin; silicic acid, silica, calcium, potassium, and phosphorus

Medicinal Uses: Horsetail is mainly a urinary tract medicine. It is soothing to the area and is of use in diminishing urinary tract irritability and painful urination. Internal preparations are mildly diuretic and will assist in eliminating fluid build up from non-organic causes around the ankles, wrists, and mid-sections of the body. Moreover, when taken as a daily tea, kidney stone formation is reduced through the plant's ability of increasing urine volume.

Horsetail is hemostatic. Although the mechanism of action is not clearly defined, the plant lessens passive hemorrhaging. Use it if there is blood in the urine from physical injury or gastrointestinal bleeding from ulceration and other non-malignant inflammatory processes. Internal preparations may even be useful if there is blood-tinged sputum from a severe cough. Topically and internally the plant facilitates wound healing and tissue repair. This is mainly due to Horsetail's flavonoid, silica, and silicic acid content. The plant is also used to strengthen the hair, nails, and skin. Connective tissues throughout the body are augmented; the plant makes a good tea for fortifying bones damaged by injury, or weakened from osteoporosis.

Indications:
♦   Painful urination, irritability
♦   Fluid retention
♦   Kidney stones, as a preventative
♦   Passive hemorrhaging, renal, lower urinary, pulmonary, and GI tract tissues
♦   Gastrointestinal ulceration
♦   Weakened hair, nails, skin, bones, and connective tissues
♦   Wounds (internal and external)

Collection: Equisetum arvense has the highest quercetin content in its new spring growth, approximately 50% of its total flavonoid content. Other species are probably similar. As spring changes to summer, the plant's quercetin content quickly diminishes. Only collect the infertile stems of E. arvense, as this will ensure the plant's sustainability. Fertile and infertile stems alike can be collected of Scouring rushes. Clip the stems at their bases. Use fresh or dry. After drying, the stems are easily separated into 1-2 inch sections for storage.

Preparations and Dosage:
♦   Fresh juice: 1 ounce 3 times daily
♦   Herb infusion: 2-4 ounces 3 times daily
♦   Poultice: as needed

Cautions: It is possible that Horsetail, exposed to common agricultural run-off, produces several toxic compounds. Do not collect and use the plant around these areas. In addition, excessive quantities of the tea or juice may irritate the kidneys.

Other Uses: The abrasive qualities of Scouring rush are practically legendary, but over-rated. It has been said that the plant has been used to sharpen knives, clean and polish pots and metals – an herbal equivalent to steel wool.

JOJOBA   *Simmondsiaceae* – Jojoba family

Simmondsia chinensis
Goatnut

Description: Jojoba is a many-branched shrub reaching 3-6 feet in height. The ovoid leaves are entire, leathery, and arranged oppositely along the stems. They are ¾-2 inches long, grayish-green, and tend to yellow with age or stress. The leaves are positioned upright so most of its exposure to the sun occurs in the morning and late afternoon; this orientation minimizes sun-stress. Jojoba is divided between male and female plants. Both flower types are inconspicuous. The seed produced from the female, the famed "goatnut", is shaped like an acorn, is dark brown when mature and surrounded by a lighter husk. At any given time, it has been placed in the Box, Spurge, or Jojoba families.

Distribution: Between 1,500-5,000 feet look for Jojoba growing on rocky slopes and hillsides throughout the Sonoran Desert and Chaparral Scrub regions of Arizona, and southern California.

Chemistry: glycosides contained within fruit: simmondsin, d-pinitol, and galactinol; leaf tannins: both condensed and hydrolyzable types

Medicinal Uses: As a tannin-containing plant Jojoba topically applied to the skin is astringent. The fresh leaf poultice, tea, or dried leaf powder will lessen surface inflammation from scrapes, rashes, and burns. The plant's tightening effect will diminish blood flow from cuts and will tend to lessen discharge from weepy rashes. Jojoba also proves to be slightly antimicrobial to surface tissues, thereby helping tissues to heal more quickly. The tea used as a mouthwash or gargle will help to resolve mouth sores, lessen bleeding from gums, and soothe sore throats. If swallowed the tea will diminish diarrhea through its astringing effects on the intestines.

Indications:
♦ Cuts/burns/rashes (external)
♦ Mouth inflammations/sore throats (gargle)
♦ Diarrhea

Collection: Trim the upper branches of the plant when new leaf growth is apparent. The leaves should be light green and hydrated.

Dosage:
♦ Leaf decoction: 4-6 ounces 3 times daily
♦ Topical preparations: as needed

Cautions: Jojoba's array of tannins can be disrupting to sensitive mucus membranes that line the gut and intestines, so keep use short term: 5-7 days at a time. Like other tannin bearing plants caution should be applied if taking Jojoba while pregnant due to its vasoconstricting effects on uterine lining.

Other Uses: Jojoba seeds are fully mature and edible from late summer through fall. They are a rich and flavorful seed, particularly if roasted. In larger amounts they tend to be tortuous on digestion. The liquid wax extracted from the seed is used widely in the natural cosmetic industry.

There is some speculation based on research that eating Jojoba seeds produces satiation through its influence on CCK (cholecystokinin); eating several seeds before meals may reduce the amount of food needed to feel full.

JUMPING CHOLLA *Cactaceae* – Cactus family

Opuntia fulgida (Cylindropuntia fulgida)
Chain-fruit cholla, Cholla brincadora, Velas de coyote

Description: Jumping cholla is a tree-like cactus that in rare circumstances can reach 12 feet in height, though normally it is between 3-9 feet tall. This cactus has a thickened and branching trunk upon which joints of varying lengths form and radiate outward. The green fruits are oval and uniquely chain downwards, one fruit growing out of the previous. As these cacti age the fruited chains become quite long; they are easily broken and seem to "jump" to anyone brushing by them. The flowers are rose-purple with pink and yellow tinges. The larger thorns, which cover the trunk, are surrounded by papery sheaths that tend to glisten with bright sunlight. Most of the fruits are sterile, which does not affect the plants successfulness, for it excels at asexual reproduction. Any joint or seedless fruit that falls to the ground will almost invariably take root.

Distribution: From sea level to 3,600 feet Jumping cholla is found on gravely and sandy soils. It inhabits flats as well as rocky foothills. From central Arizona, it ranges south.

Chemistry: similar to Prickly pear, Jumping cholla has carbohydrate-containing polymers, consisting of a mixture of mucilage and pectin; calcium oxalate

Medicinal Uses: Jumping cholla root tea is diuretic. It is soothing to urinary tract pain and irritation. The root also has a widespread reputation in diminishing kidney and bladder gravel; it is most likely of use with uric acid/ low pH urine deposits. Using the root tea as a kidney stone preventive is its optimal application.

The gum from Jumping cholla dissolved in water and drunk is soothing to gastrointestinal inflammation. Like Prickly pear, the gum augments gastric mucus making its application useful in healing peptic ulcers, gastritis, or soothing intestinal irritation associated with diarrhea. Topically the gum mixed with water is soothing to burns, bites, and rashes.

Indications:

- Urinary tract irritability, pain
- Urinary gravel preventive/uric acid stones
- Peptic ulcers/gastritis
- Diarrhea with intestinal inflammation
- Burns/skin irritation (external)

Collection: When digging Jumping cholla roots start at least 1 foot out from the central trunk as the plant sends out secondary horizontal roots close to the surface for rainfall absorption. As you dig closer to the central roots, collect the secondary roots. The main anchoring roots will be directly under the cactus trunk. These tap roots are thicker and reach deeper into the ground. The ideal sized plant to collect is 2-3 feet in height; the bigger the plant the more spines and branches there will be to navigate. After finishing spread the fruits and branches around the area, this will insure a plentiful recovery in the future.

The gum, which occasionally exudes from injuries along the trunk or joints, dries in varying sized nodules. After dislodging the gum from its anchor point, scrape off any embedded thorns or debris.

Preparations: Cut the roots into ¼-½ inch sections and dry normally. The gum can be stored as is or broken into smaller chunks for future use. In preparing the gum tea, use ½-ounce in weight of material in 1 pint of water. Simmer, stir, and strain well.

Dosage:
- Root/gum tea: 4-8 ounces 2-3 times daily
- Gum tea: apply as needed

Cautions: Consuming an excess of Jumping cholla for medicine or food, like Prickly pear, may usher in chills and attending elevated temperature.

Other Uses: Occasionally very large gum nodules can be found. Often the center part is relatively soft. This can be cut into pieces and eaten. The Seri Indians of northwest Mexico consider it a supplementary food.

The most recently developed fruits at the end of the fruit chain can be peeled and eaten. Some will be seed filled, others not. Whether eaten raw or cooked, they are mild tasting and mucilaginous. Be mindful of the very small thorns, called glochids. They cover most parts of the plant.

JUNIPER   *Cupressaceae* – Cypress family

Juniperus monosperma
One seed juniper

Juniperus communis
Common juniper

Juniperus deppeana
Alligator juniper

Juniperus scopulorum (Juniperus virginiana var. scopulorum)
Rocky mountain juniper

Description: Junipers are small shrubs or medium sized trees, often rounded or conical in shape with stringy or checkerboard-like bark. These evergreen plants have either branchlets covered by short scale-like leaves clustered in pairs (sometimes in groupings of 3) or branchlets supporting needle-like leaves in groupings of 3. Usually there is a resin gland situated on the back of each scale-like leaf. When crushed all Junipers are aromatic. Male and female flowers tend to develop on separate trees, although in rare circumstances both types can be found on the same tree. Both male and female flowers are small and unremarkable. The berries are actually specialized cones and take a season or two to mature fully. They are blue to copper in color, fleshy, sweet, and contain 1-12 hard seeds.
    Juniperus monosperma is a small tree or large shrub that branches from the ground. Typically, it has no main trunk to speak of, but if so, it is short. Its bark is light gray and shreddy. The leaf groupings of 2 or sometimes 3 are scale-like and like most Junipers are pressed against the branchlets. The mature fruit is dark blue with a fine bluish-white, waxy powder covering its surface. Normally the fruits contain 1 seed, on rare occasions 2-3. They are brown and oval. J. communis is usually a shrubby, prostrated plant, although in some areas such as in southern Illinois and northern Germany it reportedly reaches tree proportions. Beyond these exceptional cases, J. communis is usually less than 5 feet in height and sometimes double or triple that across.

Its branches tend to grow laterally and form tangled masses. The evergreen leaves are needle-like and lance shaped; they are whitish above and dark green beneath. The berries take 2 seasons to ripen fully, are bluish-black, fleshy, sweet, and contain 1-3 small hard seeds.

Juniperus deppeana is a small tree reaching 30 feet in height. This species is remarkably long-lived; some are purported to be 1500 years old. The trunks, particularly on older trees, are thickened and somewhat tortuous. The grayish bark is fissured in a checkerboard pattern, lending credence to the common name Alligator juniper. On older trees, sometimes only small strips of living bark arise from the base to enliven a full canopy. There is a noticeable resin gland on the back of each leaf. The fruits are reddish-brown and are covered by a grayish waxy coating. The berry contains 3-4 angled seeds.

Juniperus scopulorum is a large bush or small tree reaching 35 feet in height. This tree has a slender crown and drooping branches, which gives it a weeping appearance. In open areas where the crown is rounded and the branches grow upward, the plant is bush-forming. The bark is brownish-gray and pulls away in narrow strips. The small pointed leaves are scale-like and arranged in pairs. Each has a resin gland on its back. The fruits are blue and are covered by a whitish coating that is easily rubbed off. They are juicy, sweet, and contain 1-2 seeds. J. scopulorum is very closely related to J. virginiana or Red cedar of the eastern part of the country. Morphologically the two trees are almost identical. The most significant variation is that it takes one season for J. virginiana's fruits to mature, whereas it takes two for J. scopulorum to do the same.

Distribution: Juniperus monosperma is found from western Kansas and central Colorado to the Texas Panhandle, through much of New Mexico and central-eastern Arizona to southern Nevada. Look for the tree between 3,000-5,500 feet throughout the bulk of its range. It can be found also at lower elevations to the north and east. It is commonly found in rocky soils with Pinyon pine.

Juniperus communis is found throughout temperate North America. In the southwest, it is encountered at elevations of 8,000 feet and higher. It is a ubiquitous Juniper extensively found throughout Europe. J. deppeana is found throughout middle mountain elevations of 4,500-8,000 feet. Look for it in canyons and drainage areas and on hillsides. It ranges from west Texas through New Mexico to Arizona. J. scopulorum is distributed from Alberta south to western Texas. From there it is found west to British Columbia, Washington, eastern Oregon, Nevada, and northern Arizona. It is found throughout a great array of elevations - from nearly sea level along the northwest coast, to almost 9,000 feet throughout the southwest.

Chemistry: prominent essential oil content for Juniperus communis: α-pinene, β-pinene, sabinene, myrcene, delta-2-carene, α-phellandrene, β-phellandrene, delta-3-carene, limonene, bornylacetate, (e)-caryophyllene, α-humulene, α-muurolene, germacrene a, germacrene d, germacrene d-4-ol, γ-cadinene, delta-cadinene, and α-cadinol

Medicinal Uses: Juniper has centuries of cross-cultural usage behind its application as a urinary tract medicine. Through Juniper's stimulating nature it works best in alleviating low-grade, long-standing, subacute or chronic urinary tract irritability and discomfort. Use in chronic cystitis and painful urination accompanied by mucus in the urine. Although alcoholic preparations tend to extract Junipers volatile constituents more completely the leaf or berry tea is as useful is serving as a urinary tract antiseptic; most Junipers are broadly inhibiting to bacteria and fungi. Small amounts of the tea are useful in imparting cellular stimulation in low-grade, on and off again nephritis, particularly if used in formula.

Due to its aromatics, Juniper tends to be moderately carminative. Several ounces of the tea or 30-40 drops of the tincture can lessen stomach bloating and cramping. Topically Juniper oil or salve can be helpful in resolving long-standing episodes of eczema and psoriasis. Through the plant's interesting mix of antiinflammatory qualities and stimulating aromatics, it often is the right plant for long-standing, subacute problems of the urinary tract and skin.

Indications:
◆ Cystitis/urethritis, chronic
◆ Nephritis, chronic
◆ Dyspepsia
◆ Eczema/psoriasis (external)

Collection: Collect the leaves and/or fruits alone or together. Both parts are equally potent as medicine. Dry normally.

Preparations and Dosage:

♦ Leaf/berry infusion: 4-6 ounces 3 times daily
♦ FPT/DPT (75% alcohol): 30-40 drops 3 times daily

Cautions: Do not use Juniper during pregnancy due to the plant's potential of stimulating uterine vasculature. Also do not use in acute inflammatory states affecting the kidneys.

Other Uses: Termites that are force fed Juniper sawdust die prematurely.

KIDNEYWOOD   *Leguminosae* – Pea family

Eysenhardtia polystachya (Eysenhardtia orthocarpa)
Palo azul, Bura dulce

Description: Kidneywood is a large bush or small tree. Occasionally it reaches 18 feet in height, but it is usually less. The outer bark on older sections is gray and fissured and forms in a checkerboard pattern. Kidneywood's leaves, which are deciduous in response to drought stresses and low temperatures, are pinnate and are composed of numerous, small leaflets. Upon closer examination, the small dot-like resin glands are apparent on the undersides of the leaflets, young stems, and flower calyxes. A resinous odor is noticeable when the foliage is crushed. The terminal spikes are composed of small, white, delicate flowers that appear in response to warm temperatures and rainfall from early spring to late summer. They are followed by equally small, linear, clustered green seedpods. Within each pod is 1 flat seed.

Distribution: Kidneywood is found from 4,000-5,000 feet, from Pima County, Arizona, east to southern Hidalgo County, New Mexico. Typically, the plant grows on hillsides and canyons of Desert Grasslands and Oak Woodlands.

Chemistry: at least several florescent isoflavones; chalcones: coatline a and b

Medicinal Uses: As the name Kidneywood implies, the tea made from the small branches effects the kidneys and lower urinary tract. If prone to acidic, overly concentrated urine, associated kidney stones and urinary tract sediment then Kidneywood will be of use. Because of the plant's alkalinizing nature, acidic precipitants dissolve back into the urine, thereby reducing pain and urinary tract irritability associated with lithic deposits. Kidneywood is diuretic and soothing to kidney and urinary tract irritability. Its mild antimicrobial activity further helps to explain its usefulness to this area of the body.

Indications:
♦ Urinary tract gravel
♦ Acidic, overly concentrated urine
♦ Upper and lower urinary tract irritability and pain

Collection and Preparations: After pruning a number of smaller secondary branches from several large plants cut them into small ½-¼ inch sections; the leaves also can be used. The branch/bark decoction makes a pleasant tasting, slightly astringent tea.

Dosage:
♦ Branch/bark decoction: 4-8 ounces 3 times daily

Cautions: The heartwood should not be collected in the United States given the significant impact it would have on our limited but locally available populations. Moreover, there is not a great medicinal advantage over utilizing these parts over the smaller branches.

Other Uses: Of historical interest is that sixteenth and seventeenth century Western European practitioners and lay people alike employed the plant, then known as Lignum nephriticum, for issues formerly mentioned. Also during the same period, the chemist Richard Boyle used preparations of the heartwood as an acid - base indicator. Considered a scientific break through at the time, the process gained a wider acceptance in measuring pH until export of Kidneywood became unstable and fell into neglect.

LEADWORT

Plumbaginaceae – Plumbago family

Plumbago scandens
Pitillo, Hierba de alacran

Description: This perennial is often found prostrated along the ground or weakly growing up through bushes that it is sheltered under. The leaves form alternately along the stems; they are entire with wavy margins. The flowers cluster in spike-like racemes at branch ends; they are white, tubular, and have 5 petals. The small seed capsules have numerous thickened hairs on their surfaces. They easily stick to clothes and animal fur, making transport easy. Plumbago capensis, which is cultivated as an ornamental in warmer parts of the country, has sky-blue flowers; it can serve as a substitute for our own native variety.

Distribution: In southern Arizona Leadwort is mainly isolated to Pima and Pinal Counties. It is also found in southern Florida. Between 2,500-4,000 feet look for the plant in ravines, canyons, and gullies where rain run-off frequently courses by. Ideally, Leadwort grows under larger shrubs and trees where it gains some protection from intense sunlight. Look under Acacia, Mesquite, and Hackberry trees. The plant does not have a wide range but it is locally abundant, robust, and is easily propagated.

Chemistry: plumbagic acid, naphthoquinones: plumbagin, chitranone, maritinone, elliptinone, isoshinanolone, and epiisoshinanolone, coumarins: seselin, 5-methoxyseselin, suberosin, xanthyletin, and xanthoxyletin

Medicinal Uses: There are numerous species of Leadwort currently used in TCM (Traditional Chinese Medicine) and Ayurveda; also throughout Tropical America, these plants are used medicinally. Although internal uses differ to some degree according to what therapeutic system is used, external uses coincide and are practical and safe. Topical preparations stimulate tissue healing. The plant has a stimulatory effect on parenchymal and connective tissue cells, collagenation, and other factors, all augmenting the healing process. Tissue macrophage activity is also stimulated, which not only accounts for the plant's indirect antimicrobial activity but also further complements its wound healing properties. Use Leadwort much like Copperleaf. Apply topically when wounds, ulcers, cuts, and abrasions have become subacute. In other words, use Leadwort when the inflammation has diminished somewhat and tissues are lax and slow to heal. Topically Leadwort also speeds the time it takes abscesses to come to a head and is of use in splinter removal.

Indications:
- Wounds/ulcers/cuts, that are slow to heal (external)
- Edema, disorganized tissue fluid build-up with tissue laxity (external)
- Abscesses/splinters, to bring to a head (external)

Collection: When sufficiently leafed-out, in flower or not, collect the herbage of the plant.

Preparations and Dosage:
- Dried leaf poultice/fomentation/salve/oil: topically as needed

Cautions: Since Leadwort is a cellular stimulant there is a slight possibility of external preparations causing redness and inflammation. Discontinue use if this occurs.

LIMBERBUSH
Euphorbiaceae – Spurge family

Jatropha cardiophylla
Heartleaf limberbush, Sangre de drago, Sangre de cristo

Jatropha cinerea (Jatropha canescens, J. giffordiana)
Ashy limberbush, Sangre de drago, Lomboy

Jatropha cuneata (Jatropha spathulata)
Limberbush, Leatherplant, Sangre de drago, Torote

Jatropha macrorhiza
Nettlespurge

Description: Jatropha cardiophylla is a curious appearing plant, as are most others of the genus. This small bush has numerous, extremely flexible, wand-like stems arising from its base. Typically, the stem bark is reddish-brown. The heart-shaped, triangular leaves form in groupings along the stem. They are shiny, wider than long, and have rounded teeth. The small, white tubular flowers hang delicately from the upper stems; they are followed by a small, rounded, encased seed. Quite possibly the most unique characteristic of many Jatrophas throughout the southwest is their distinctive sap. When a branch is clipped at the base, a deep reddish-brown sap exudes covering the wound, looking surprisingly blood-like.

Jatropha cinerea is a tall plant with yellowish-brown stem bark. When young the undersides of the ovate leaves are felty. J. cuneata is also a stout, many-branched shrub; unlike J. cardiophylla and J. cinerea, its leaves are wedge-shaped but like the others, its sap is blood red. J. macrorhiza, technically not a Limberbush-type, represents an entirely different growth morphology. Whereas the other Jatrophas are semi-woody perennials, J. macrorhiza is herbaceous. Yearly, the plant's above ground foliage dies back to the ground. From a large, thickened taproot, several 1-2 foot tall stems arise supporting large, palmately lobed dark green leaves. A 3-celled fruit follows the small rose-pink flowers.

Distribution: Jatropha cardiophylla reaches its northern most limits just north of Tucson, Arizona. From 2,000-3,000 feet look for the plant on rocky hillsides and foothills. In southern Arizona's Senita basin, J. cinerea is found in isolated pockets. From this point, the plant is found south to Mexico, between sea level and 2,400 feet, on plains, hills, and along washes. It is not recommended to collect this species in the United States because of its limited distribution. J. cuneata is found along with the previously described species, but it is of larger distribution. Look for the plant among gravelly flats and slopes from southern Yuma to southwestern Pima County, Arizona. Look for J. macrorhiza from 3,500-7,500 feet throughout southern Arizona and New Mexico. Antelope horns is a common companion plant.

Chemistry: condensed and hydrolyzable tannins

Medicinal Uses: All varieties of Limberbush are extremely astringent. The roots by weight contain approximately 5% tannic acid. The dominant phenol group, which tannic acid belongs to, is generally called hydrolyzable tannins. They are the reason why these plants are able to tan hides. When in contact with cellular protein structures hydrolyzable tannins constrict, tighten, and alter these surfaces. Like Desert rhubarb, therapeutic use of Limberbush is somewhat limited, due to its drastic effect on cell surfaces.

Externally use the fresh sap or stem poultice to soothe and astringe burns, bites, and stings. Its use on weepy rashes and hive outbreaks is also of some value. Internally Limberbush tea is used to quell acute diarrhea; it is a purely symptomatic gastrointestinal astringent. The tea can also be gargled for mouth sores and spongy and bleeding gums.

Jatropha macrorhiza has a similar array of tannins, but also it contains strongly purgative compounds. Liken its effect to very strong Rhubarb. Enough J. macrorhiza to provide a laxative effect will almost surly elicit rebound constipation. Consider recognizing this species for its visual beauty and not as a medicine.

Indications:
◆ Diarrhea
◆ Skin eruptions/burns/cuts/stings (external)
◆ Mouth sores/spongy and bleeding gums (gargle)

Collection: Clip several stems at the plant's base; apply the sap as needed or cut into small ½-inch sections and dry.

Preparations and Dosage:
◆ Stem decoction: 2-4 ounces 2-3 times daily
◆ Sap/stem poultice: externally as needed

Cautions: Use Limberbush internally for several days at a time. If used longer the plant may irritate the kidneys. Do not use during pregnancy due to the plants potential vasoconstrictive effect on uterine lining.

Other Uses: Like Desert rhubarb, it is a plant to know about if attempting to tan hides the old way.

MALLOW

Malvacea – Mallow family

Malva neglecta
Common mallow, Cheeseweed

Malva parviflora
Little mallow

Description: Mallow is a clump-forming, spreading annual, or short lived perennial with a thickened, short taproot. The plant increases in size quickly even in the presence of modest rainfall. The large 5-7 lobed leaves are heart-shaped at their bases and have serrated margins; they are attached to long petioles that connect to the main spreading stems. Typically, the 5-petaled flowers are inconspicuous, white to pale lavender or pinkish, cleft, and, ¼-2/3 of an inch long. The fruit is round, flattened, and button-like; the 5 sepals that remain after the other flower parts drop off surround it. The round seed disk separates into 10-12 sections or carpels, each of these contain 1 seed. Throughout parts of the southwest that have winter-spring influenced Pacific rains, Mallow is an initiatory plant that when at its peak literally can cover anything in its path that is not moved.

Distribution: This European native is commonly found throughout the United States. It is here to stay and is thriving in the west. Look for the plant anywhere the ground has been disturbed, but particularly around edges of building and structures, irrigated lands, yards, and roadsides.

Chemistry: polysaccharides: arabinogalactans, β-d-glucan, l-arabinose, d-xylose, l-rhamnose, d-galactose, d-galacturonic acid, and d-glucuronic acid

Medicinal Uses: Mallow has several distinct medicinal effects practically identical to Marshmallow, Hollyhock, and Globemallow. The tea is soothing to a dry, irritative cough and bronchial irritation present typically in the beginning or ending stages of a lung cold or bronchitis. Mallow's polysaccharides are stimulating to innate immunity; leukocyte activities are enhanced. The plant's effect is not necessarily strong but it is helpful during the wintertime cold and flu season to combat immune depression.

Some of these Mallow family constituents are excreted through the kidneys and out the urinary tract. The change in quality of urine that follows has a soothing, antiinflammatory effect on the area. Lower urinary tract irritation is lessened, as is episodic kidney inflammation. Mallow has an age-old use as a kidney stone preventive. So drink a cup of tea daily if prone to lithic deposits. Its taste is pleasant enough to warrant long-term use without revulsion. If suffering from gastritis from stress reactions or poor dietary choices Mallow is soothing to inflamed gastric mucosa. It is well combined with Artemisia douglasiana or A. filifolia in healing peptic ulcers. Like Globemallow, the fresh or dried plant can be used as a drawing poultice. The tissue stimulating and softening effect provided by Mallow is of use in resolving boils, abscesses, and removing splinters. Combine with other immune stimulating or circulation enhancing herbs for a more profound effect.

Indications:
♦   Bronchitis with an irritative cough
♦   Cystitis/urethritis
♦   Kidney irritation
♦   Urinary tract gravel, as a preventive
♦   Gastritis
♦   Boils/abscesses/splinters (internal and external)

Collection: The entire plant – leaves, stems and roots – are useable. In loose, moist soils, the taproots pull up easily; when split they are starchy and white.

Preparations and Dosage:
♦   Leaf infusion/root decoction: 4-8 ounces 3 times daily

Cautions: None known.

MANZANITA

Ericaceae – Heath family

Arctostaphylos spp.
Big bearberry, Manzanilla, Coralillo

Description: Manzanita is an evergreen bush or small tree reaching 3-18 feet in height. The outer red bark is thin and visually striking, on some varieties peeling freely and on others remaining smooth and intact. The forked branches form in tangles at branch ends making these plants practically impenetrable when growing in thickets. The leaves are usually ovoid, thickened, and often point upwards. The small, pink, urn-shaped flowers form in clusters at branch ends and then transition into small 4-10 seeded tan fruits.

Distribution: Coastal mountainous regions of California have the densest populations of the plant. From this area, they radiate south and eastward to Texas. Typically, a mid-mountain plant throughout the southwest, look for Manzanita with other Chaparral Scrub plants, such as Silk tassel and Scrub oak. It is found on exposed hillsides and rocky slopes.

Chemistry: phenolic glucosides: arbutin, methylarbutin and hydroquinone; tannins: caffeic acid, gallic acid, catechol and ellagic acid; triterpenoids: uvaol, ursolic acid, lupeol, α-amyrin, β-amyrin, erythrodiol and oleanolic acid; anthocyanidins: delphinidin and cyanidin; quercetrin and quercetin

Medicinal Uses: Manzanita inhibits lower urinary tract bacteria that thrive in alkaline urine. In the presence of alkaline urine, arbutin, a main constituent of Manzanita, is broken down into hydroquinone and subsequently is responsible for the plant's antibacterial qualities. Escherichia coli, a typical urinary tract pathogen, thrives in alkaline urine. In the presence of normal acidic urine, or Manzanita acidified urine, the bacterium finds attachment to cell walls difficult. Combining the use of Manzanita or most other Heath family urinary tract acidifiers, such as Madrone or Cranberry, with diet changes that include more animal source proteins, along with limiting simple carbohydrates, can promptly resolve alkaline urinary tract infections.

Manzanita is also a urinary tract astringent. The plant's tannin complexes responsible for this tone lax urinary tract tissues by imparting a local tightening effect. Use when there is dragging urinary pain in combination with dribbling of urine and mucus discharge.

As a post-partum sitz bath, Manzanita is useful in tonifying and soothing vaginal and cervical tissues. Since Manzanita is moderately inhibiting to Candida albicans it is well worth combining topical applications with internal use of Desert willow, Trumpet flower, or Trumpet creeper.

Indications:
- Lower urinary tact infection with alkaline urine
- Vaginitis with or w/o Candida involvement
- As a post-partum sitz bath

Collection: Gather Manzanita leaves during late spring through summer after flowering when the ripe fruit is present. The arbutin content is most concentrated at this time, less so when the plant is in flower.

Preparations: Several things can be done to facilitate the breakdown of arbutin and methylarbutin into hydroquinone, therefore increasing its effectiveness. Simply drying the leaf starts the conversion. The hydroquinone content is also increased by rehydrating the leaves in a small amount of water for 3-4 hours. After this initial soak, decoct normally.

Dosage:
- Leaf decoction: 4-6 ounces 3-4 times daily
- DPT (50% alcohol): 30-60 drops 3-4 times daily
- Sitz bath: as needed

Cautions: Manzanita may have a vasoconstricting effect on uterine lining, so it is contraindicated during pregnancy. The plant's tannins can have an irritating effect on gastric mucosa and the kidneys; limit consecutive use to two weeks. With the addition of most Mallow family plants, i.e. Globemallow and Marshmallow, or Cornsilk length of usage can be increased.

Other Uses: The fruits are edible; although seed filled and mealy, they have an apple-like taste. They are good for making jams and jellies.

MARSH FLEABANE   *Compositae* – Sunflower family

Pluchea camphorata (Pluchea purpurascens)
Salt-marsh fleabane

Pluchea sericea (Pluchea purpurascens var. purpurascens)
Arrowweed, Cachanilla

Description: Pluchea camphorata is a tall, herbaceous annual. Its upper, multi-branched portion accentuates its robust appearance. With age, the stems become reddish-brown. The leaves are large, serrated, and ovoid. They are of varying sizes and alternate along the stem; the lower leaves are petioled. The mature flower clusters form in large corymbs and are purplish-pink. The whole plant is somewhat sticky to the touch and has a strong camphor-like odor. When not in flower the plant may easily be confused with Camphorweed. The reddish stems are a useful distinguishing characteristic in that they are absent in Camphorweed.

Pluchea sericea is a thicket-forming shrub. Its wand-like stems can reach 10 feet in height, but usually are less. The leaves are lanceolate, have a prominent mid-vein, and alternate along the upper stems. There is a very distinctive coating of leaf and twig hairs on the newer branch growth. These appressed hairs coat the plant making it somewhat silvery in appearance. The flower clusters are situated at the branch ends and are reddish-purple to lavender. Moreover, like others in the Sunflower family, the mature seeds are wind carried by their delicate tufts.

Distribution: Pluchea camphorata grows throughout most of the United States. In the west it is typically found in low-elevation, saline-alkaline moist soils. Look to the edges of slow moving rivers, around ponds, lakesides, and on moist alluvial fans.
   Pluchea sericea is found in low-lying moist soils, along drainages, streams, and on river and pond sides. It is well distributed throughout the low elevation southwest. It is found throughout southern California, east to southern Nevada, Utah, southern Colorado, south through much of Arizona, along the Rio Grande in New Mexico, and finally to the Trans-Pecos region of Texas. Often both species are found side by side.

Chemistry: flavonoids, triterpenes and sesquiterpenes

Medicinal Uses: The uses of Pluchea camphorata and P. sericea generally overlap, although different parts of the plants are used. P. camphorata, being the more stimulating of the two, moves blood to surface tissues more so than P. sericea. The roots of P. sericea and the herb portion of P. camphorata made into various topical preparations are decidedly antiinflammatory and antioxidant to damaged tissues. Both plants are well applied to wounds. They facilitate healing, and resolve fluid build up and swelling.

Internally both plants are sedating to gastrointestinal tract cramps associated with diarrhea. The tea, used longer-term, is diminishing to irritative-inflammatory conditions of the gastrointestinal tract walls, such as gastritis or colitis. If feverish, the hot tea of P. camphorata is diaphoretic; as a cold tea, it is diuretic. The plant may also stimulate menses as well as sedate period cramps.

Indications:
♦   Wounds/cuts/abrasions (external)
♦   GI tract cramps with associated diarrhea
♦   GI tract inflammation
♦   Fevers, dry

Collection: Gather the roots of Pluchea sericea and the herbage of P. camphorata, minus the flowers if allergic to Sunflower family pollen.

Preparations and Dosage:
♦   FPT/DPT (60% alcohol): 30-60 drops 3 times daily
♦   Leaf/root tea: 4-6 ounces 3 times daily
♦   External preparations: as needed

Cautions: Do not use either plant internally during pregnancy since fluid dynamics and uterine vascularity are shifted by the plant.

MESQUITE

Leguminosae – Pea family

Prosopis velutina (Prosopis juliflora var. velutina)
Velvet mesquite

Prosopis pubescens
Screwbean mesquite, Tornillo

Prosopis glandulosa var. torreyana (Prosopis juliflora var. torreyana)
Western honey mesquite, Algarroba, Chachaca

Prosopis glandulosa (Prosopis juliflora var. glandulosa)
Honey mesquite

Description: Depending on soil and water conditions, Velvet mesquite can be a large shrub, or a small or large tree. Older Velvet mesquites found along bottomlands and riversides have large, multi-branched trunks and can reach 50-60 feet in height. The same tree growing in less hydrated soils, along secondary drainages or on hillsides, are 10-20 feet tall. The older bark is fissured and dark and where the tree has sustained some injury from insects or branch damage a light brown sap weeps from the area. Composing each leaf is 1 or 2 sets of primary leaflets; each contains 9-30 sets of secondary leaflets. They are small and densely pubescent. Velvet mesquite, like most other Mesquites, has paired spines formed at leaf nodes. The spines tend to be more abundant on younger branches. The 2-5 inch long yellow flower spikes are cylindrical in shape. Numerous small flowers compose the spikes. The seedpods are 4-8 inches long, narrow, and tend to gently curve in one direction or another. Like the leaves, the outer pod covering is also pubescent, and is light tan in color when mature.

Screwbean mesquite is a large spiny shrub or small tree. The bark on older trunks is fibrous and stringy. The primary leaflets develop in sets of 1 or 2. Secondary leaflets number 5-9 sets, are small and covered with a dense coating of hairs. The pale gray spines develop from leaf nodes. The cream-colored flower spikes are 1½-2 inches long, and are typical for the genus. Without a doubt, the most characteristic part of the plant is its tightly spiraled, tan seedpods. These natural corkscrews are 1-2½ inches long and encase small tan seeds.

Western honey mesquite, a large shrub or small tree, reaches 20 feet in height. Its pinnate leaves are composed of 1 set of primary leaflets and 8-20 sets of secondary leaflets. They are between ½-1 inch in length and are typically hairless or have hairs only along the leaflet's margins. The large spines form in pairs at leaf nodes. The cream colored-yellow flower spikes are 2-5 inches long. When mature the seedpods are tan and are 4-10 inches long. Honey mesquite is similar in appearance to Western honey mesquite, although this species' larger leaves lend it a weeping appearance – a kind of weeping mesquite. It is an attractive small tree.

Distribution: From 1,000-4,500 feet Velvet mesquite is found just south of the Mogollon Rim in central Arizona and continues south through the bulk of the state. The tree is found along washes, drainages, rich bottomlands, and increasingly on drier slopes and mesas. Look for Screwbean mesquite from sea level to 3,000 feet along major drainages throughout most of our southwestern deserts. In Arizona, the tree is found along the Colorado, Gila, Bill Williams, and Santa Cruz Rivers. In New Mexico look along the southern expanse of the Rio Grande and continuing in Texas until Devils River. In southern Utah, southern Nevada and southern California the tree is also common along major drainages.

Western honey mesquite grows from sea level to 6,000 feet throughout much of southeastern California, southern Nevada, and in a small segment of Utah's Washington County. In Arizona look along practically the entire length of the Colorado and Gila Rivers, in isolated pockets in Cochise County, to southwestern New Mexico, particularly along the Rio Grande. It follows this course into Texas and reaches its eastward limit at Corpus Christi. Honey mesquite begins where Western honey mesquite leaves off. From southeastern New Mexico the tree covers much of Texas, southeastern Colorado, Kansas, Oklahoma, and finally to the Shreveport area of Louisiana. It is a tree of Desert Grasslands, plains, and prairies.

Chemistry: condensed and hydrolyzable tannins

Medicinal Uses: Like other Pea family plants, namely Acacia and Mimosa, Mesquite leaf powder can be applied to cuts and scrapes to lessen superficial inflammation and astringe minor bleeding. The leaf tea is used to soothe sunburn, rashes, bites, and most other red and weepy conditions. The tea can also be gargled for sore throats and mouth sores.

The liquid or hardened sap, mixed with water and salt is soothing to conjunctivitis. Mixed equally with Prickly poppy tea will increase the solutions antimicrobial activity. Even though the sap has some inherent mucilage, over time, the tannins can prove drying to the eyes, therefore it is best to use for several days at a time, then alternate to Prickly poppy or Desert anemone alone. Mesquite is also a valuable food plant, as described below.

Indications:
♦ Cuts/scrapes/inflammations (external)
♦ Sore throats/mouth sores (gargle)
♦ Conjunctivitis (eyewash)

Collection: From late spring to early summer, gather the leaves when they are fully mature. On larger trees, during the spring and summer, a pan can be set out, under the tree's wounds, to catch the weeping sap. Older nodules of hardened sap are also collected; they are found on older and younger trees alike. Gather Mesquite pods from mid to late summer, still on the tree when they are tan and brittle.

Preparations: The collected liquid sap is strained and diluted with 5 parts of distilled water; the entire solution is made isotonic by adding salt. See directions under eyewash. By applying low heat, the liquid sap can also be dehydrated for future use. The hardened sap is slowly simmered in 32 parts of distilled water. After it has been completely dissolved strain well through a paper towel. 1 teaspoon of salt is then added. After cooling to room temperature, use as needed.

If not using immediately, store the pods in a refrigerator or freezer, as every bean potentially has a small insect growing inside of it. If there is a sudden occurrence of winged creatures flying around indoors, look to the bucket of Mesquite pods sitting forgotten in the corner – that is their source.

Dosage:
♦ Leaf infusion, topically or as a gargle: as needed
♦ Eyewash: 2-3 times daily for 2-3 days, then rotate to a tannin free solution

Cautions: None known.

Other Uses: ½-1 pound of dried, mature pods are put into 2-3 gallons of water and boiled. After a time strain this Mesquite pod tea, and simmer down alone. Reduce until a thickened consistency is reached. You now have a tasty, sweet syrup that can be used on pancakes, desserts, and other similar things.

Using an electric or hand grinder, the dried pods are made into a meal or flour. All types of baked goods, cookies, breads, etc. can be made with the meal-flour.

MIMOSA   *Leguminosae* – Pea family

Mimosa dysocarpa
Velvet-pod mimosa, Gatuno

Mimosa biuncifera
Wait-a-minute bush, Catclaw mimosa

Description: Mimosa dysocarpa is a 3-6 foot high perennial bush. The plant's thorns are spaced alternately along its branches. The smaller stems are distinctive in that they are 5-ridged. The leaves are doubly compound; they are composed of 5-10 sets of primary leaflets and 6-12 sets of smaller secondary leaflets. The pink to rose-colored flowers form in cylinder-like spikes and are about an inch long. With age, the flowers become lighter in color giving them a distinctive 2-toned appearance. The 1-2 inch long seedpods contain numerous light brown seeds. The plant is called Velvet pod mimosa because the seedpods (and stems) are covered with fine appressed hairs making them velvety to the touch.

Mimosa biuncifera is also between 3-6 feet tall but occasionally it becomes larger, particularly if it has access to moister soils. It is a many-branched shrub that can grow in dense or open groupings. The branches have 2 recurved thorns per node, unlike Catclaw acacia, which has alternating thorns along its stems. The leaves are bipinnate; the primary leaflets are composed of 4-7 sets, secondary leaflets have 6-13 sets. The small ball-like flower clusters are typically cream-colored, but occasionally are pink or lavender. The reddish-brown pods have weak thorns on their margins. The seeds are smooth, dark brown, and almost a ¼-inch long.

Distribution: Look for Mimosa dysocarpa between 4,000-6,500 feet in canyons, along hillsides and slopes from southern Arizona, east to New

Mexico and western Texas. M. dysocarpa prefers upper Desert Grasslands and Oak Woodlands as its primary habitat. M. biuncifera is found between 3,000-6,000 feet throughout Arizona, New Mexico, and a large extent of Texas. Look for the plant in middle mountain drainages and along hillsides.

Chemistry: hydrolyzed and condensed tannins

Medicinal Uses: Use Mimosa like most other southwestern legume shrub-trees. These plants are mildly astringent due to their tannin content. Topical preparations are soothing to abraded tissues and scraped skin. Compounding this effect with Mimosa's mild antimicrobial qualities makes the plant equally useful in diminishing the chances of superficial cuts becoming infected. A wash made from Mimosa leaves is also well applied to sunburned skin. It is soothing and cooling to these inflamed tissues. As a gargle, Mimosa is useful in astringing bleeding gums and is soothing to canker sores and sore throats.

Indications:
♦ Scrapes/cuts/skin abrasions/burns (external)
♦ Mouth sores/sore throats (gargle)

Collection: When Mimosa has fully leafed-out, usually after mid-spring, clip the branch ends from the plant. Dry these whole, then strip the leaves from the branch ends. Keep the leaves as medicine.

Preparations and Dosage:
♦ Leaf wash/powder/poultice: apply as needed
♦ Leaf infusion: gargle as needed

Cautions: None known.

Other Uses: The dried beans can be cooked and eaten.

MORMON TEA

Ephedraceae – Joint-fir family

Ephedra spp.
Mexican tea, Brigham tea, Joint fir, Popotillo, Tepopote, Canatillo

Description: Depending on species, Mormon tea varies in size. Some species are low-growing and often prostrate. Others like Ephedra trifurca can develop sizable trunks and attain heights of 6-7 feet. Mormon tea's thin, wand-like branches are its most visible identifying feature; they look to be large clumps of stiff-spiny grasses. Mormon tea's branch color varies depending on species and season. Some are bluish-green, others are yellowish-green and so on. At each branch node, small leaves oppositely paired or in sets of 3 form virtually unnoticed. In the spring, small male and female cones are produced on separate plants; they are clustered around branch nodes. After the female cone is successfully pollinated 1-3 small seeds are produced.

Distribution: At varying elevations, Mormon tea is common throughout our western deserts. Look for the plant in many different topographies. Flats, basins, rocky slopes, and hillsides are some typical habitats for the plant.

Chemistry: flavonoids: lucenin 1, vicenin 2, and an array of tannins

Medicinal Uses: Even though our western Mormon tea contains no ephedrine and only traces of pseudoephedrine, the plant still is useful as a sinus passage decongestant, and in a limited capacity, as a bronchial dilator. Apparently, Mormon tea contains enough "sub-ephedrines" to make this effect noticeable. In addition, the plant's flavonoid content may contribute to these properties. Take the tea or tincture throughout allergy season for hayfever. Moreover, used before allergy season Mormon tea reduces allergic tendencies by strengthening mucus membranes.

Traditionally, Mormon tea has been used to soothe urinary tract irritability. The tea tends to calm bladder and urethral irritation and can be useful in diminishing kidney irritability through its soothing diuretic properties. In addition, the tea is astringing to mouth, esophageal, and upper stomach irritations. This attribute is common in many plants with substantial flavonoid-tannin contents. Surface membranes tend to be strengthened and inflammation is sedated through Mormon tea's interaction with cell walls.

Indications:
♦ Rhinitis
♦ Urinary tract irritation
♦ Upper gastric irritability

Collection: Throughout mid to late spring when new branch growth is at its peak snip the last foot of green growth. Chop these branch ends into smaller sections for tea or tincture.

Preparations and Dosage:
♦ Branch decoction: 4-6 ounces 3 times daily
♦ DPT (50% alcohol): 30-60 drops 3 times daily

Cautions: Use in moderation during pregnancy. Due to the plant's substantial tannin concentration, it has potential as a uterine wall vasoconstrictor.

MOUNTAIN MARIGOLD   *Compositae* – Sunflower family

Tagetes lemmoni
Lemmon's marigold

Description: Mountain marigold is an herbaceous perennial that freezes back to the ground in the winter months. In mid-summer when at the peak of its growth it usually stands 3 feet tall by 3 feet wide with an array of yellow daisy-like flowers suspended at its branch tips. If the leaves are closely examined oil glands can be clearly seen. The same volatile oils the glands contain are responsible for the mint-anise, slightly skunky odor that permeates the air if the plant is brushed against.

Distribution: Mountain marigold is a mid-mountain plant of southeastern Arizona and northern Mexico. It is found from 4,000-8,000 feet among Oaks and Conifers in canyon bottoms where the soil is more apt to be nutrient rich and moist.

Chemistry: acetylenic thiophenes, flavonoids, benzofurans, and carotenoids: lutein and zeaxanthin

Medicinal Uses: Mountain marigold tea is soothing to stomach and upper small intestinal irritation. If the upper gastrointestinal tract is inflamed from emotional or physically derived stresses, this plant offers relief through its mild antiinflammatory and analgesic properties. Use if suffering from gastritis, pre-ulcerous conditions, and gas pains.

The plant has an interesting effect on the nervous system and corresponding emotional outlook. Shortly after 30 drops of the fresh plant tincture is taken, a calming quality can be felt along with a lightness of mind, sometimes to the extent of giddiness. I have seen the effects of this plant useful in times of fixated emotional morbidity.

If feverish, the hot tea is a reliable way to initiate sweating. Mountain marigold is predictably vasodilating. The plant's aromatics shift blood flow to the surface of the body, dilating the pores of the skin, therefore facilitating diaphoresis. An oil or salve can be made from the dried flowers and applied to poorly healing skin, cuts, and scrapes. It is nutritive to tissues and will expedite healing.

Indications:
♦ Gastric irritation/gas pains
♦ Dry fevers
♦ Poorly healing tissues/scrapes (external)

Collection: From late spring to late summer collect the upper foliage with or without the flowers (the flowers are rich in carotenoids and flavonoids).

Preparations: Tincture fresh, or dry the leaves and flowers for tea or topical use.

Dosage:
♦ FPT: 30-60 drops 3-4 times daily
♦ Leaf infusion: 4-8 ounces 3-4 times daily
♦ Oil or salve made from the flowers: topically as needed

Cautions: None known.

NIGHT BLOOMING CEREUS *Cactaceae* – Cactus family

Selenicereus grandiflorus (Cereus grandiflorus, Cactus grandiflorus)
Sweet scented cactus, Queen of the night

Peniocereus greggii (Cereus greggii)
Queen of the night, Reina de la noche

Description: Selenicereus grandiflorus is a thin stemmed cactus that creeps along the ground and climbs into surrounding vegetation. The fleshy stems have 5-6 ridges that extend along its length and are lined with small groupings of spines. The white-cream colored flowers are large, showy, and fragrant. They are 8-10 inches wide with thin, linear sepals surrounding the larger petals. They open in the evening and close with the morning sun. The small fruits are orange-red and contain numerous small seeds.

Peniocereus greggii is a weak-stemmed, thin cactus growing up among other small bushes and trees for support. Typical support-protection plants are Creosote bush, Catclaw, and other desert shrubs. The weakly spined branches are usually 4-5 ribbed, grayish-green, and somewhat branched. They are easily mistaken for dead sticks so a trained eye is often needed to find the plant when not in flower. The above ground stems occasionally die back each year only to grow anew from a large tuber. The flowers, similar to Selenicereus grandiflorus', are very large, fragrant, and open for one night only in the spring. A group of plants in a local vicinity has an uncanny ability of flowering during the same night. The fruits are small and ovoid, similar in most respects to S. grandiflorus'.

Distribution: Selenicereus grandiflorus is indigenous to the West Indies but is widely cultivated as an ornamental and occasionally can be found in nurseries in warmer parts of the country. It grows well as an indoor potted cactus. Peniocereus greggii is found throughout lower elevations in western Texas, southern New Mexico, and Arizona. Look to Creosote bush mesas and hillsides; it is never an easy plant to locate in the wild but once you do, there will probably be others close by.

Chemistry: Selenicereus grandiflorus: hordenine; roots of Peniocereus greggii: peniocerol, desoxyviperidone, viperidone, viperidinone, and β-sitosterol

Medicinal Uses: Therapeutic applications of Selenicereus grandiflorus and Peniocereus greggii generally overlap, although P. greggii is considered the weaker of the two. S. grandiflorus has a well-documented western tradition, which spans more than 150 years. First used by Homeopathic practitioners, then by Eclectics and finally some non-conformist, standard-practice doctors, all agreed, Cactus (as S. grandiflorus was formerly called) was a useful cardiovascular medicine. Traditional Mexican use of P. greggii appears to be similar, although specific differences are not known. Both species will be referred to as Night blooming cereus.

Use Night blooming cereus in heart irregularities resulting from deficiency. The plant is well suited in slowing and strengthening a rapid, thready, excitable pulse. Individuals who tend to be of a nervous temperament and who are prone to palpitations, shortness of breath and weakness, resulting from over work or emotional upset will benefit from Night blooming cereus. Similar to Hawthorn, a gloomy, dark emotional outlook accompanying the above symptoms makes Night blooming cereus indicated. As a heart tonic for older individuals with mild to moderate heart enlargement or weakness from tobacco use, the cactus is warranted.

Just how Night blooming cereus enlivens the heart is still under debate, but it appears that it may augment adrenergic-sympathetic responses affecting the organ. The plant combines well with thyroid sedating herbs such as Lycopus or Leonurus in diminishing hyperthyroidal heart palpitations. Fluid retention tends to be lessened around the extremities, particularly around the ankles if dependant upon weak cardiac action. Unlike Digitalis, Night blooming cereus does not have a cumulative effect, so there is no danger of build-up toxicity. The plant best suits functional disturbances but is of moderate value in organic valvular irregularities such as mitral and aortic regurgitations.

Indications:
- Cardiac irregularities dependant upon weakness
  - Tachycardia/arrhythmia/palpitations

Collection and Preparations: Unless island hopping in the Caribbean, collecting Selenicereus grandiflorus, will probably be from a potted plant. Clip several stems and/or flowers from the plant, cut into small ¼-½ inch pieces and tincture fresh. If a group of Peniocereus greggii is found in the desert, be light-handed about collection. Clipping several branches from a plant will not have a detrimental effect on it due to the plant's massive storage root capable of re-sprouting stems the next year. If in flower, leave it to set seed. Do not collect the root in the wild, as the plant is endemic and isolated in the United States. Occasionally P. greggii can be found propagated at native plant nurseries throughout the southwest, if so using the root is permissible. Process and tincture the stems and/or roots the same as S. grandiflorus. Drying either plant voids their medicinal activities.

Dosage:
♦ FPT of Selenicereus grandiflorus: 5-15 drops 1-4 times daily
♦ FPT of Peniocereus greggii: 10-25 drops 1-4 times daily

Cautions: Do not use Night blooming cereus if there is a strong, bounding, full pulse, typically exhibited in robust individuals with strong temperaments. In these individuals, Night blooming cereus may raise blood pressure; inversely in asthenic types, the plant typically lowers blood pressure or will have no effect on the matter. Do not use while pregnant or nursing.

OCOTILLO   *Fouquieriaceae* – Ocotillo family

Fouquieria splendens
Coachwhip, Candlewood, Jacob's staff

Description: Like many plants of the Southwestern Deserts, Ocotillo is semi-succulent and appears bizarre at first sighting. It is a multi-stemmed long lived perennial often living to be 150 or 200 years old. A mature, well-nourished plant can produce upwards of 100 spiny stems that rise vertically from its base. The stem bark is distinctly patterned into living material, which is yellowish and waxy, and non-living material, which is grayish and serves a protective function. The oval green leaves are waxy as well. Depending on rainfall, Ocotillo abundantly produces leaves and correspondingly loses them in drier times. This cycle can occur a half-dozen times a year. At the branch ends conical red flower spikes are followed by valved seed capsules.

Distribution: Ocotillo is typically found from 6,000 feet and lower throughout the Sonoran, Mojave, and Chihuahuan Deserts. Look for the plant on mesa tops, rocky slopes, and plains.

Chemistry: dammarenediol and its triterpenes derivatives; iridoid glucosides: galioside, splendoside, asperocotillin, adoxoside, adoxosidic acid, and loganin; kaempferol, quercetin, isoquercetin, rutin, cinnamic acids, caffeic acids, scopoletin, leucocyanidin, and ellagic acid

Medicinal Uses: Ocotillo tends to be a mild expectorant. It increases bronchial secretion somewhat, making it easier to dislodge impacted phlegm. The plant is also sedating to a dry, spasmodic cough; a useful combination of activities used in wintertime lung afflictions.

Ocotillo has a general decongesting effect on lymphatic and venous circulation of the pelvic area. This use is well applied to hemorrhoids, pelvic lymph enlargements and prostatitis. It is speculated that Ocotillo clarifies lipid-lymph uptake via the portal circulation. Overall, this enhances extracellular fluid movement of the area, lessening trunk-pelvic congestion. Traditional use of Ocotillo among Hispanic New Mexicans has been for sore throats, tonsillitis, and to simulate menses.

Indications:
♦ Dry cough with impacted phlegm
♦ Hemorrhoids, pelvic lymph enlargements/prostatitis

Collection: After finding a many-branched, healthy Ocotillo, select a thick limb close to the outside circumference of the plant. Pull down on the limb until it snaps off at its base. With a knife, strip the spiny bark off the core wood. The leaves can be collected with the bark as well.

Preparations: Because of Ocotillo's nonpolar constituents, the plant is extracted well with alcohol. Although a vita-mix blender works well the dried bark can be difficult to powder. The fresh plant tincture tends to be the most efficacious preparation.

Dosage:
♦ FPT/DPT (70% alcohol): 30-60 drops 3 times daily
♦ Bark decoction: 4-6 ounces 3 times daily

Cautions: Do not use during pregnancy.

Other Uses: Cut branches stuck in the ground and watered root easily. Living Ocotillo fences can be made or rather assisted; they are functional and change with the seasons. A beverage tea is made with the flowers.

PASSIONFLOWER   *Passifloraceae* – Passionflower family

Passiflora mexicana
Mexican passionflower

Passiflora foetida
Corona de cristo

Passiflora incarnata
Maypop, Purple passionflower

Description: All Passionflowers share a majority of unifying characteristics. They are vining plants that trail on the ground or climb into supporting vegetation. The anchoring tendrils are opposite the deeply lobed leaves, which alternate along the stem. The flowers form on axillary peduncles of varying length; depending on species, they are generally a showy affair of different color. Normally there is a base of 5 or 10 tepals. Resting on top of this arrangement is a fringed corona, comprised of numerous filaments. Above this are 5 stamens and 3 styles in whorled patterns. The fruits are many seeded and depending on variety can be sweet and aromatic.

Passiflora mexicana's leaves are deeply 2-lobed, appearing like a pair of pants. The mid-vein area traversing each lobe can have a whitish coloration. The corona is purplish-pink. P. foetida has 3-5 lobed leaves; they are grayish-green and felty. Its corona is lilac-colored. P. incarnate has 3-lobed leaves with pale blue-violet filaments.

Distribution: Look for Passiflora mexicana throughout southeastern Arizona between 2,500-5,000 feet. The plant is commonly found growing up among Mesquites along streams and gullies that run with seasonal water. P. foetida ranges from southern Arizona and southern New Mexico to Texas. It is considered a weed throughout much of the tropical world. P. incarnate grows in warmer temperate regions. It is found throughout the southeast and as far west as Texas. Other species are planted as ornamentals throughout warmer parts of the west. The bulk of over 300 species exist throughout Tropical America.

Chemistry: for Passiflora incarnata: indole alkaloids: harman, harmine, harmalin, harmol, and harmalal; flavonoids: orientin, isoorientin, vitexin, and isovitexin; cyanogenic glycosides

Medicinal Uses: Passionflower is a multi-faceted sedative. It is applicable to several different stress patterns and if used properly can take the place of herbal regimens that comprise a number of herbs. Firstly, use Passionflower to take the edge off anxiousness and tension from daily stresses. Stronger doses of 1 teaspoon of tincture taken before bed can be quite effective in alleviating insomnia; Passionflower works best in thin, easily stressed, nervous individuals. Other more robust body types may respond well to Passionflower but less predictably. If timed well Passionflower diminishes mild seizure activity; take the herb before an episode fully manifests. The plant is also indicated in diminishing tics and muscle spasms from fright, anger, and other vicissitudes of life.

Passionflower tends to be one of the most reliable herbs in curbing cravings and anxiety in substance withdrawal. Make Passionflower a primary herb if quitting Cannabis, opiates, alcohol, or nicotine habits. It is calming to the nerves and soothing to the mind when the body is crying out to be re-intoxicated. It is of particular use in the tremors of alcohol withdrawal.

The plant fits individuals with excessive cardiac force that have a strong, bounding pulse, hypertension, and noticeable surface vasodilation – blood movement – around the upper chest and neck. Use Passionflower to lower blood pressure and slow the heart rate. It is one of the best remedies in aborting tachycardia. The plant is underrated in its application to bronchial complaints when there is an irritative, spastic cough that is difficult to stop. The spasmolytic effect of Passionflower is serviceable in bronchial constriction and shortness of breath when nervousness is exacerbating the episode. The plant is calming to griping and spasmodic diarrhea from food reactions or the catch all – irritable bowel syndrome.

Indications:
♦   Anxiety/tension/muscle spasm
♦   Insomnia
♦   Mild seizure activity/tics

- ◆ Substance withdrawal
- ◆ Tachycardia with hypertension and forceful pulse
- ◆ Spasmodic cough/bronchial constriction
- ◆ Spasmodic diarrhea

Collection: Passiflora mexicana and P. foetida are summer bloomers and are collected from late summer to early fall when in full flower. Ideally, prune the whole vine with leaf, flowers, and immature fruits. Also, collect the cultivated varieties in bloom. Passionflowers that are medicinally potent stink when in flower or when their foliage is crushed. Let their rank smell be an indicator to different variety's potency.

Preparations and Dosage:
- ◆ FPT/DPT (50% alcohol): 60-90 drops 3-4 times daily or 1 teaspoon in acute situations
- ◆ Fluidextract: 30-60 drops 3 times daily
- ◆ Herb infusion: 4-8 ounces 3 times daily

Cautions: Do not use Passionflower during pregnancy due to a weak contractile inhibition on uterine smooth muscle. Although the plant has use in replacing anti-anxiety or sedative pharmaceuticals, full doses of both simultaneously will prove synergistic and will leave the recipient overly sedated.

Other Uses: Passiflora edulis is primarily cultivated in warmer parts of the world for its edible fruits. As a medicine, the plant is inferior. Inversely the other varieties, principally the southwestern natives, will have semi-edible fruits with medicinal/sedative overtones.

PENSTEMON

Scrophulariaceae – Figwort family

Penstemon spp.
Beardtongue

Description: Depending on species, Penstemon generally takes on three varying morphologies; it is either small, delicate and ground hugging, upright and herbaceous, or robust and shrub-like. Whatever the shape these perennials have opposite leaves; the upper ones are sessile and tend to clasp the stem. The lower leaves are petioled. Often the leaves are somewhat thickened, lance or ovoid shaped, smooth and glaucous. The flowers form in racemes and are found in a wide array of colors: reds, pinks, and purples are common. The tubular flowers have 5 united petals and are often 2-lipped. The oval seed capsules contain many small brownish seeds.

Distribution: With over 200 species worldwide, most occur in the American West. Penstemon frequents varying elevations; from low elevation arid desert, to high mountains with Conifers and Aspen, some variety of Penstemon will probably be close by. Look to the edges of draws, gullies, rocky hillsides, meadows, and along trail and roadsides. It is a common plant.

Chemistry: iridoid glycosides, phenolic acids, and anthocyanines

Medicinal Uses: Penstemon is largely unexplored as a plant medicine. Other Figwort family plants of medicinal note are Figwort (Scrophularia spp.) and Devil's claw (Harpagophyton procumbens). There is some suggestion that Penstemon may also have inflammatory sedating qualities, as these other plants do, but more experimentation is needed. For now Penstemon used topically is a mild therapy for stings, bites, rashes, and poorly healing tissues. Penstemon's structure-enhancing anthocyanines, mainly responsible for the flower's coloration, are very useful in augmenting the skins repairing process. This makes the plant applicable in cut and wound healing. Combined with Penstemon's soothing and cooling attributes makes it a worthy application to many conditions.

Indications:
♦ Rashes/bites/stings (external)
♦ Wounds/cuts (external)

Collection: When in flower clip the upper herbage and use fresh or dry. Emphasis on tissue repair can be increased by collecting more flowering racemes.

Preparations and Dosage:
♦   Oil/salve/poultice: as needed

Cautions: None known.

PEPPERGRASS   *Cruciferae* – Mustard family

Lepidium thurberi
Thurber's peppergrass

Description: Peppergrass is a small, 1-2 foot tall annual. From its base, the stems are many branched, long, and narrow. They are covered with short flattened hairs. The 1-3 inch long leaves are variable in shape and are usually pinnately lobed or pinnatifid. After maturing, the leaves typically fall off, leaving the upper stems covered with seedpods. The flowering racemes are formed of small, white, 4-petaled inflorescences. The small seedpods are oval, notched at the top, and narrowed towards the base. Each seedpod contains 2 seeds; they are reddish and oval.

Distribution: Peppergrass ranges in Arizona and New Mexico. From 5,000 feet and lower the plant is wildly distributed in sandy and disturbed soils. Look along trailsides, roadsides, vacant lots, and rocky slopes.

Chemistry: benzyl glucosinolate, glucotropaeolin, and undoubtedly other Mustard family constituents

Medicinal Uses: Peppergrass, like many other Mustard family plants tends to be hot and expanding. A fresh or dry seed poultice applied to painful, arthritic joints is a useful approach in limiting those distresses. Known as a counterirritant, Peppergrass redirects circulatory emphasis, blood movement, and pain sensitivity to the surface. The poultice or plaster can diminish headaches particularly if the pain feels deep-seated.

Internally peppergrass is carminative and warming to the stomach. Its dilatory effect on vasculature increases blood movement to the stomach walls, improving digestive response and food assimilation. Not only is Peppergrass a diuretic it also is stimulating to menses. Use when menstruation is suppressed due to cold and poor uterine circulation.

Lepidium thurberi is only one Peppergrass species out of dozens that can be used medicinally. It is easy to determine what varieties are good medicines: after chewing, if the seeds are hot and pungent then they will be effective.

Indications:
♦ Indigestion, with bloating and feeble stomach circulation
♦ Amenorrhea
♦ Arthritis (external)
♦ Headache (external)

Collection: strip the small green seedpods from the plant, lay out to dry or use fresh.

Preparations and Dosage:
♦ FPT/DPT (60% alcohol): 30-40 drops 3 times daily
♦ Seed infusion: 2-4 ounces 3 times daily
♦ Poultice/plaster: as needed

Cautions: Remove the plaster or poultice when increased heat and circulation is felt. If left too long on the skin it can cause the area to blister. Although somewhat unpredictable, Peppergrass (as well as most other Mustard family plants) contains compounds that can be mildly sedating to thyroid function. This is usually not a problem in individuals with normally functioning thyroids, but may exert some suppressant effect if consumed regularly by hypothyroidal individuals. Do not use during pregnancy due to the plant's menses stimulating ability.

Other Uses: Peppergrass can be used as garnish or added to salads and the like for its hot, pungent taste.

PERIWINKLE

Apocynaceae – Dogbane family

Vinca major
Big leaf periwinkle

Description: Periwinkle is a trailing perennial with dark green, ovate-pointed leaves. They are 2-3 inches long, opposite, waxy, and have wavy margins. The non-flowering stems grow close to the ground and root profusely at the nodes. The showy, solitary purple flowers form from leaf axils; the corolla is 5-lobed and fused at the base. Like many other Dogbane family plants when a leaf or stem is broken a milky latex exudes from the wound. The plant in the west does not reproduce sexually but by spreading rhizomes.

Distribution: Periwinkle is originally native to southern Europe and northern Africa. In warmer areas throughout the United States, it is found as an ornamental escapee. From pockets in the northwest part of the country, it is found in horseshoe pattern – down the west coast through most of California, throughout the southwest and southeast to the mid-eastern states. Temperature extremes, sun exposure and lack of moisture limit the plant's expanse. Look to shaded streamsides and around old farms and homesteads.

Chemistry: alkaloids: majvinine, reserpinine, vincamajoreine, vincawajine, majoridine, methoxyvellosimine, and lochvinerine

Medicinal Uses: Through Periwinkle's vasoconstricting effect on peripheral blood vessels, like caffeine, it can be useful in diminishing pain and sensitivity in the acute stages of a migraine headache. Systemically as well, the plant lessens passive hemorrhaging. Use it to quell mild bleeding from hemorrhoids, nosebleeds, and urinary tract injury. Profuse menstruation, as well as mid-cycle bleeding, diminishes under use of the plant.

Indications:
♦ Migraines, acute pain
♦ Bleeding hemorrhoids/nosebleeds/urinary tract passive hemorrhaging
♦ Menorrhea/mid cycle-bleeding

Collection: Gather the leafing vine with or without flowers. Tincture fresh, or dry for other preparations.

Preparations and Dosage:
- FPT/DPT (50% alcohol): 20-40 drops 3 times daily

Cautions: Do not use during pregnancy or while nursing. Periwinkle may slightly lower blood pressure, so it is not recommended if taking cardiovascular medications.

PLANTAIN   *Plantaginaceae* – Plantain family

Plantago major
Broadleaf plantain, Ribwort

Plantago lanceolata
Buckthorn plantain

Plantago purshii (Plantago patagonica)
Wooly plantain

Description: Broadleaf plantain is a small, low-growing perennial. The leaves are distinct in that they originate from the stalkless center of the plant. They are ovoid, dark green, hairless, pleated, and have wavy margins with or without serrations. The flowers are inconspicuous and small; they are clustered in elongated spikes, typically rising upward from the center of the plant. The seedpods contain numerous, small, reddish-brown seeds. Like Dandelion, Broadleaf plantain and others are notorious for maneuvering their flower spikes so they are just missed by lawn-mower blades.

Buckthorn plantain also has pleated, wavy leaves but they are more lance-shaped. The flowers are clustered towards the tips of the flower stalks. Generally, it is a larger, upright plant. Woolly plantain is a small 3-10 inch annual. All above ground parts of the plant are hairy. The linear leaves stand upright, are several inches long, and originate from the base of the plant. The whitish, small flowers, cluster in spikes much like Broadleaf plantain.

Distribution: Broadleaf and Buckthorn plantain are European natives that have naturalized here extensively. Look for them where the soil has been disturbed and is moist. Places like lawns, gardens, and roadsides usually host these plants in abundance. Wooly plantain is a fairly ubiquitous native that is found throughout the country, but it prefers drier and sandy soils. Look for the plant on rocky slopes and basins. It too will be found in abundance throughout disturbed soils and rangelands.

Chemistry: mucilage composed of polysaccharides; tannins; iridoid glycosides: aucubin and catalpol; silicic acid; protocatechuic acid; flavonoids: apigenin and luteolin

Medicinal Uses: The fresh plant chewed or crushed and then placed on insect bites or stings is one of the better "bush medicines" for these conditions. Like Chickweed, it is also soothing to heat rashes and burns, and will help in wound healing. Internally Plantain is mild; it is not a major medicine but it is multifaceted. The tea or fresh juice diminishes mucus membrane heat. Use it for intestinal inflammation with compounding diarrhea. Plantain is a soothing diuretic that lessens urinary tract irritation and burning upon urination. In addition, the plant reduces bronchial irritation particularly when the lungs feel hot and dry. Well-hydrated Plantain growing along streamsides contains more mucilage whereas desert growing Plantago purshii is higher in tannin content; uses will vary slightly in accordance with different constituent make-ups.

Indications:
- Skin inflammations from bites, stings, and rashes (external)
- Tissue injury (external)
- Intestinal inflammation with diarrhea
- Painful urination
- Bronchial irritation

Collection: Gather the herbage of all three plants. Use fresh or dry.

Preparations and Dosage:
- Fresh plant poultice/oil/salve: as needed
- Cold infusion/standard infusion: 4-8 ounces 2-3 times daily
- Fresh juice: 1-2 ounces 3 times daily, topically as needed

Cautions: None known.

PRICKLY PEAR

Cactaceae – Cactus family

Opuntia engelmannii (Opuntia phaeacantha, Opuntia discata)
Nopal, Nopalitos, Tunas

Description: By nature, this cactus is succulent and at maturity stands 4-6 feet tall by 8-10 feet wide. The bulk of the plant is composed of connected pad-like stems that arise from a thickened base. The green, pancake-like, elliptical pads have clumps of thorns spread throughout their surfaces. Smaller thorns, called glochids are intermingled with larger thorns; they are particularly abundant on the circumference of the pad. New flower bud and pad growth commences in mid-spring. The bright yellow flowers bloom in late spring to early summer. Each flower only lasts one day; they open early in the morning and close at midday when it is the hottest. Early to mid-summer the burgundy, pear-shaped fruits develop.

Distribution: From south-central California Prickly pear is found eastward to central Texas, as far north as South Dakota, south through Colorado, Arizona, and New Mexico. The plant thrives in numerous ecosystems including dry deserts, grasslands, and Juniper-Oak Woodlands. Look for Prickly pear on hillsides, canyon bottoms, and lower desert basins. From coast to coast, there are dozens of species of Prickly pear of similar morphology, but primarily this species is a plant of the arid west.

Chemistry: carbohydrate-containing polymers, consisting of a mixture of mucilage and pectin; betalains: betaxanthin, betanin, vulgaxanthin, miraxanthin, and portulaxanthin; rhamnose, galactose, galacturonic acid; calcium oxalate

Medicinal Uses: Many other varieties of Prickly pear (collectively called Platyopuntia) can be used as well. Taken before meals, Prickly pear reduces blood sugar concentrations by 20-30% in individuals with NIDDM (non-insulin dependent diabetes mellitus). This effect is achieved through the plant's soluble fiber, which slows down the uptake of dietary sugars, and through its ability to increase cellular sensitivity to insulin. Prickly pear also lowers plasma LDL (low density lipoprotein) levels. The plant's soluble fiber has a propensity to bind with cholesterol-containing bile acids, limiting their re-uptake by the portal circulation. This effect limits the liver from overproduction of these "bad" cholesterols. Several ounces of pulp mixed with a small amount of water have a cooling effect on esophageal and stomach irritation, be it from acid reflux or gastritis. Its antiinflammatory effect soothes irritated gastric membranes nicely. Not only does Prickly pear mucilage serve as a protectant to damaged stomach lining it also has the ability of augmenting the quality of gastric mucus making it useful in most ulcer healing approaches.

Externally slices of Prickly pear pad applied to acute injuries, such as contusions and sprains, reduce inflammation and keep unorganized cellular fluids from building up in damaged tissues. On separate occasions, I have broken several toes in the desert clambering around on rocks with inadequate footwear. Each time Prickly pear was abundant and I applied pad slices on the toes until they healed fully. The swelling and discoloration was reduced, as was the pain. It is a simple remedy that works.

Applied externally to burns and inflammations, the pulp makes an excellent healing poultice. Consider it a good equivalent to Aloe Vera.

The flower's of Prickly pear, and most other Opuntias for that matter, are high in flavonoids. The flower infusion, taken internally and applied topically is good for fortifying tissues that are slow to heal and that have difficultly maintaining connectivity. In addition, flower preparations strengthen fragile capillaries and minimize varicosity development. The flower tea tends to be diuretic and stimulates the kidneys excretion of uric acid. Use as a preventive therapy to lessen uric acid kidney stones and gouty conditions.

Indications:

Pad:
♦ NIDDM
♦ Elevated LDL levels
♦ Acid reflux/gastritis/gastric ulcers
♦ Burns (external)
♦ Swellings/contusions (external)

Flowers:
♦ Poorly healing tissues (internal and external)
♦ Fragile capillaries/varicosities (internal and external)
♦ Water retention
♦ Uric acid kidney stones/gout

Collection and Preparations: When harvesting, stay mindful of the very small thorns or glochids; they may not be seen but they can certainly be felt. Find a sizable Prickly pear, one that looks healthy and has no signs of environmental stress or insect damage. Locate one pad in the bunch that is sticking slightly out from the others. Take two good-sized rocks that fit well into your hands and scrape the larger thorns off the pad. When this is complete, cut along the outer circumference of the pad, removing the thorns that were missed. Hold the pad with a gloved hand and cut it from the plant. Now cut it down the middle as if you are cutting open a bagel. Scrape the pulp from the pad's center into a bowl. This will keep in the refrigerator for at least one week. Repeat this process as needed when stores get low.

For internal use, start by mixing several ounces of Prickly pear pulp with several ounces of water. Drink as needed. Blending the mixture can help in liquefying the combination so it is easier to drink. Store-bought prickly pear slices are not as effective as our freshly made, native preparations. Indian-fig or Mission prickly pear (Opuntia ficus-indica), which has soluble fiber content but is also high in glucose, is not as helpful to those who tend toward hyperglycemia. In addition, Prickly pear fruit juice, which can be bought at many health food stores, is lower in soluble fiber and is high in simple-sugar content.

Dosage:
- Pulp slurry/cooked pad: 1-2 ounces before meals
- External pulp/flower infusion/salve: apply as needed
- Internal flower infusion: 4-8 ounces 2-3 times daily

Cautions: Do not use in IDDM (insulin dependent diabetes mellitus). Eating excessive amounts of the raw pad or fruit has been known to cause Prickly pear syndrome, a feverish state with accompanying chills. It is self-resolving but has been known to give people a scare who are attempting to exist solely from the plant.

Other Uses: The young pads can be eaten raw or cooked after the thorns are removed by boiling, brushing, or roasting. The tart taste is from calcium oxalate acumination. For a tasty treat, the ripe fruit is split down the middle and the inner pulp is eaten, with or without the seeds. They are not as refined as Saguaro fruits but are sweet and usually abundant. Prickly pear fruits are a popular base for making juices, jellies, and wine.

Prickly pear is a host plant for Cochineal (*Dactylopius coccus*), a small, cottony-web forming insect. Although not popular today because of displacement by synthetic dyes, years ago the British used the pigment derived from the insect to dye their army's coats red, hence "Red coats". Crushed and applied to cuts and scrapes Cochineal is significantly antimicrobial.

PRICKLY POPPY   *Papaveraceae* – Poppy family

Argemone spp.
Cowboys' fried egg, Chicaolte, Cardo santo

Description: Prickly poppy stands about 2 feet tall with clasping bluish-green leaves rising up along the stem at alternately spaced intervals. The 2-3 inch diameter flowers develop from spring through summer. The large, white, paper-thin petals surround a core of orange stamens, which seem to be always alive with insects of all types. The oblong, spiky seedpods start to appear in mid-summer. After beginning to dry, these capsules open and release miniscule dark black-brown seeds. When young Prickly poppy has some superficial likenesses to Wild lettuce, the similarities end when a leaf or stem is broken. A yellow-orange sap weeps from the wound, very unlike the milky sap that exudes from Wild lettuce.

Distribution: Prickly poppy is found throughout the west. It frequents disturbed soils such as roadsides, dry riverbeds, and overgrazed land.

Chemistry: major alkaloids: dihydosanguinarine, sanguinarine, berberine, protopine, cheletrythine, and coptisine

Medicinal Uses: As a sedative, Prickly poppy works best when there is pain from acute injury making sleep difficult. Its quieting effect on afferent pain signals gives some relief particularly if the acuity of the situation is dependent upon muscular rigidity. Prickly poppy is also useful in sedating smooth muscle constriction of bronchial and intestinal tissues. The herb fits when there is a hectic, spasmodic cough with bronchial heat and hyperactivity. Likewise, the herb has value if there is intestinal cramping with associated bouts of diarrhea.

Externally the oil or salve made from the seeds makes an excellent burn dressing. It is soothing and pain relieving to inflamed and abraded tissues.

An externally applied tea is antimicrobial, assisting cuts and broken skin in staying free of pathogens. An isotonic tea of the herb, strained well of very small leaf and stem hairs, makes a soothing eyewash; it reduces conjunctiva inflammation. Styes also diminish with its use. The plant can be likened to a combination of Bloodroot, Desert barberry, and California poppy.

Indications:
- Muscular pain
- Insomnia, restlessness
- Spasmodic cough
- Intestinal cramps
- Bacterial infections (external)
- Burns, abrasions (external)
- Conjunctivitis (eyewash)

Collection: Collect Prickly poppy throughout the spring and summer. With pruners snip the upper half of the plant, including leaf, flower, and seedpods. Wear gloves while collecting the plant. The fine hairs of the plant are sharp and stiff.

Preparations: After drying the uncut herb, garble everything from the stems. Chop the stems into ¼-½ inch pieces. Use both parts for medicine.

Dosage:
- Herb infusion: 2-4 ounces 2-3 times daily
- DPT (50% alcohol): 20-40 drops 2-3 times daily
- Eyewash: 3-4 times daily

Cautions: Even in moderate quantities, problems can potentially develop when the seeds or particularly the refined seed oil is ingested regularly. In northern India Mustard seed oil, adulterated with Prickly poppy seed oil (Argemone mexicana) has been the cause of numerous deaths. Individuals succumb as a result of massive interstitial fluid disorganization, vascular deterioration, and subsequent edema. It is important to note that ingesting a refined seed oil, which by its nature is a highly potentiated substance, is very different from ingesting crude seed-herb preparations used here.

Although seed preparations of Prickly poppy have been used as a mildly stimulating laxative, it is best to err on the side of caution and not use these preparations internally, or at least not by themselves. If seed preparations are used, keep their use short term, 2-3 days at a time. The internally used whole herb is less toxic. Short-term use of 2-3 weeks at any one time is relatively safe. Individuals taking this plant should be strong, healthy, and currently not on any major pharmaceutical regimens. Do not use while pregnant or lactating.

PUNCTUREVINE   *Zygophyllaceae* – Caltrop family

Tribulus terrestris
Goathead, Sandbur, Bullhead

Description: Puncturevine grows mat-like and covers expansive stretches. The entire plant is hairy, including the leaves, which are composed of 4-7 small compound leaflets. They are borne on long horizontal stems sometimes reaching 7-8 feet in length, though normally they are only 2-3 feet long. In the summer, the small, 5-petaled, bright yellow flowers open in the morning and close soon after when confronted by the hot sun. The seed capsules are 5-sectioned and break apart at maturity; each section is double-spined and contains several seeds. They are viable for at least five years, making eradication next to impossible. The seed capsules or goatheads as they are "affectionately" called are legendary for the discomfort they cause to bare feet.

Distribution: A non-native from southern Europe, Puncturevine now is distributed widely throughout the west. Look for the plant in disturbed areas such as roadsides, vacant lots, and along fields and pastures.

Chemistry: sapogenins: terrestrosin, ruscogenin, and hecogenin; harmine and nor-harmine; flavonoids: quercetin and rutin

Medicinal Uses: Although terminology and descriptions of effects differ, western perspectives and more ancient systems such as Traditional Chinese Medicine and Ayurveda coincide on Puncturevine use. On its relationship to the cardiovascular system, the plant fits individuals with moderately elevated blood pressure who suffer from angina pectoris. The coronary artery, which supplies blood to the heart, is dilated through Puncturevine's effect, therefore quenching the heart's literal cry for oxygen. Compounding this with Puncturevine's slowing and force-lessening effect on the cardiac muscle makes the plant very useful for hypertensive, middle-aged individuals whose lifestyle has become sedentary and diet is caloricly burdensome.

Puncturevine is useful in diminishing the formation of both uric acid and oxalate based kidney stones, be it from injury, dehydration, or metabolic excesses. In addition, its tendency to dilute the urine through its diuretic action, combined with the plant's soothing effect on urinary tract mucus membranes, makes the plant's application to urinary irritability well suited.

It is known that Puncturevine augments androgens, particularly DHEA (dehydroepiandrosterone) and testosterone within the body. Although the mechanism is still unclear, the effects are noticeable in that libido is increased, and in men, erectile response is heightened, as is the quantity and quality of sperm. Nocturnal emissions or spermatorrhea lessens under its use. Many men using the plant often notice a related sense of increased physical strength and will – a good tonic for older men and the metrosexual alike.

Traditionally Puncturevine is used for skin outbreaks that exhibit redness and heat – the typical eczematous rash. Since the plant is significantly antiinflammatory and hence somewhat mediating to allergic reactivity, topical and internal use of Puncturevine is of value in treating eczema and psoriasis. Of interest also is the plant's stimulatory effect on melanocyte proliferation, making external therapies of use in treating vitiligo.

Indications:
♦ Essential hypertension with fluid retention
♦ Angina pectoris
♦ Kidney stones, as a preventative, both uric acid and oxalate types
♦ Decreased libido/low sperm count and poor quality
♦ Allergic skin conditions/eczema/psoriasis (internal and external)
♦ Vitiligo

Collection: Collect Puncturevine from mid to late summer after it responds to seasonal rains. The plants are easily pulled up, roots and all; be mindful of the seed capsules or goatheads as they can gouge hands easily if aggressively handled. Collect the seed capsules in the late summer to early fall.

Preparations: The whole plant is active, although the mature, dried capsules with seeds are traditionally used. Puncturevine lends itself to most preparations.

Dosage:
- Herb-seed infusion: 2-4 ounces 3 times daily
- FPT/DPT (60% alcohol): 30-40 drops 3 times daily
- Topical preparations: as needed

Cautions: Most reports of Puncturevine toxicity have been though observations of the effects on sheep from grazing areas where the plant is in great abundance. Cases of liver and kidney problems and sun-sensitivity do arise in these circumstances. With this in mind, prudence suggests if the herb is to be used as a simple, keep the duration short term (several weeks). In formula, long-term use is acceptable. Do not use during pregnancy, while nursing, or with liver or kidney disease.

PURPLE GROMWELL   *Boraginaceae* – Borage family

Lithospermum multiflorum
Stoneseed, Puccoon

Description: Purple gromwell is a small, herbaceous perennial. Vertical stems, reaching 1-2 feet in height, arise from the root crown. The leaves and stems are verdant and somewhat hairy. The leaves form alternately along the stem and are narrow and elongated. Each leaf has a prominent mid-vein. The yellow flowers form in terminal clusters and are scorpioid shaped. Each tubular flower has 5 small petaled lobes. The small seeds are white and very hard, hence the name Litho-spermum (stone-seed). The plant's taproot is long and slender. Purplish splotches are evident on the root's crown.

Distribution: From Wyoming, the plant grows south to Arizona and New Mexico. Throughout the southwest, it can be found from 6,000-9,500 feet. Look to Pine and Juniper Woodlands. The plant is fond of flats and slopes.

Chemistry: naphthoquinone, hydroxycinnamic acid ester: rosmarinic acid; γ-linolenic acid; pyrrolizidine alkaloids, chlorogenic acid, succinic acid, and lithospermic acid

Medicinal Uses: The medicinal potency of Purple gromwell is largely due to the purplish-red pigments contained in the roots. Surely, many species not profiled here are as medicinally potent. These pigments, largely composed of naphthoquinone, are also pronounced in Lithospermum erythrorhizon, a much-researched Chinese species.

Topically the plant has use in wound healing, mainly through its curbing effect on erratic, yet typical, inflammatory-oxidative states normally associated with wound and cuts. Furthering this effect is Purple gromwell's moderate antibacterial quality. Purple gromwell is also inhibiting to various fungal strains, so its application is warranted in topical skin and nail funguses. There is also promise in the plant sedating the excesses of psoriasis and eczema.

Although lately Lithospermum ruderale has been shown to be broadly sedating to gonadotropic and thyroid stimulating hormone activity, because of the presence of pyrrolizidine alkaloids, internal use of the plant should be avoided. Incidentally, this hormonal altering activity coincides with the Shoshone's sterility inducing/contraceptive use of the plant. The roots and seeds of L. virginianum were once used by the Eclectic physicians and lay practitioners alike as a soothing diuretic. The tea was also indicated in dissolving urinary tract gravel.

Indications:
- Wounds/cuts/scrapes (external)
- Bacterial and fungal infections (external)
- Psoriasis/eczema (external)

Collection: Gather the plant in the spring or summer using the foliage or flowers as an indicator. The roots are small but older plants can produce sizable woody taproots. After the roots are dug, discard the foliage.

Preparations and Dosage:
- Root decoction: topically as needed
- DPT (50% alcohol): topically as needed
- Oil/salve/poultice: as needed

Cautions: As previously mentioned Purple gromwell contains liver-toxic pyrrolizidine alkaloids, as do many other Borage family plants (particularly the Amsinckia and Cryptantha genuses) in the southwest. Internal use is to be avoided.

Other Uses: Purple gromwell has potential as a dye plant as the Chinese variety, Lithospermum erythrorhizon, was used in silk staining.

RATANY

Krameriaceae – Ratany family

Krameria grayi
White ratany, Chacate

Krameria parvifolia
Range ratany, Chacate

Krameria secundiflora (Krameria lanceolata)
Three fans, Prairie bur

Description: These low-growing shrubs form into mound-like clumps. They are densely branched and in the case of Krameria grayi, are somewhat spiny. The herbage is grayish-green and hairy. The small linear leaves, particularly on younger branches, hug the stem and point upwards. The crimson-purple flowers are composed of 3-5 petals and can appear strangely beak-like. The seedpods, the size of a cultivated cherry, are inflated, oddly shaped globes surrounded by small barbed spines. On closer examination they do look like something out of a science fiction novel – fact stranger than fiction. Krameria is a reputed partial root parasite. Creosote bush and Triangle-leaf bursage are typical hosts.

Distribution: Generally, these three species overlap in habitat. Both Krameria grayi and K. parvifolia are found from 5,000 feet and below through much of Arizona, southeastern California, and southern Nevada, to western Texas. They are common to desert mesas, foothills, and alluvial fans where soils are rocky. K. secundiflora, found from 4,000-7,000 feet, ranges from southeastern Arizona east to Florida.

Chemistry: catechin and epicatechin; proanthocyanidin derivates: procyanidin and propelargonidin; neolignans and norneolignans: ratanhiaphenol 1 and 2

Medicinal Uses: Many species of Ratany, some not profiled here, have a rich western medicinal history. These plants were widely used in Western Europe and later here in the United States up until the early twentieth century, when many other botanical medicines were promptly dropped and replaced with new-generation isolated substances.

Above all else, Ratany is astringent. Virtually all of its medicinal benefits derive from this fact. The tea used as a mouthwash is tonifying to gums and can be used with Ginger or Prickly ash for added tissue stimulation. It is of use in periodontitis, spongy and receding gums, and relieving to aphthous stomatitis, or canker sores as they are commonly called.

Ratany diminishes diarrhea by its astringent effect on the gastrointestinal tract and its contents. Moreover, passive hemorrhaging, be it bronchial, uterine, urinary or gastrointestinal tract centered, is diminished. Menorrhea, or excessive menstruation dependent upon perimenopause or subnormal levels of reproductive hormones, is often diminished by Ratany, albeit symptomatically. The plant serves as a tissue and capillary bed constrictor and does not affect circulating hormone levels. Colliquative sweating may be lessened with Ratany. The addition of Sage may augment the effectiveness of treatment.

Topically Ratany is applied to weepy sores, cuts, rashes, and stings to astringe, lessen inflammation, and facilitate healing. The salve is employed topically to shrink hemorrhoids and diminish associated bleeding. Rectal suppositories made with Ratany oil are used to encourage healing of anal fissures.

Indications:
- Periodontitis/spongy and bleeding gums/canker sores (mouthwash)
- Diarrhea
- Menorrhea
- Passive hemorrhaging of urinary tract, GI tract, lungs, uterus
- Colliquative sweating
- Hemorrhoids/anal fissures (external)

Collection and Preparations: From mid-spring through summer, the herbage is relatively hydrated and pickable. Although the root bark was the article of choice in the past, there is really no need to dig up these long-lived, slow-growing perennials. The herb preparations are not quite as strong, but slightly higher doses will compensate for this.

Dosage:
- FPT/DPT (50% alcohol, 10% glycerin): 30-60 drops 3 times daily
- Cold infusion: 2-6 ounces 3 times daily, topically as needed
- Suppositories: 1-2 daily (one being used before bed)

Cautions: Like most tannin plants internal use should be limited to short term: 2-3 weeks concurrently, or else gastric and/or renal irritation may result. Ratany is not recommended during pregnancy due to its vasoconstricting effect on uterine lining.

RAYWEED   *Compositae* – Sunflower family

Parthenium incanum
Mariola, Crowded rayweed

Description: Rayweed is a small, woody-based perennial shrub 2-3 feet in height. The plant is densely branched and when fully leafed out occasionally droops with abundant leaf mass. The leaves themselves are grayish-green, lobed, and are alternately arranged along the stems. The small cream flowers form in flattop panicle groupings above the foliage.

Distribution: From 2,500-5,000 feet Rayweed is found from the Grand Canyon area in northern Arizona to Pima and Cochise Counties in southern Arizona, east to central New Mexico, and finally to the Edwards Plateau and Rio Grand Plain in Texas. Typical locations for it are along rocky hillsides and on the edges of gullies. It prefers alkaline, calcrete-laden soils and is most abundantly found throughout the Chihuahuan Desert.

Chemistry: sesquiterpene lactones: tetraneurin, fruticosin; triterpenoids; flavonoids: quercetin, penduletin, quercetagetin, polycladin, and artemetin

Medicinal Uses: A ½-cup of Rayweed tea before meals is a stimulating bitter. It stimulates an array of digestive secretions that augment protein and fat digestion. It, like other bitters, can be used before a meal to restore appetite and proper digestive response to food. In time, this will provide better assimilation of nutrients. The plant to some degree is a bile stimulant, as are most plant bitters. Some individuals may find Rayweed mildly laxative making the plant indicated in constipation dependent upon stress, poor eating habits, and a suppressed urge to defecate.

Indications:
♦ Indigestion
♦ Liver sluggishness

♦   Mild constipation

Collection: From early to mid-summer, gather the leaves of Rayweed before the plant flowers.

Preparations and Dosage:
♦   Leaf infusion: 2-4 ounces 3 times daily

Cautions: Do not use during pregnancy and while nursing due to the plants bioactive chemistry.

Other Uses: Like its relative Guayule (Parthenium argentatum) which grows in Mexico, Rayweed also has substantial, although smaller, rubber content. It was once cultivated during WWI and WWII for this purpose when other rubber containing plants were difficult to procure.

SAGE   *Labiatae* – Mint family

Salvia columbariae
Chia

Salvia lemmoni (*Salvia microphylla var. wislizeni*)
Little leaf sage

Salvia apiana
White sage

Salvia carnosa (*Salvia dorrii*)
Purple sage, Desert sage

Salvia mohavensis
Mojave sage

Salvia clevelandii
Cleveland sage, Chaparral sage

Description: All Salvias have square stems, opposite leaves, and to varying degrees are aromatic. The flowers form in whorls around the upper stems, but also, depending on variety, develop interrupted spikes. Each calyx and corolla is 2-lipped. The flowers are generally tubular.

Salvia columbariae is a small annual that responds to winter-spring rains. The plant's basal leaves are 1-4 inches long, pinnatifid, toothed, and felty. The blue flowers form in whorls around the upper flower stems. The stiff calyxes are somewhat spiny. S. apiana is a 3-5 foot tall perennial. The petioled leaves are oblanceolate and 1-3½ inches long. The leaves and upper stems are made silvery-white by a covering of appressed hairs. The whorled flower clusters develop on the upper stem sections. They are white or speckled with lavender. S. carnosa is a highly variable species with many varieties exhibiting leaf and flower differences. This small shrub is less than 3 feet high. The leaves are spatula shaped, linear, or obovate. They are covered with a fine layer of appressed hairs making their appearance silvery. The whorled flowers form on upper branch stems and are blue.

Salvia mohavensis is a small, many-branched shrub generally 3 feet tall. Leaf blades are oblanceolate or deltoid, green, and covered with short leaf hairs. The whorled flowers are pale blue or lavender. S. clevelandii is also about 3 feet in height. The leaves are ½-1½ inches long, oblong, and coated with a grayish pubescence. Flowers are blue-lavender. The whole plant is extremely fragrant. S. lemmoni is 3 feet tall by the same wide. The plant's leaves are green, ovate, and when young, sticky with leaf oils. Flowers are typically crimson-pink in color.

Distribution: From 4,000 feet and below Salvia columbariae is common in sandy washes, drainages, and disturbed areas. It ranges from southern California to southern Nevada, Utah, and Arizona. S. apiana is found in California from coastal ranges in Santa Barbara and San Diego Counties, east to the desert's edge, and south. Look to dry slopes in Chaparral Scrub areas. From Washington to Arizona, S. carnosa is extensively distributed throughout the desert west. Look to Juniper-Pinyon Woodlands and Sagebrush Deserts.

Salvia mohavensis is found from 1,000-5,000 feet in desert regions of southern Nevada, southeast California, and western Arizona. Look to dry rocky slopes and canyon walls. S. clevelandii is found on dry slopes, below 3,000 feet in Chaparral Scrub areas, and coastal mountains of southern California. S. lemmoni ranges in southern Arizona. Look for it throughout Pima and Cochise Counties. This high elevation Sage can be found on mountainsides and rocky slopes from 6,000-8,000 feet. It has a limited distribution, but is locally abundant.

Chemistry: volatile oil content for Salvia columbariae (others are similar): α-pinene, camphene, β-pinene, myrcene, α-phellandrene and β-phellandrene, 3-carene, p-cymene, 1,8-cineole, limonene, cisocimene, transocimene, γ-terpinene, terpinolene, linalol, camphor, borneol, 4-terpineol, α-terpineol, bornylacetate, β-caryophyllene, γ-cadinene, α-cadinene, and farnesol; diterpenes: carnosic acid, carnosol, rosmanol, epirosmanol, isorosmanol, salvicanol, and rosmadial

Medicinal Uses: Salvia's medicinal potency is greatly dependent upon its strong aromatic smell. Like most other Mint family plants, the stronger the smell, the stronger the medicine. If there is a fever, the skin is hot and dry, and there is a strong determination of blood a hot cup of Sage tea is diaphoretic. The room temperature tea or tincture curbs colliquative sweating, particularly when body temperature is low to normal, the skin is soft and relaxed, and the extremities are cool. Internally Sage is decidedly carminative. It is useful taken as a spasmolytic for gas pains and flatulence. Its dilatory nature moves blood, hence activity to the stomach walls.

Applied externally Sage is strongly antiinflammatory and antioxidant. It is efficacious in relieving pain and redness from burns and other injuries. Its use rivals Lavender in these conditions. The steam can be inhaled from a cup or pot of hot tea for Strep throat. This process concentrates the antimicrobial aromatics to the back of the throat where most of the bacterial colonization takes place. This done for five minutes three times a day, along with internal immune stimulating herbs such as Baptisia, Echinacea, or Bursera, combined with rest, is a useful plan.

Several different varieties of Sage have been used in English herbal medicine for memory loss, forgetfulness, and to "strengthen the brain". Lately it has been discovered that the essential oil of several varieties of Sage, namely Salvia lavandulaefolia, inhibits AchE (acetylcholinesterase) in cholinergic neuronal synapses of the brain. This has promise in diminishing the dementia and cognition loss of alzheimer's. Even in non-alzheimer's study subjects improved attention and recall has been shown. Apparently, Sage blocks AchE from breaking down acetylcholine into inactive choline and acetate, therefore keeping the compound in the synapse longer. This then improves brain nerve transmission. AchE inhibition through pharmaceuticals is the primary conventional treatment for alzheimer's. The plant's monoterpene content, which is largely responsible for this effect acts strongest as a whole complex. The plant's aromatics are much less potent taken out of context and used in an isolative fashion, even if recombined to mimic the plant's natural essential oil ratios. This is not a new phenomenon. Most plants work best as whole herbal medicines, not standardized extracts.

For ages, Salvia officinalis has been used to decrease milk production in mothers needing to wean their children. Other varieties may be as useful.

Indications:
♦ Fever, dry, moderate temperature
♦ Colliquative sweating
♦ Burns (external)
♦ GI tract gas and spasm
♦ Strep throat/sore throat
♦ Memory loss/poor cognition
♦ Alzheimer's
♦ To lessen breast milk

Collection: Gathering Sage is always a pleasant experience due to the plant's characteristic smell. Collect the leaves and flowering parts only, as these have the greatest concentration of aromatics. Without distillation/extraction equipment Sage essential oil can not be procured. It is best purchased.

Preparations: For internal use of Sage essential oil use 1 part essential oil to 1 part olive oil, so for every 10 drops of Sage essential oil, 10 drops of olive oil is used. Mix together and in each capsule put 4 drops of combined oil. Use this same mixture topically. If it is agreeable, try applying undiluted for a stronger effect.

Dosage:
♦ Herb infusion: 4-8 ounces 3 times daily
♦ FPT/DPT (50% alcohol): 30-60 drops 3 times daily
♦ Steam inhalation: 3 times daily
♦ Capsules of essential oil: 1 capsule 3 times daily
♦ Essential oil: topically as needed

Cautions: Do not use the essential oil during pregnancy or while nursing.

Other Uses: Use as a seasoning. Southwestern Sages, particularly Salvia apiana are used extensively ceremonially, ironically more so now by Whites than by the American Indian originators of the tradition.

SAGEBRUSH   *Compositae* – Sunflower family

Artemisia tridentata
Big sagebrush, Mountain sagebrush

Description: This moderately sized evergreen bush varies in size depending on rainfall and soil conditions. In ideal circumstances where the winters are cold and there is adequate precipitation the plant can reach 9-10 feet in height, but 3-4 feet is more common with average soil, rainfall, and warmer temperatures. The trunk of Sagebrush is woody, thickened, and on older plants, is covered by grayish-brown stringy bark. The leaves are wedge-shaped and typically have 3 blunt teeth. However, they sometimes have 4-9 teeth, and occasionally are completely lacking teeth and are entire. The leaves' silvery-blue appearance results from the plant's dense coating of leaf hairs. When the aromatic leaves are crushed, a distinctive sage-like smell is apparent; the plant's pungency is also evident when it is well hydrated and daytime temperatures are high. In the fall, the small yellow flowers form in panicles at branch ends. Throughout most of its range Sagebrush is a prolific seeder, demonstrated by various removal programs designed to clear western grazing lands of the plant.

Distribution: Sagebrush is a dominant plant throughout western rangelands. It can be found from British Colombia and South Dakota south to the Rocky Mountains, New Mexico, central Arizona, and California.

Chemistry: artemeseole, camphor, carvacrol, 1-8-cineol, α-pinene, β-pinene, thujol, and thujone, among many other constituents

Medicinal Uses: Not only is Sagebrush a strong, multi-faceted medicinal plant, it is also ubiquitous in large expanses enabling wider use with little ill effect on plant populations as a whole. The plant affects numerous organ systems more profoundly than the best Mugwort, a closely related herb. Residents of the Great Basin Desert, the Paiutes, Hopi, Hispanic New Mexicans and American pioneers, have all used Sagebrush medicinally.

When drunken cold, Sagebrush tea is an aromatic bitter. It is stimulating to hydrochloric acid, pepsinogen, and other gut secretions (as are most other Artemisias). This compounded with its carminative and bile stimulating effects increases digestive prowess. Proteins and fats are digested and assimilated more efficiently with less gas and cramping associated with gastrointestinal tract weakness. The cold tea is diuretic, whereas drunk hot it is strongly diaphoretic, particularly when the skin is hot and dry, the pulse is strong and there is a general feeling of contained body heat. The plant can break the most stubborn of fevers.

Sagebrush is broadly antimicrobial and anti-parasitic. It lends itself well as a treatment for some food and water borne illnesses. It inhibits Salmonella spp. and Escherichia coli, among other pathogenic organisms responsible for food poisoning. Modern findings and traditional use also support the plant being used in amebic infections, i.e. montezuma's revenge-traveler's diarrhea, and as a broad-spectrum vermifuge. Pinworms and roundworms are the surest parasites Sagebrush will eliminate.

The plant is stimulating to menses mainly through its essential oil and thujone content. The hot tea or tincture put in hot water is particularly useful in dilating uterine capillary beds, therefore delivering more blood and activity to the area. This usually is enough to stimulate menses if it is slow to start from recent viral infections or even from moving to a colder locale.

When applied topically, Sagebrush is significantly antimicrobial and antifungal. Various external preparations are all useful in inhibiting numerous Staphylococcus, Streptococcus and fungal varieties. From ringworm and athlete's foot to wounds and ulcers that need some infection fighting help, the plant is powerful. Compounding this effect is Sagebrush's analgesic effect. Acute pain from contusions, sprains, and blows along with chronic pain from rheumatoid arthritis or bothersome old sport injuries, are all quieted.

A warm poultice or fomentation is decidedly sedative to menstrual, intestinal, and stomach cramps. Moreover, the plant makes a strong antimicrobial respiratory tract medicine. Inhaling the volatile oil filled steam of the tea is useful in bronchitis, especially when mucus is impacted and difficult to expectorate. The inhaled steam rivals White sage and Eucalyptus in treating strep throat and sinusitis.

Indications:
♦ Indigestion with upper and lower GI tract cramps and flatulence
♦ Liver, bile sluggishness, from non-organic causes

- Fevers, dry skin, strong determination of blood
- Food poisoning
- Amebic diarrhea
- Pinworm/roundworm worm infestation
- Amenorrhea with water retention and feelings of coldness
- Fungal infections (external)
- Wounds/blows/contusions (external)
- Menstrual cramps (external)
- GI tract cramps (external)
- Bronchitis with impacted mucus and dry cough (inhaled steam)

Collection and Preparations: In the spring, before flowering, snip the last 8-10 inches of new growth from the branch ends. These clippings can either be wrapped in small bundles or chopped into smaller manageable pieces for drying.

Dosage:
- Leaf infusion: 2-4 ounces 3 times daily
- FPT/DPT (60% alcohol): 10-30 drops 3 times daily
- Inhaled steam: 2-3 times daily
- External preparations: as needed

Cautions: Due to Sagebrush's thujone and related essential oil content, do not use during pregnancy or while nursing. Discontinue use if there are sensations of dizziness, nausea, or headache. Internally use Sagebrush consecutively for 1-2 weeks or less.

Other Uses: Although the smoke is harsh on the eyes and respiratory tissues, Sagebrush smudge has a rich historical and present day ceremonial use. It is known as the "other" Sage.

SENNA
Leguminosae – Pea family

Senna leptocarpa var. glaberrima (Cassia leptocarpa var. glaberrima)
Slimpod senna

Senna armata (Cassia armata)
Spiny senna

Senna covesii (Cassia covesii)
Desert senna

Description: Senna leptocarpa var. glaberrima is a 2-3 foot tall, herbaceous bush. When fully leafed-out and in flower the plant's sub-tropical look is distinctive. The leaves are deeply green and usually between 4-7 inches long. They are pinnately divided into 4-8 sets of long triangular leaflets. The leaves alternate along the branched stems and progressively diminish in size as they terminate inter-spaced with the flowers. Towards the outer reaches of the plant, the large, deep yellow-orange flowers have 5 petals and are quite noticeable in the summer. As its name implies the pods are thin and narrow but long, usually 6-10 inches in length, brown and formed in clusters of 2-3. The encased, small brownish seeds are tightly packed together in 1 long row.
  Senna armata is a low-growing, deciduous bush usually 1-2 feet in height. Much of the year it is leafless, only to break the trend and form leaves in response to winter rains. The leaf axes, which the pinnate leaflets attach themselves to, terminate pointedly as spines. The bright yellow flowers are followed by tan, inflated seedpods. S. covesii is a small, semi-herbaceous bush. In drier winters, the spring-formed leaves are very compact and hairy, giving the plant a greenish-sliver coloration. As with other Sennas this plant also has characteristic yellow flowers followed by elongated small pods.
  Unknown to the plant, the genus has had a troubled botanical past. Originally classed as Senna, then Cassia, it is now designated as Senna again. Thankfully, the plant's medicinal qualities are unchanging.

Distribution: Look for Senna leptocarpa var. glaberrima along wash embankments, roadsides, and drainage areas. From southeastern Arizona, this plant is found east to New Mexico and south through Mexico, Central America, to South America. Look for S. armata in the western desert of southern California, the extreme southern tip of Nevada and along parts of the

Colorado River Drainage in western Arizona. Typically, it can be found along washes and drainages in sandy soils. From 1,000-4,000 feet look for S. covesii along gravely wash sides, hillsides, and roadsides throughout southeastern California, southwestern Arizona, southern Nevada, and southern New Mexico.

Chemistry: hydroxyanthracene glycosides: sennosides; naphthalene glycosides; flavonoids; mucilage (galactose, arabinose, rhamnose, and galacturonic acid)

Medicinal Uses: Senna is a straightforward stimulant laxative. A cold infusion made with the pods is the choice preparation; although the leaves can be used as well, they are considered harsher in activity. Similar to Aloe, Senna's anthraquinones affect the small and large intestines. By increasing transit time, peristalsis, and decreasing intestinal fluid absorption Senna is a reliable laxative. Mixing Senna with a carminative herb such as Ginger, Peppermint, or Dogweed will limit the plant's potential to cause griping. Taken before bed and dosed properly Senna will soften the stool and stimulate bowel movement for the next morning. Some of Senna's glycosides are broken down in the colon by bacterial activity. The resulting metabolites, particularly rheinanthrone, are responsible for much of the plant's effect.

Because the pods contain polysaccharide-starches the rate at which Senna delivers its stimulant-anthraquinones is somewhat slowed, making the pods gentler in effect. The leaves' lack of these substances is the main reason why they tend to be more irritative in nature, sometimes causing griping and flatulence.

Use Senna in obstinate constipation. It is particularly useful if constipation is dependent upon stress and anxiety. It is also important to address dietary and constitutional factors for long-term relief. Fiber and water intake, upper gastrointestinal and hepatic response to food, and psychosomatic responses are all important issues to address when resolving chronic constipation.

Indications:
♦ Constipation

Collection: The leaves, flowering racemes, seedpods, and immature seeds are all active. The leaves are the most purgative in nature. The fully mature

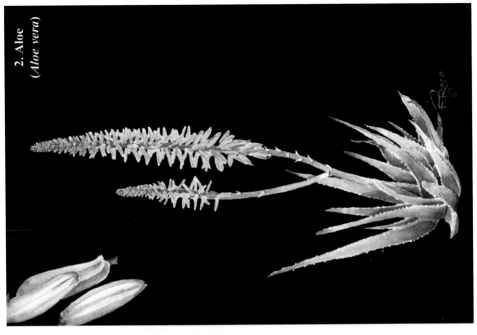

2. Aloe
(*Aloe vera*)

ALOE

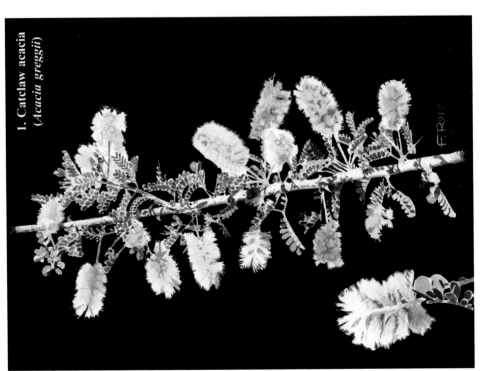

1. Catclaw acacia
(*Acacia greggii*)

ACACIA

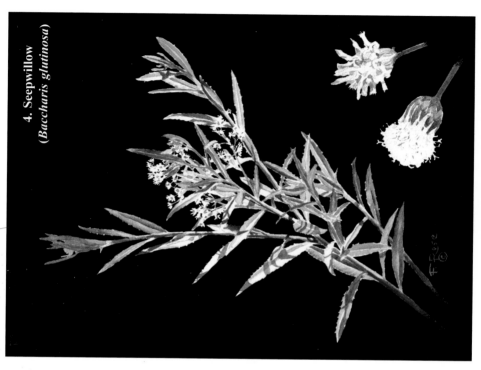

3. Antelope horns
(*Asclepias asperula*)

ANTELOPE HORNS

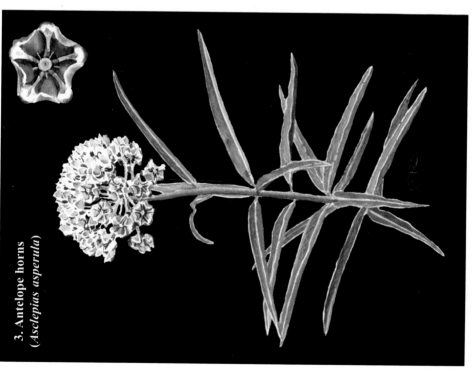

4. Seepwillow
(*Baccharis glutinosa*)

BACCHARIS

6. Red bird of paradise
(*Caesalpinia pulcherrima*)

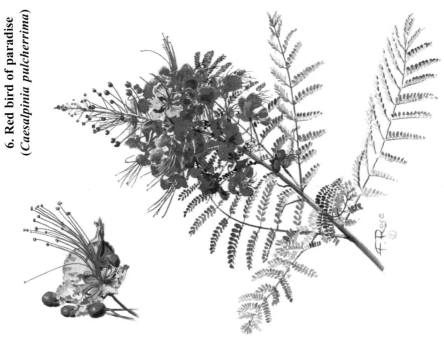

BIRD OF PARADISE

5. Beargrass
(*Nolina microcarpa*)

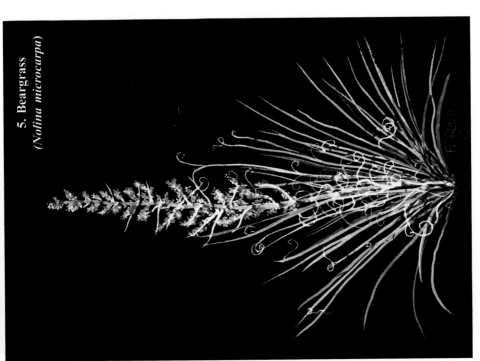

BEARGRASS

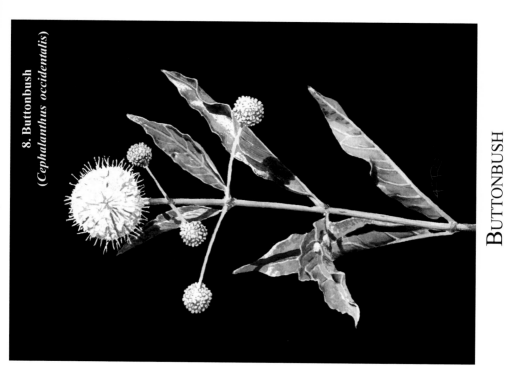

8. Buttonbush
(*Cephalanthus occidentalis*)

BUTTONBUSH

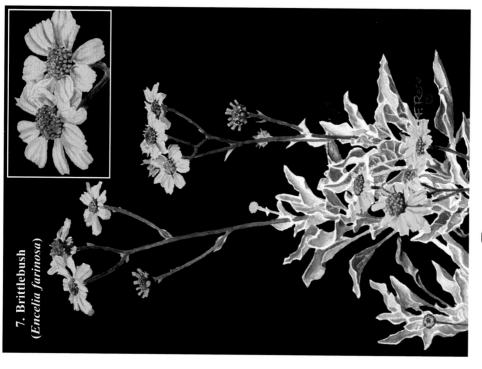

7. Brittlebush
(*Encelia farinosa*)

BRITTLEBUSH

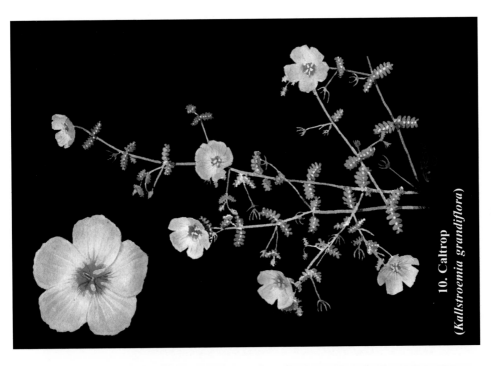

10. Caltrop
(*Kallstroemia grandiflora*)

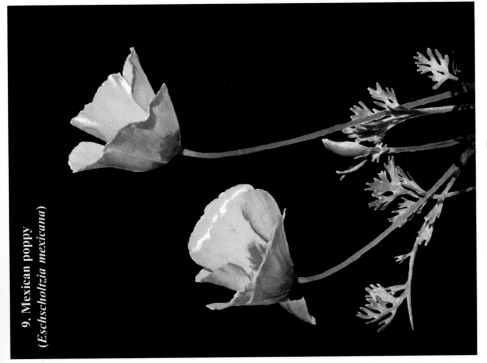

9. Mexican poppy
(*Eschscholtzia mexicana*)

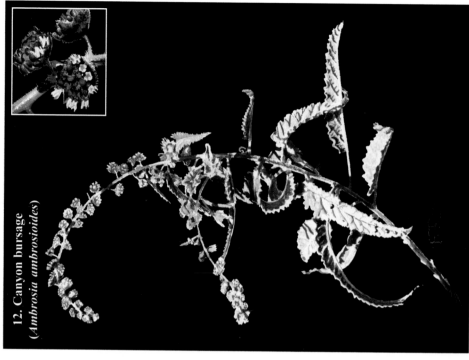

11. Camphorweed
(*Heterotheca subaxillaris*)

CAMPHORWEED

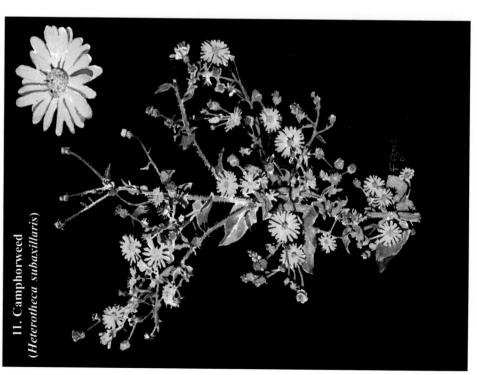

12. Canyon bursage
(*Ambrosia ambrosioides*)

CANYON BURSAGE

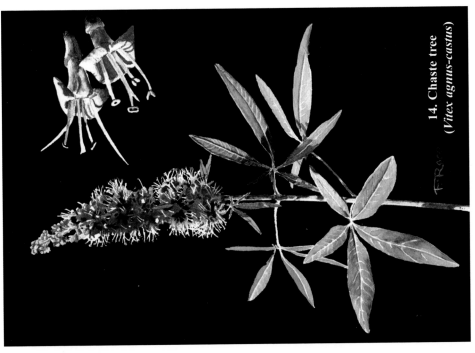

14. Chaste tree
(*Vitex agnus-castus*)

CHASTE TREE

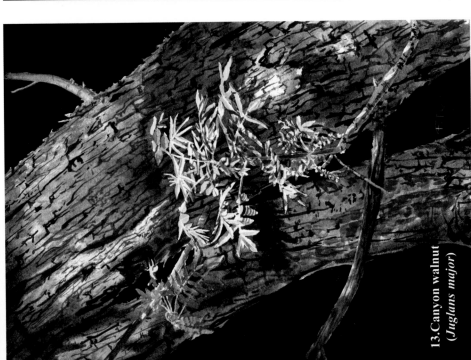

13. Canyon walnut
(*Juglans major*)

CANYON WALNUT

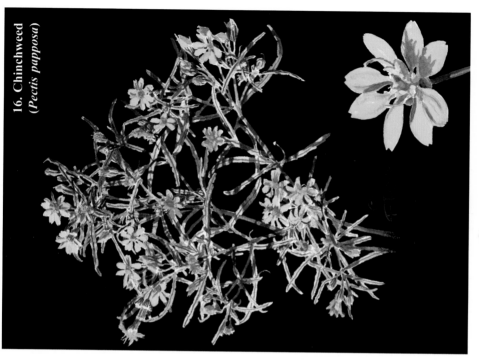

16. Chinchweed
(Pectis papposa)

CHINCHWEED

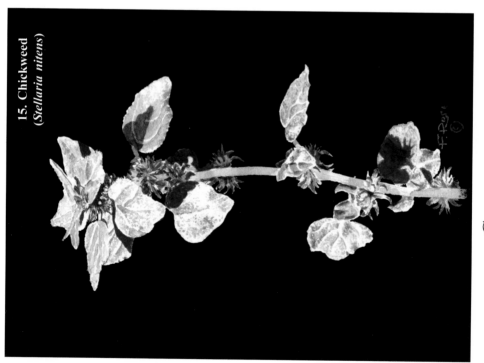

15. Chickweed
(Stellaria nitens)

CHICKWEED

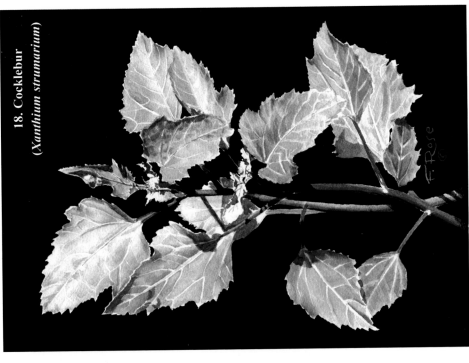

18. Cocklebur
(*Xanthium strumarium*)

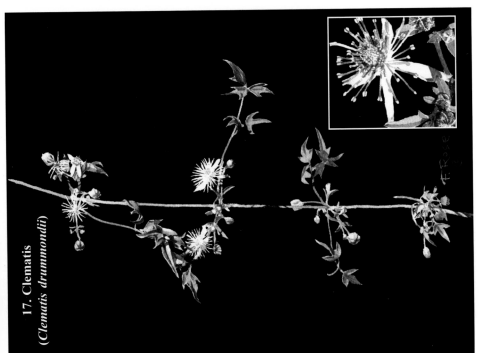

17. Clematis
(*Clematis drummondii*)

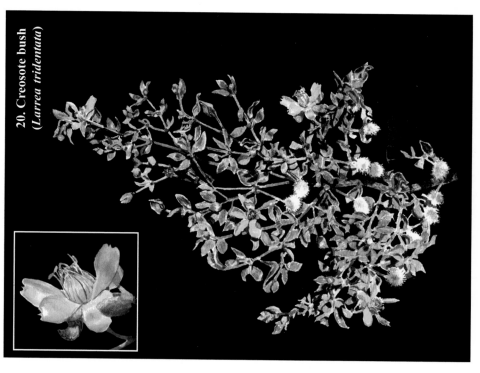

20. Creosote bush
(*Larrea tridentata*)

CREOSOTE BUSH

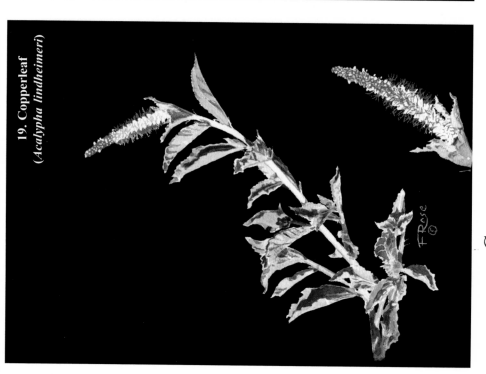

19. Copperleaf
(*Acalypha lindheimeri*)

COPPERLEAF

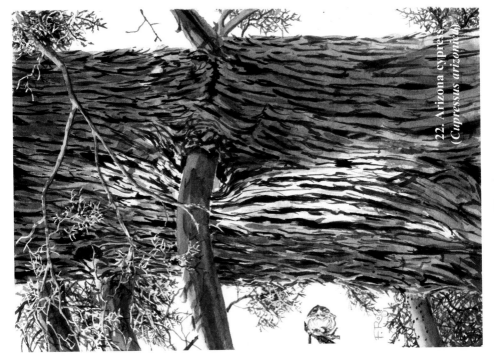

CYPRESS

22. Arizona cypress
(*Cupressus arizonica*)

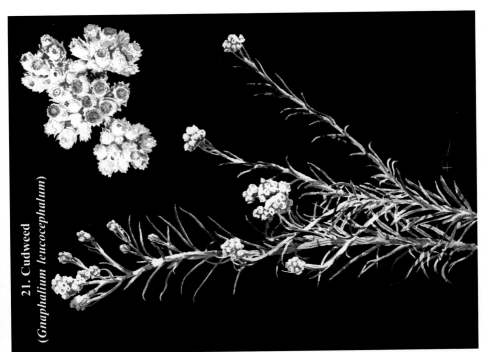

CUDWEED

21. Cudweed
(*Gnaphalium leucocephalum*)

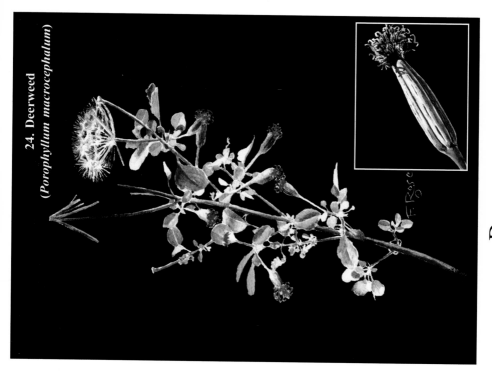

24. Deerweed
(Porophyllum macrocephalum)

DEERWEED

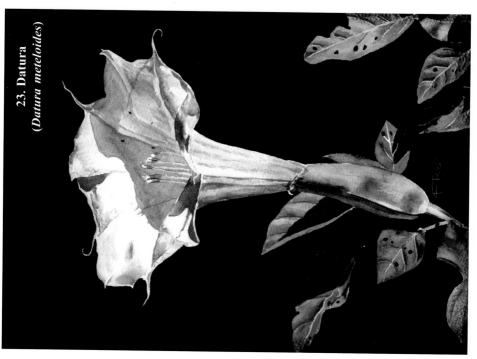

23. Datura
(Datura meteloides)

DATURA

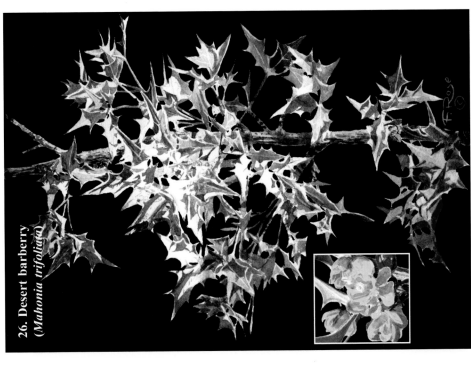

26. Desert barberry
(*Mahonia trifoliata*)

DESERT BARBERRY

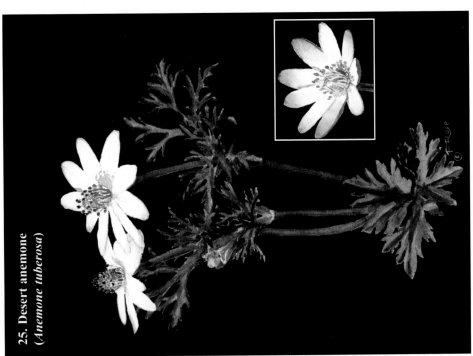

25. Desert anemone
(*Anemone tuberosa*)

DESERT ANEMONE

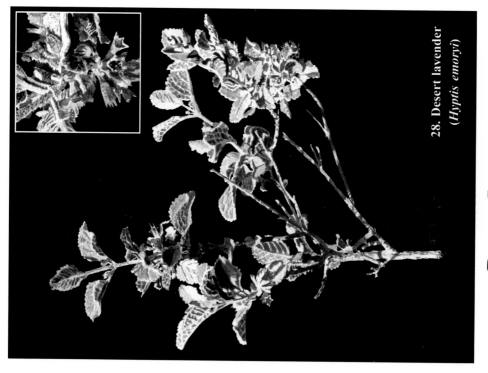

28. **Desert lavender**
(Hyptis emoryi)

DESERT LAVENDER

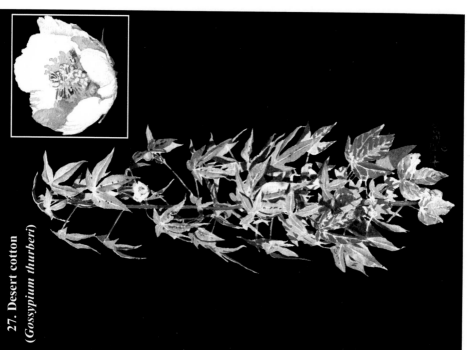

27. **Desert cotton**
(Gossypium thurberi)

DESERT COTTON

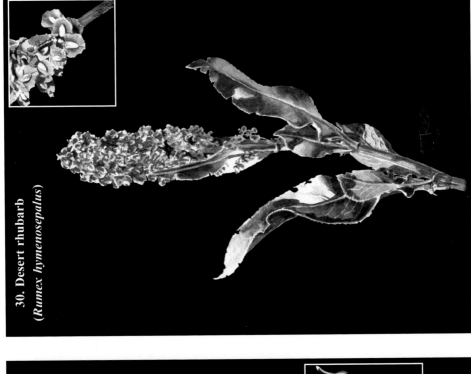

30. Desert rhubarb
(Rumex hymenosepalus)

DESERT RHUBARB

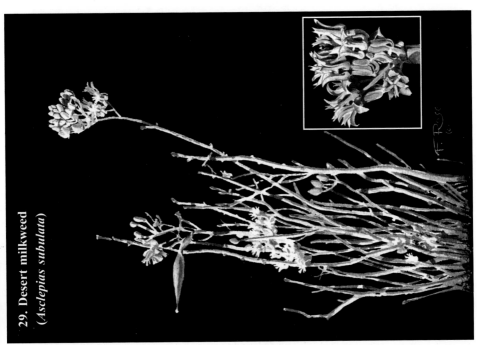

29. Desert milkweed
(Asclepias subulata)

DESERT MILKWEED

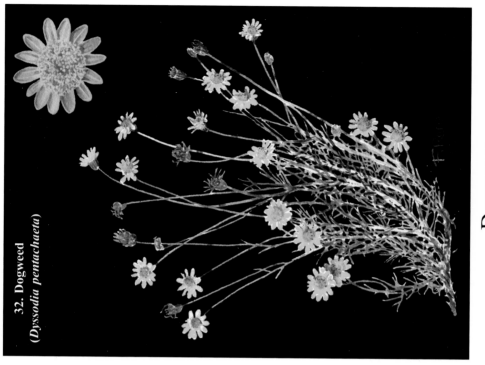

32. Dogweed
(*Dyssodia pentachaeta*)

DOGWEED

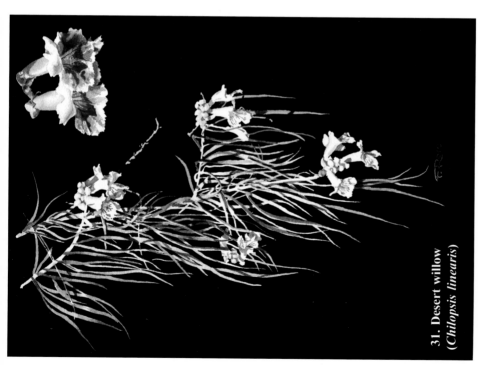

31. Desert willow
(*Chilopsis linearis*)

DESERT WILLOW

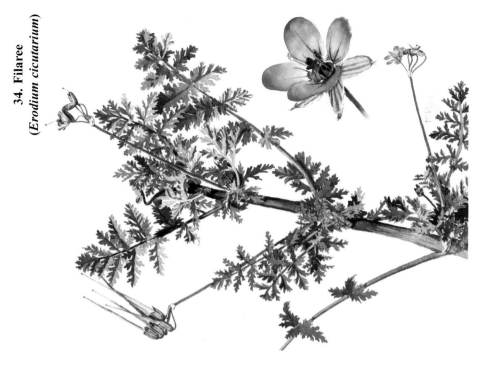

34. Filaree
(Erodium cicutarium)

FILAREE

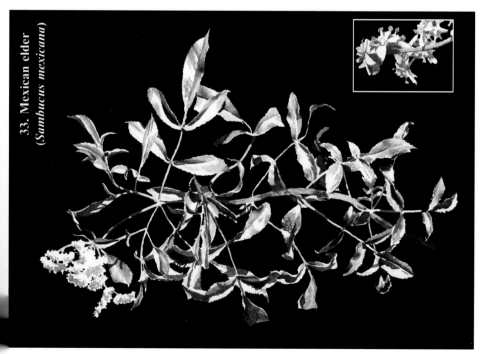

33. Mexican elder
(Sambucus mexicana)

ELDER

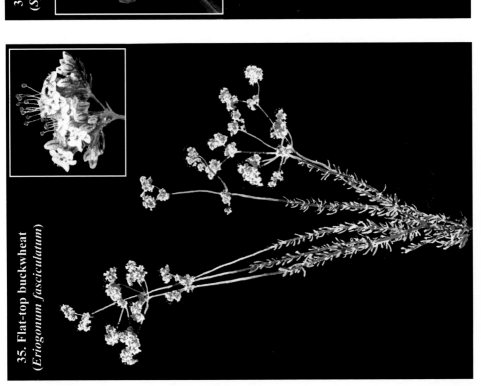

36. Globemallow
(*Sphaeralcea laxa*)

35. Flat-top buckwheat
(*Eriogonum fasciculatum*)

GLOBEMALLOW

FLAT-TOP BUCKWHEAT

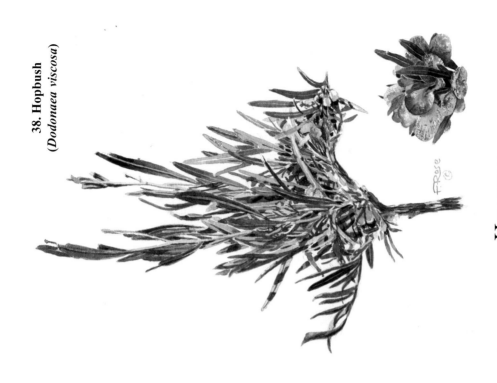

38. Hopbush
(Dodonaea viscosa)

HOPBUSH

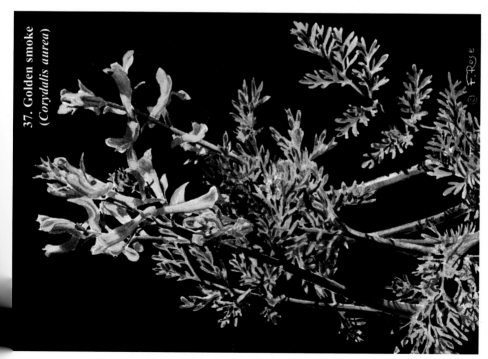

37. Golden smoke
(Corydalis aurea)

GOLDEN SMOKE

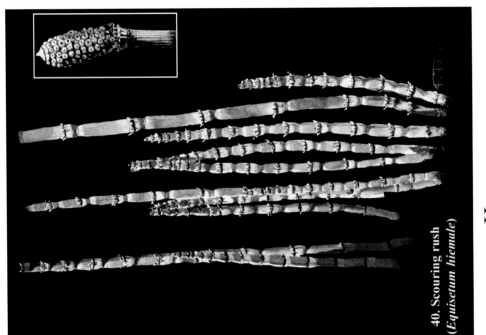

40. Scouring rush
(*Equisetum hiemale*)

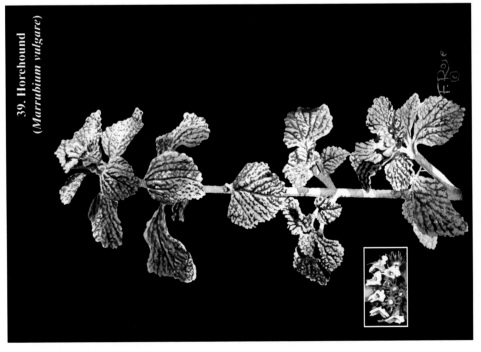

39. Horehound
(*Marrubium vulgare*)

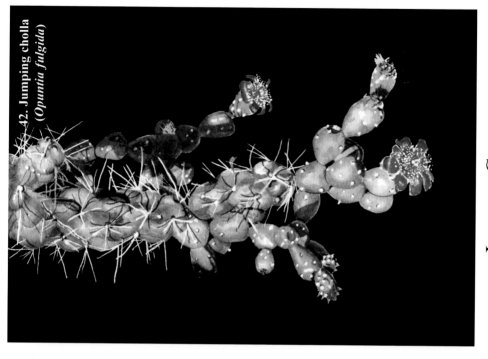

42. Jumping cholla
(*Opuntia fulgida*)

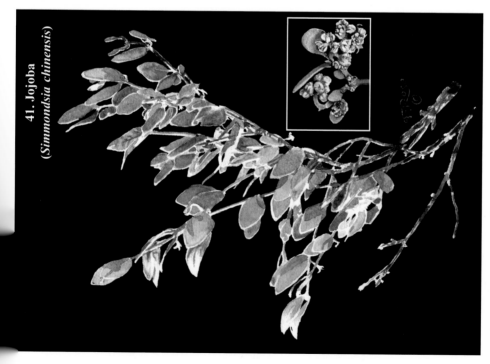

41. Jojoba
(*Simmondsia chinensis*)

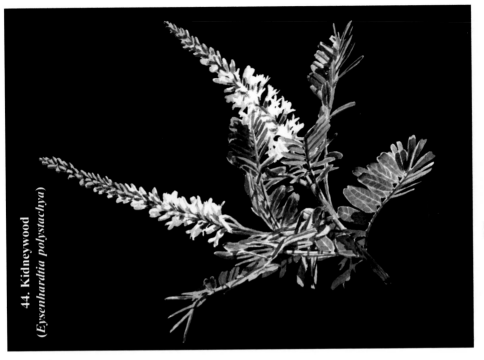

44. Kidneywood
(Eysenhardtia polystachya)

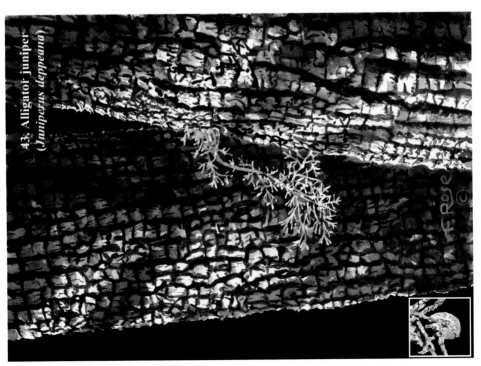

43. Alligator juniper
(Juniperus deppeana)

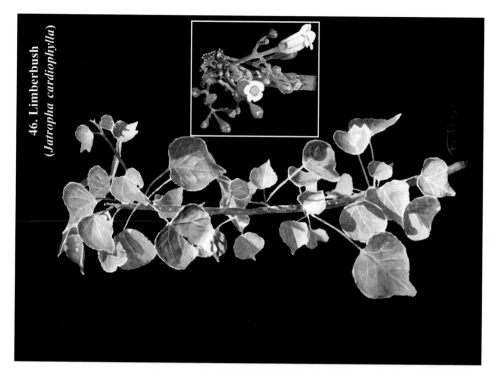

46. Limberbush
(*Jatropha cardiophylla*)

LIMBERBUSH

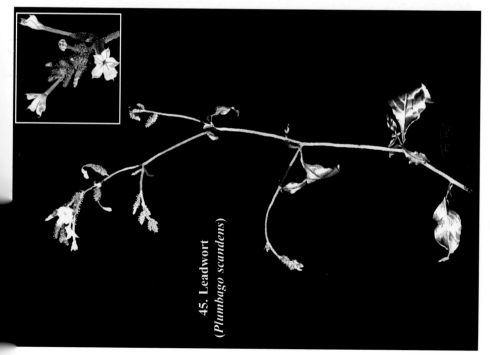

45. Leadwort
(*Plumbago scandens*)

LEADWORT

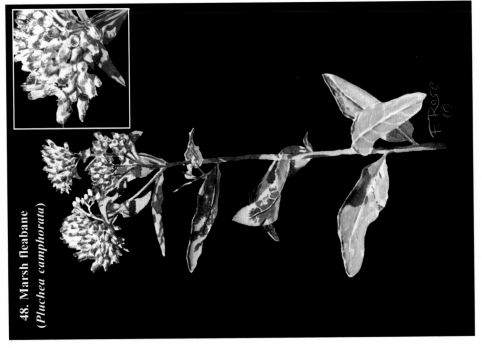

48. Marsh fleabane
(*Pluchea camphorata*)

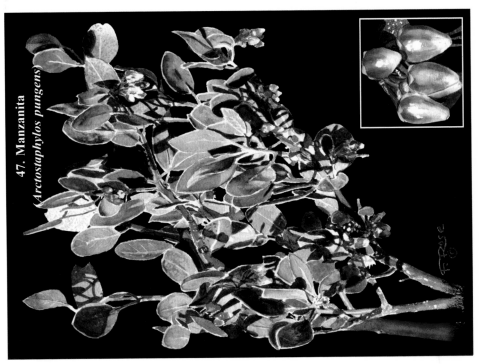

47. Manzanita
(*Arctostaphylos pungens*)

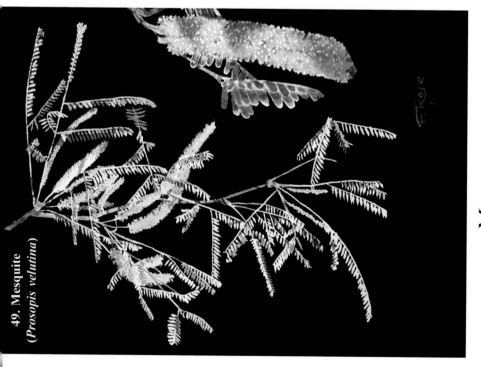

50. Mimosa
(Mimosa biuncifera)

49. Mesquite
(Prosopis velutina)

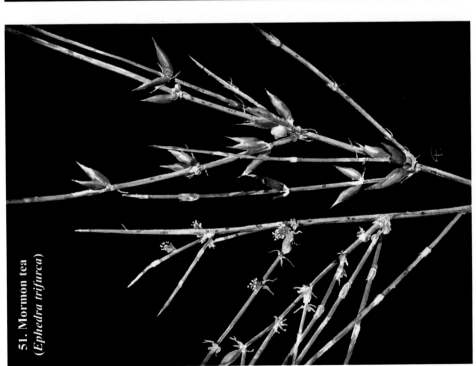

52. Mountain marigold
(*Tagetes lemmoni*)

51. Mormon tea
(*Ephedra trifurca*)

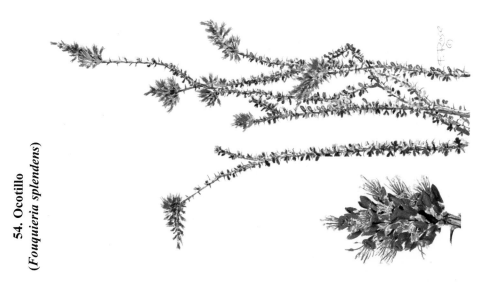

54. Ocotillo
(*Fouquieria splendens*)

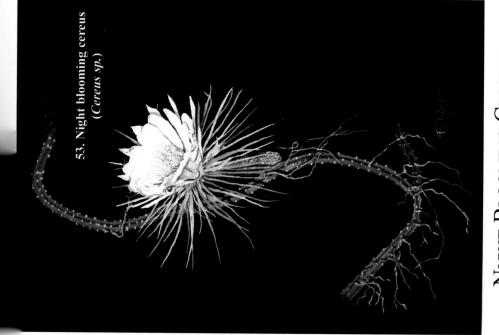

53. Night blooming cereus
(*Cereus sp.*)

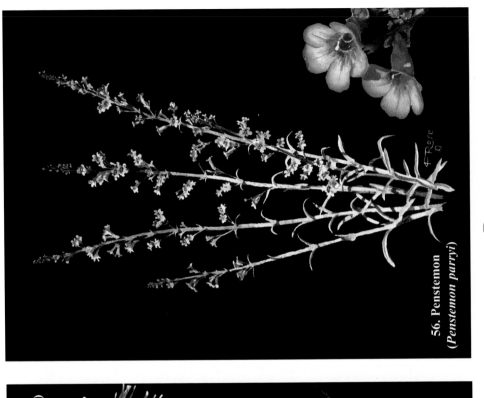

56. Penstemon
(*Penstemon parryi*)

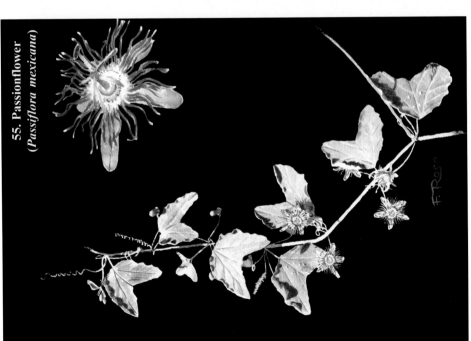

55. Passionflower
(*Passiflora mexicana*)

PASSIONFLOWER

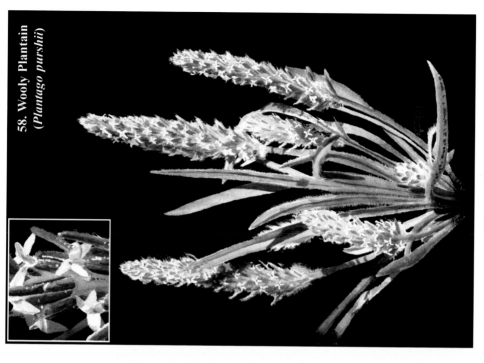

58. Wooly Plantain
(*Plantago purshii*)

PLANTAIN

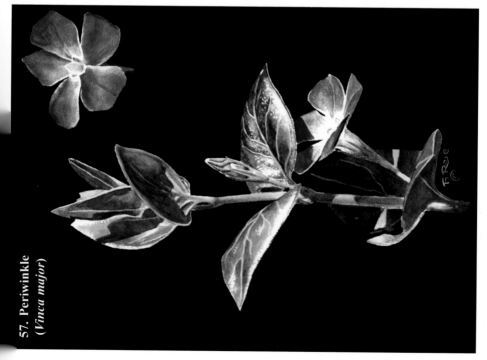

57. Periwinkle
(*Vinca major*)

PERIWINKLE

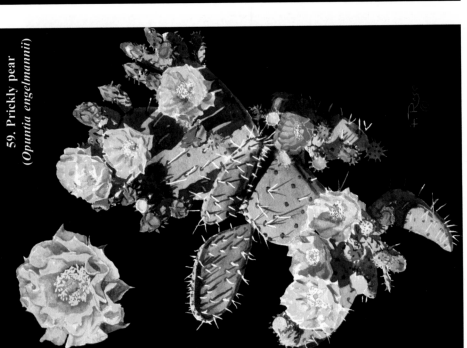

60. Prickly poppy
(*Argemone pleiacantha*)

59. Prickly pear
(*Opuntia engelmannii*)

PRICKLY POPPY

PRICKLY PEAR

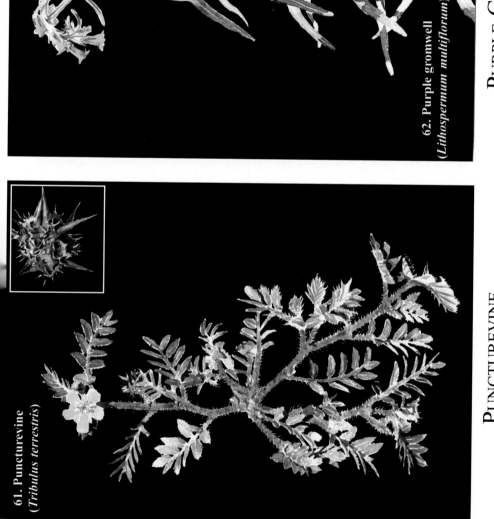

PURPLE GROMWELL

62. Purple gromwell
(*Lithospermum multiflorum*)

PUNCTUREVINE

61. Puncturevine
(*Tribulus terrestris*)

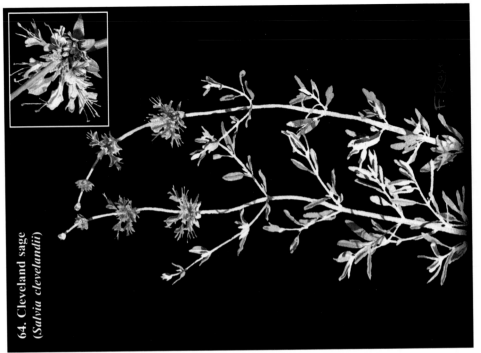

64. Cleveland sage
(*Salvia clevelandii*)

SAGE

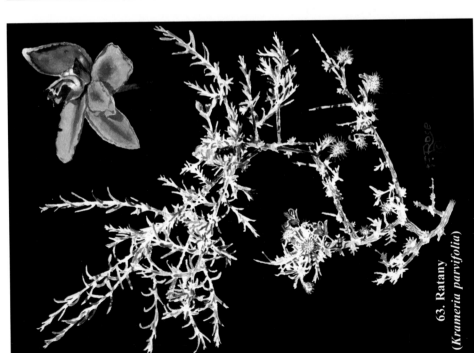

63. Ratany
(*Krameria parvifolia*)

RATANY

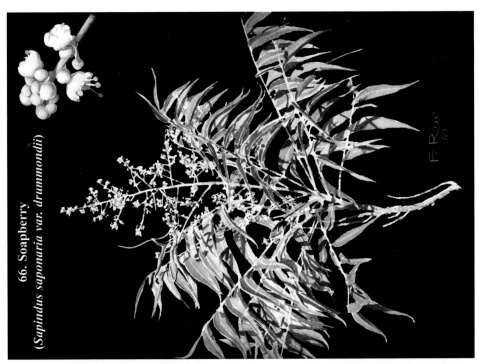

66. Soapberry
(Sapindus saponaria var. drummondii)

SOAPBERRY

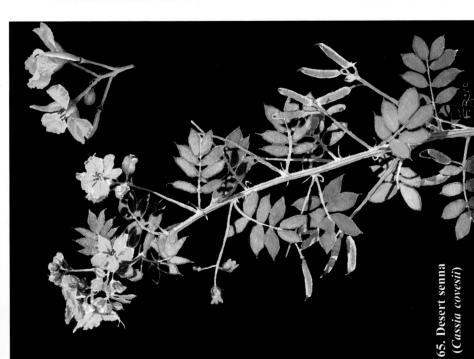

65. Desert senna
(Cassia covesii)

SENNA

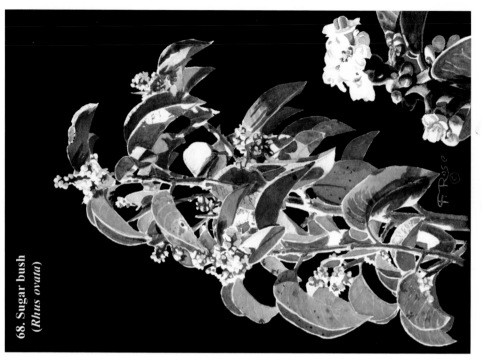

68. Sugar bush
(Rhus ovata)

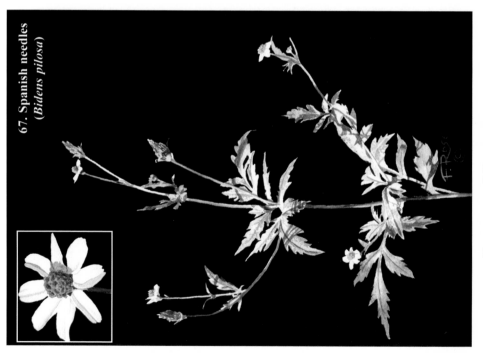

67. Spanish needles
(Bidens pilosa)

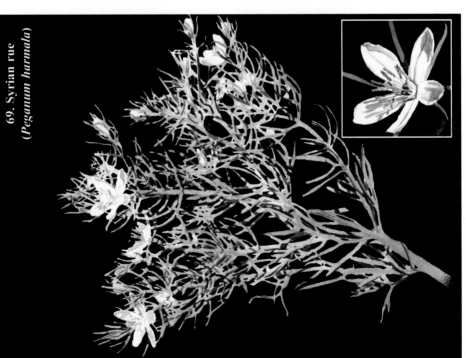

70. Desert tobacco
(*Nicotiana trigonophylla*)

69. Syrian rue
(*Peganum harmala*)

TOBACCO

SYRIAN RUE

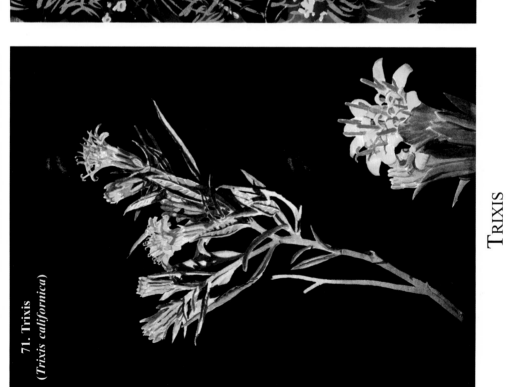

71. Trixis
(*Trixis californica*)

72. Trumpet flower
(*Tecoma stans var. angustata*)

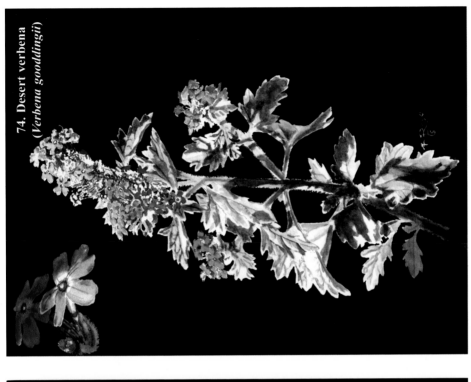

74. Desert verbena
(*Verbena gooddingii*)

VERBENA

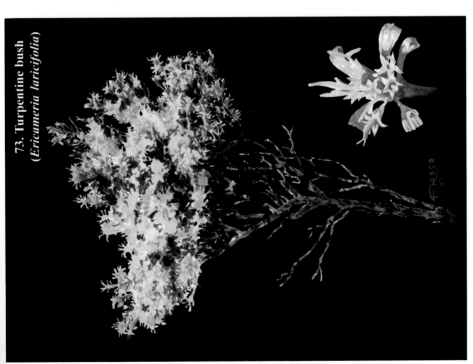

73. Turpentine bush
(*Ericameria laricifolia*)

TURPENTINE BUSH

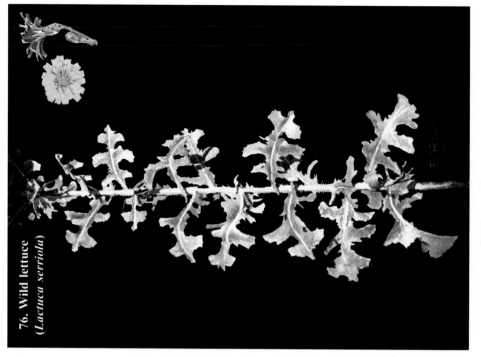

76. Wild lettuce
(*Lactuca serriola*)

WILD LETTUCE

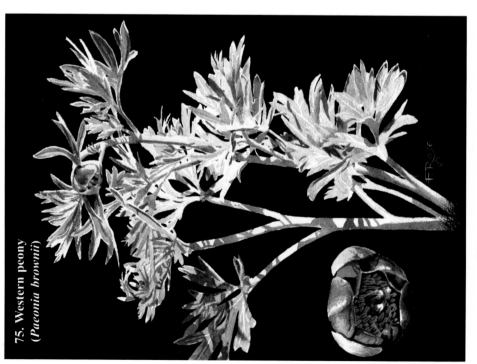

75. Western peony
(*Paeonia brownii*)

WESTERN PEONY

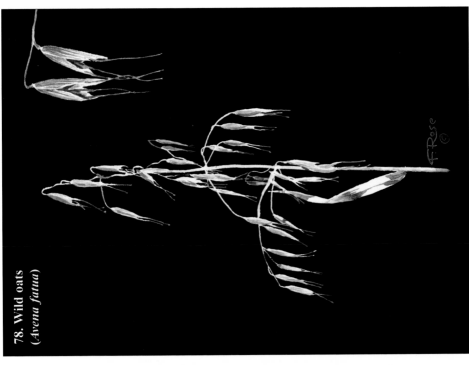

78. Wild oats
(*Avena fatua*)

WILD OATS

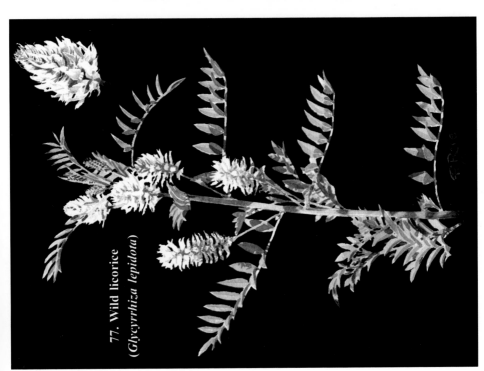

77. Wild licorice
(*Glycyrrhiza lepidota*)

WILD LICORICE

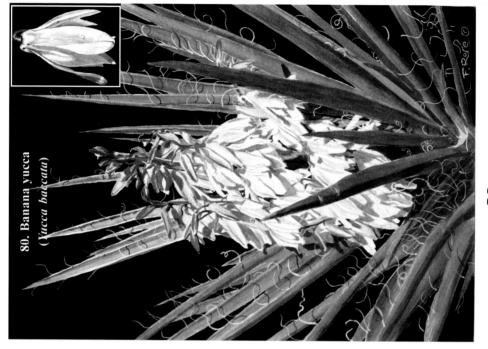

80. Banana yucca
(*Yucca baccata*)

YUCCA

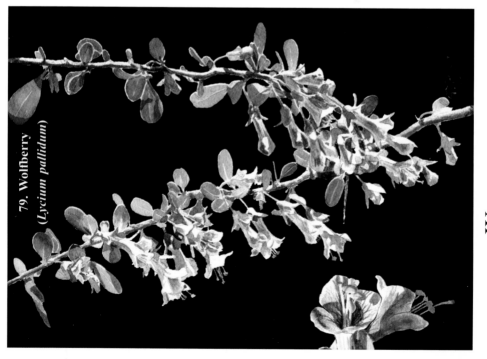

79. Wolfberry
(*Lycium pallidum*)

WOLFBERRY

ACACIA

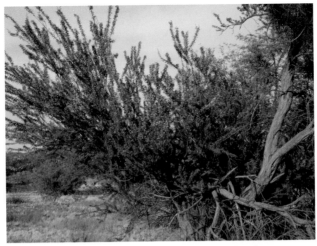

1. Catclaw acacia (*Acacia greggii*)

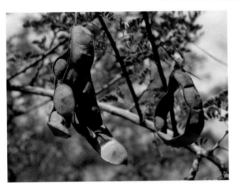

2. Catclaw acacia (*Acacia greggii*), seedpods

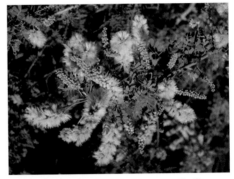

3. Catclaw acacia (*Acacia greggii*), flowers

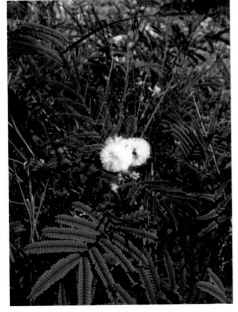

4. Fern acacia (*Acacia angustissima*)

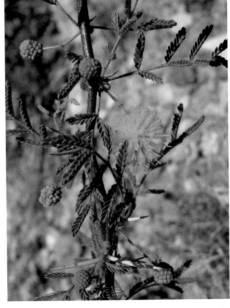

5. White thorn acacia (*Acacia constricta*)

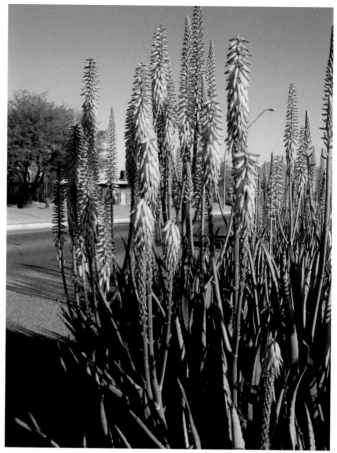

6. Aloe (*Aloe vera*)

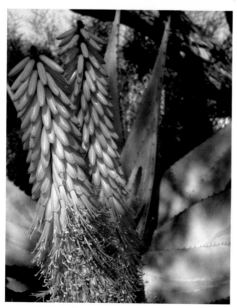

8. Cape aloe (*Aloe ferox*)

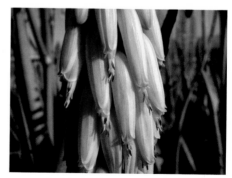

7. Aloe (*Aloe vera*), flowers

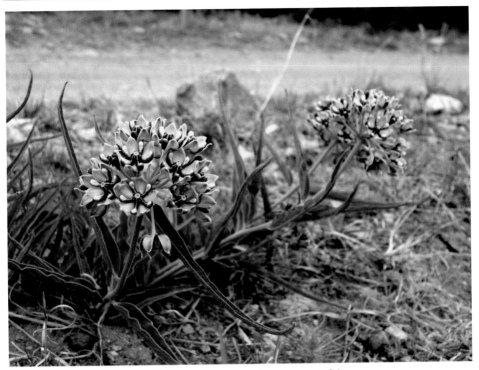

9. Antelope horns (*Asclepias asperula*)

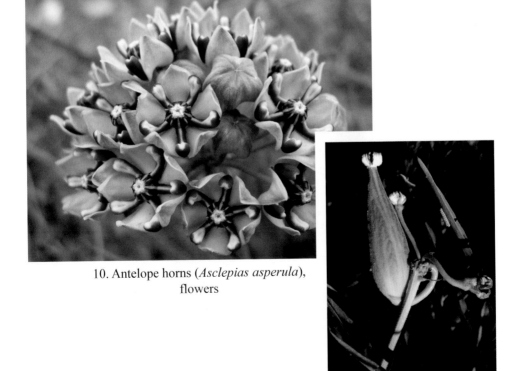

10. Antelope horns (*Asclepias asperula*),
flowers

11. Antelope horns (*Asclepias asperula*), seedpod

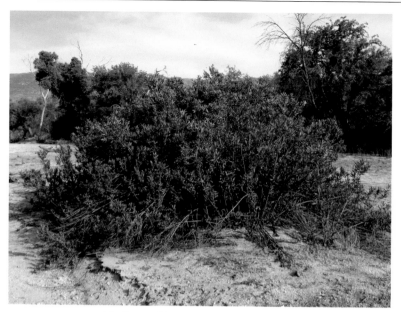

12. Seepwillow (*Baccharis glutinosa)*

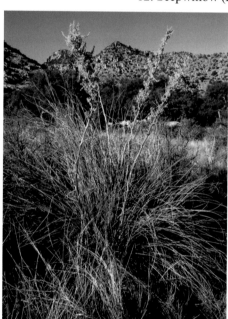

15. Beargrass (*Nolina microcarpa*)

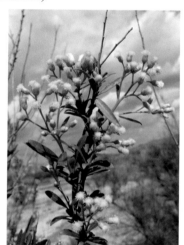

13. Seepwillow (*Baccharis glutinosa)*
female flowers

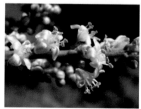

16. Beargrass (*Nolina microcarpa*),
flowers

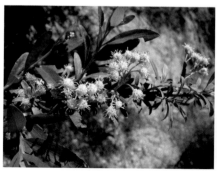

14. Seepwillow (*Baccharis glutinosa*),
male flowers

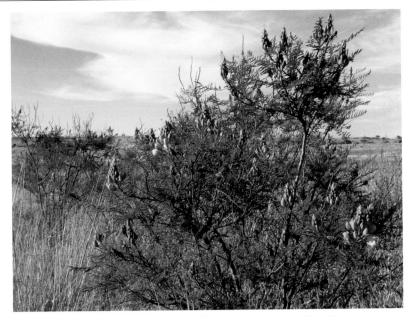

17. Yellow bird of paradise (*Caesalpinia gelliesii*)

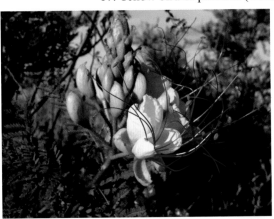

18. Yellow bird of paradise
(*Caesalpinia gelliesii*)

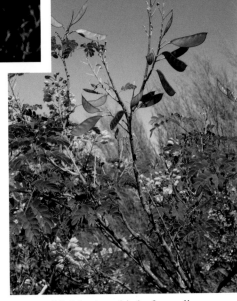

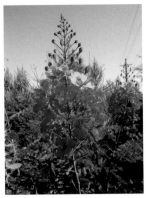

19. Red bird of paradise
(*Caesalpinia pulcherrima*)

20. Mexican bird of paradise
(*Caesalpinia mexicana*)

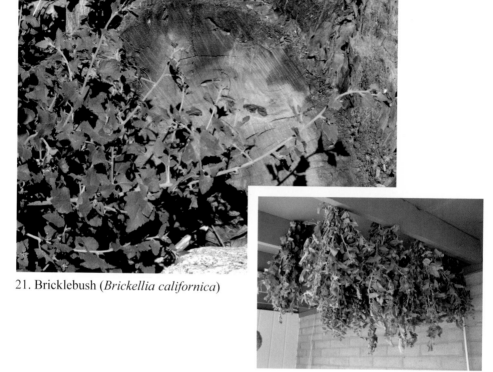

21. Bricklebush (*Brickellia californica*)

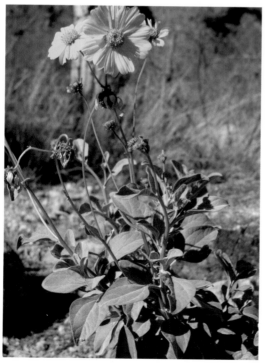

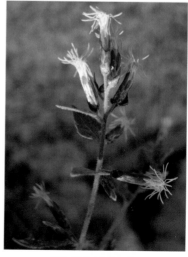

22. Bricklebush (*Brickellia californica*), hanging herb

23. Bricklebush
(*Brickellia californica*), flowers

24. Brittlebush (*Encelia farinosa*)

BURROBRUSH

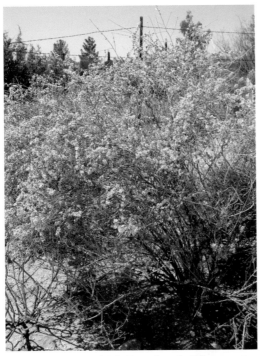

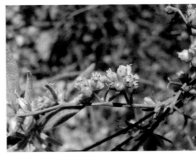

27. Burrobrush (*Hymenoclea salsola*), male flowers

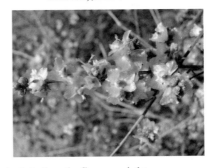

25. and 26. Burrobrush (*Hymenoclea salsola*), female flowers right

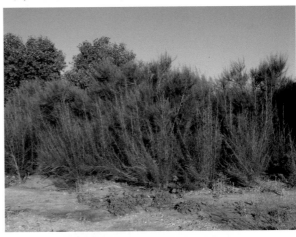

28. Burrobrush (*Hymenoclea monogyra*)

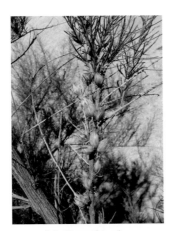

29. Burrobrush
(*Hymenoclea monogyra*),
female flowers

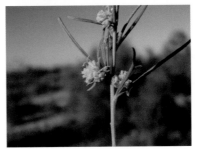

30. Burrobrush
(*Hymenoclea monogyra*), male flowers

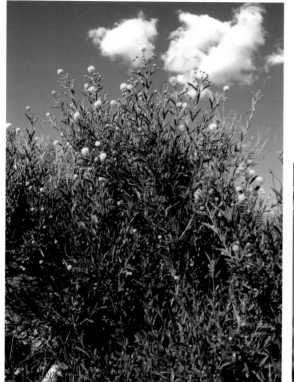

31. Buttonbush (*Cephalanthus occidentalis*)

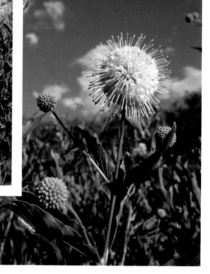

32. Buttonbush (*Cephalanthus occidentalis*), flowers

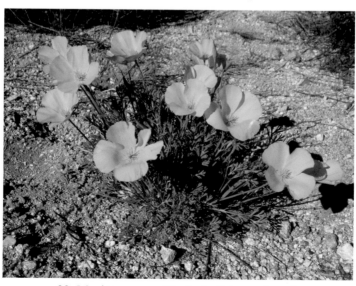

33. Mexican poppy (*Eschscholtzia mexicana*)

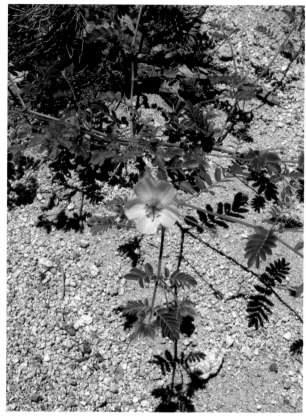

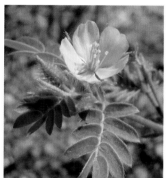

34. Caltrop
(*Kallstroemia parviflora*)

35. Caltrop (*Kallstroemia grandiflora*)

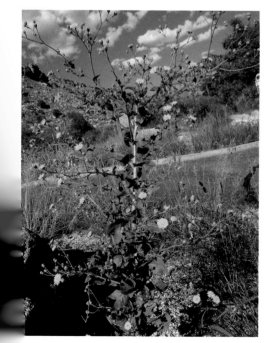

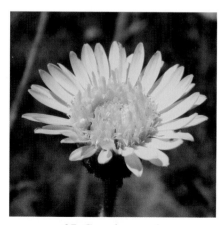

37. Camphorweed
(*Heterotheca subaxillaris*), flowers

36. Camphorweed (*Heterotheca subaxillaris*)

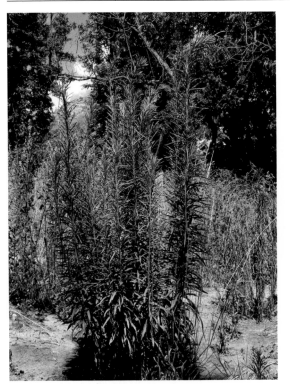

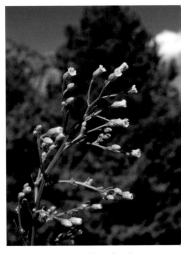

39. Canadian fleabane (*Conyza canadensis*), flowers

38. Canadian fleabane (*Conyza canadensis*)

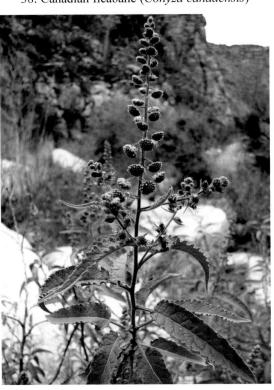

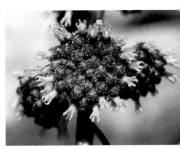

41. Canyon bursage (*Ambrosia ambrosioides*), male flowers

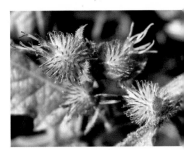

42. Canyon bursage (*Ambrosia ambrosioides*), female flowers

40. Canyon bursage (*Ambrosia ambrosioides*)

CANYON WALNUT

CHASTE TREE

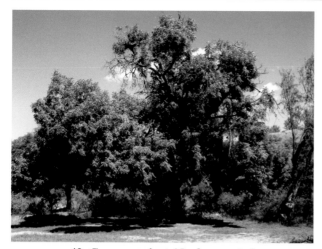

43. Canyon walnut (*Juglans major*)

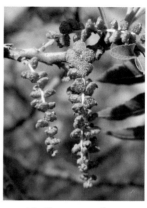

44. Canyon walnut (*Juglans major*), male flowers

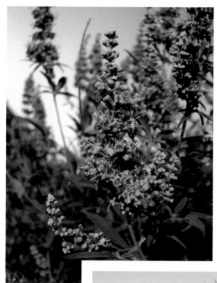

Chaste tree (*Vitex agnus-castus*), flowers

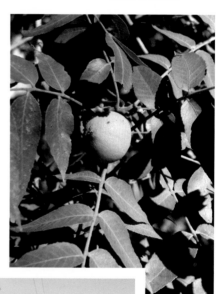

45. Canyon walnut (*Juglans major*), fruit

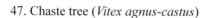

47. Chaste tree (*Vitex agnus-castus*)

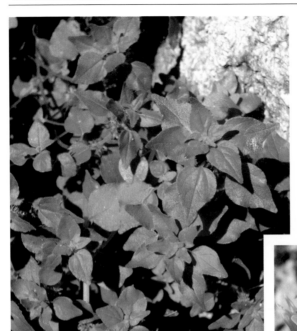

48. Chickweed (*Stellaria nitens*)

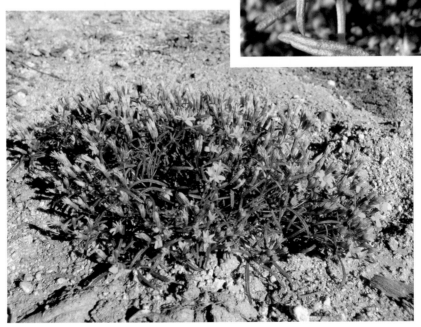

49. and 50. Chinchweed (*Pectis papposa*), flowers above right

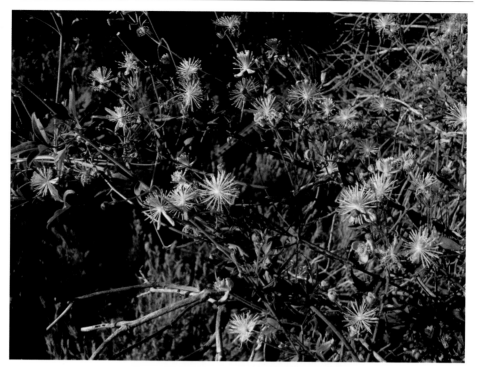

51. Texas virgin's bower (*Clematis drummondii*)

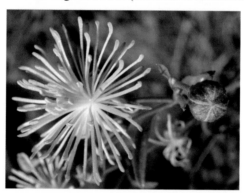

52. Texas virgin's bower (*Clematis drummondii*), flower

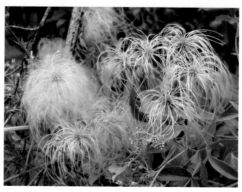

53. Texas virgin's bower (*Clematis drummondii*), mature seeds

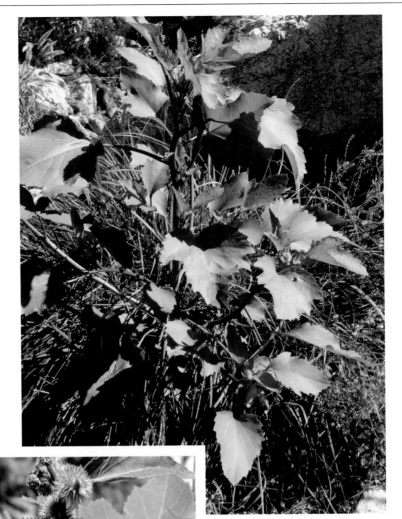

54. Cocklebur
(*Xanthium strumarium*)

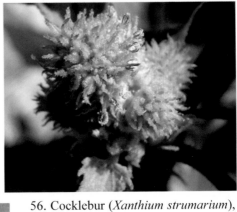

56. Cocklebur (*Xanthium strumarium*),
male flowers

55. Cocklebur (*Xanthium strumarium*),
seedpods

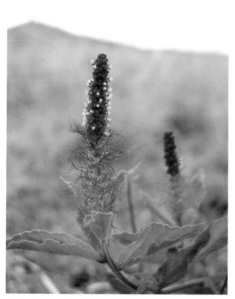

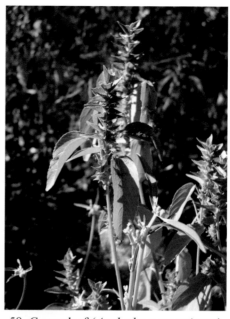

57. Copperleaf (*Acalypha lindheimeri*)

58. Copperleaf (*Acalypha neomexicana*)

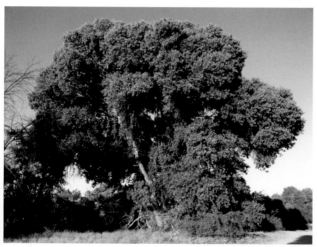

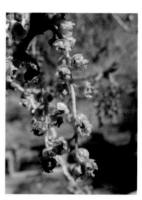

59. Cottonwood (*Populus fremontii*)

60. Cottonwood
(*Populus fremontii*),
male flowers

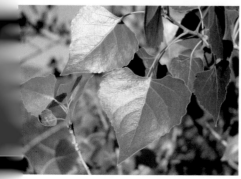

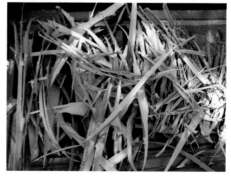

61. Cottonwood (*Populus fremontii*),
leaves

62. Cottonwood (*Populus fremontii*),
collected bark

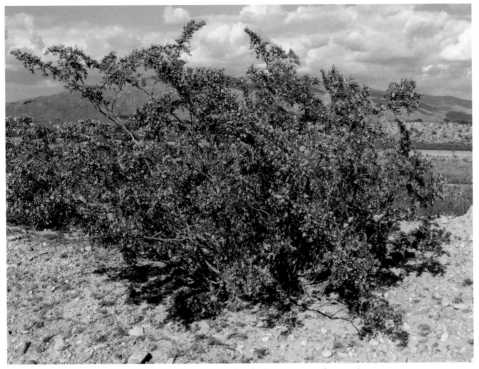

63. Creosote bush (*Larrea tridentata*)

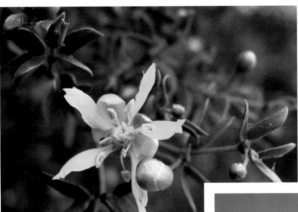

64. Creosote bush (*Larrea tridentata*),
flower

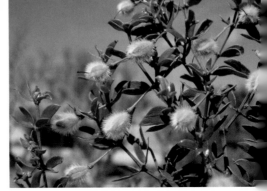

65. Creosote bush (*Larrea tridentata*), seeds

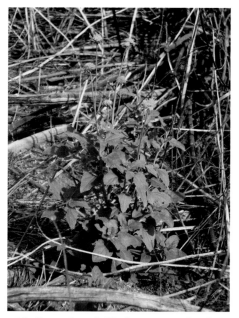

66. Crownbeard (*Verbesina encelioides*)

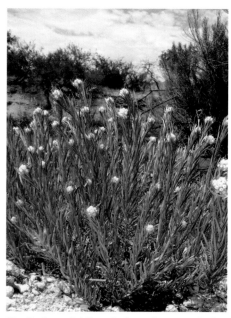

68. Cudweed (*Gnaphalium leucocephalum*)

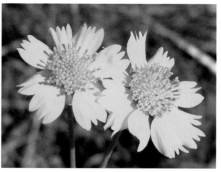

67. Crownbeard (*Verbesina encelioides*), flowers

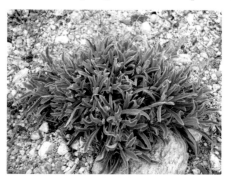

69. Cudweed (*Gnaphalium leucocephalum*)

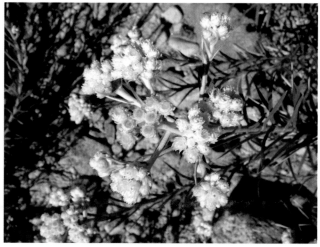

70. Cudweed (*Gnaphalium leucocephalum*), flowers

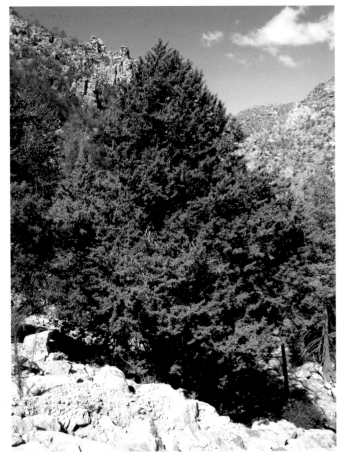

71. Arizona cypress (*Cupressus arizonica*)

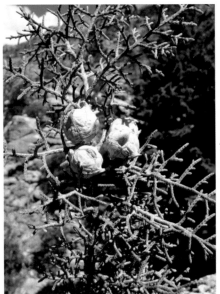

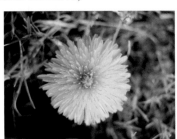

73. Dandelion (*Taraxacum officinale*), flo

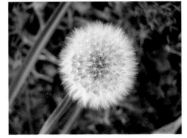

72. Arizona cypress
(*Cupressus arizonica*), cones

74. Dandelion (*Taraxacum officinale*), se

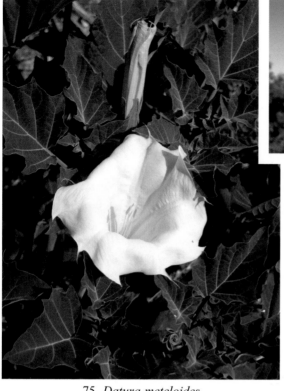

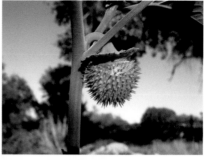

76. *Datura meteloides*, seedpod

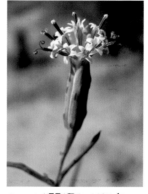

75. *Datura meteloides*

77. Deerweed
(*Porophyllum gracile*), flowers

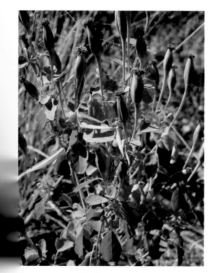

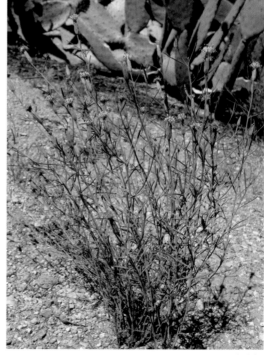

79. Deerweed
(*Porophyllum macrocephalum*)

78. Deerweed (*Porophyllum gracile*)

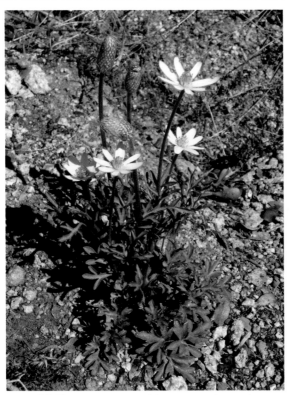

80. Desert anemone (*Anemone tuberosa*)

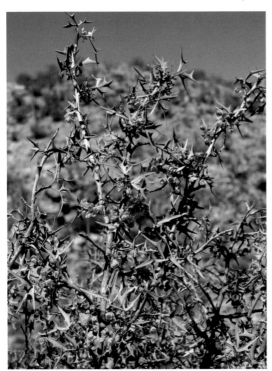

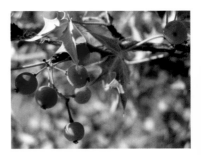

82. Desert barberry
(*Mahonia trifoliata*), fruit

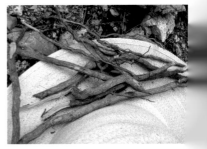

83. Desert barberry
(*Mahonia trifoliata*),
collected roots

81. Desert barberry (*Mahonia trifoliata*)

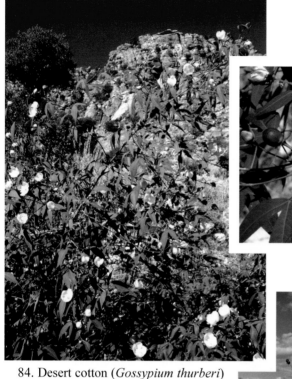

85. Desert cotton
(*Gossypium thurberi*), flowers

84. Desert cotton (*Gossypium thurberi*)

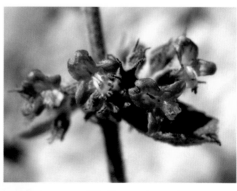

86. Desert cotton
(*Gossypium thurberi*), seedpods

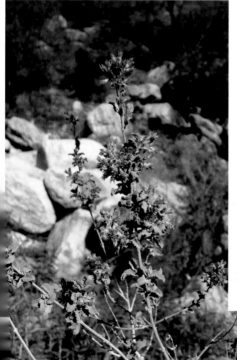

88. Desert lavender
(*Hyptis emoryi*), flowers

87. Desert lavender (*Hyptis emoryi*)

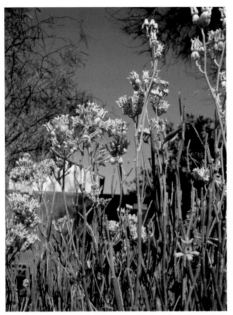

89. Desert milkweed (*Asclepias subulata*)

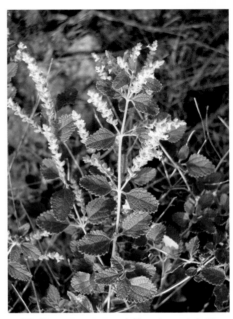

91. Desert oregano (*Aloysia wrightii*)

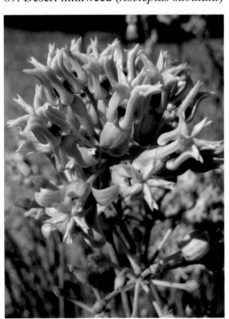

90. Desert milkweed
(*Asclepias subulata*), flowers

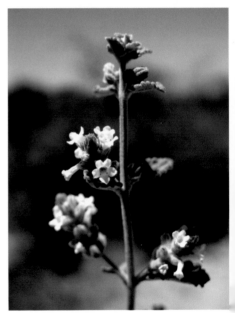

92. Desert oregano
(*Aloysia wrightii*), flowers

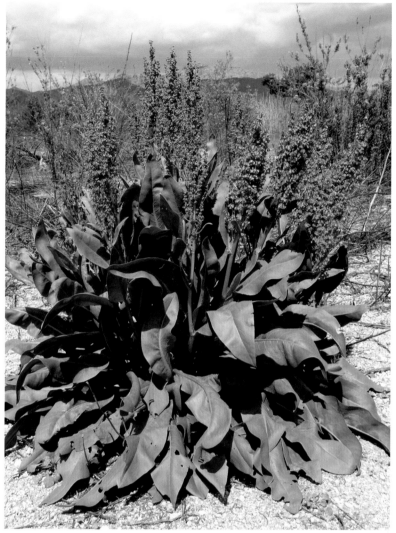

93. Desert rhubarb (*Rumex hymenosepalus*)

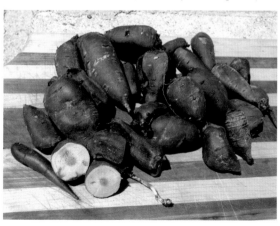

94. Desert rhubarb (*Rumex hymenosepalus*),
collected roots

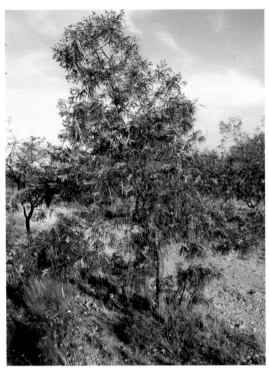

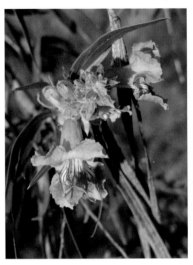

96. Desert willow
(*Chilopsis linearis*), flowers

95. Desert willow (*Chilopsis linearis*)

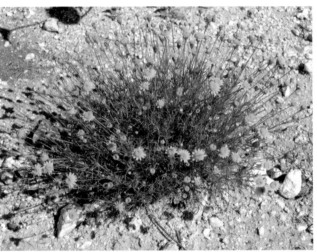

97. Dogweed (*Dyssodia pentachaeta*)

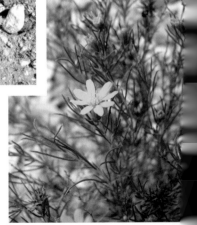

98. Dogweed (*Dyssodia acerose*

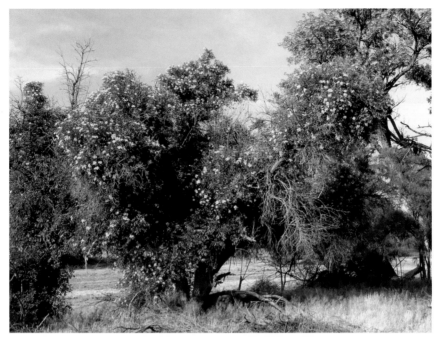

99. Mexican elder (*Sambucus mexicana*)

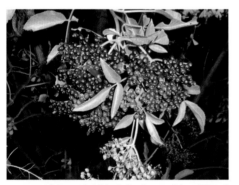
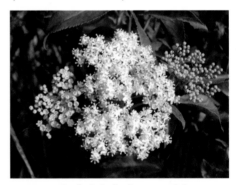

100. and 101. Mexican elder (*Sambucus mexicana*), fruit left, flowers right

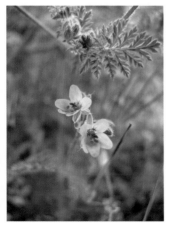
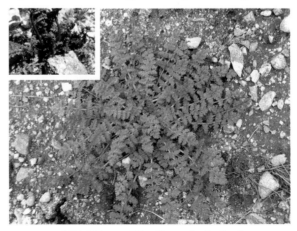

102. Filaree
(*Erodium cicutarium*), flowers

103. Filaree (*Erodium cicutarium*)
104. Filaree with *Synchytrium papillatum* (insert)

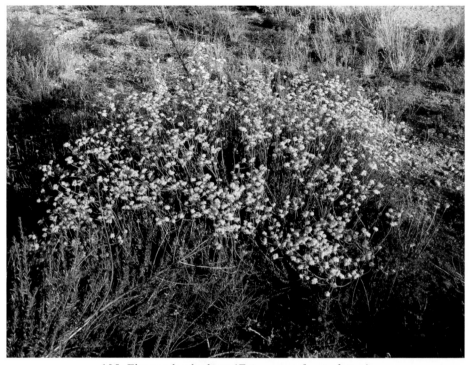

105. Flat-top buckwheat (*Eriogonum fasciculatum*)

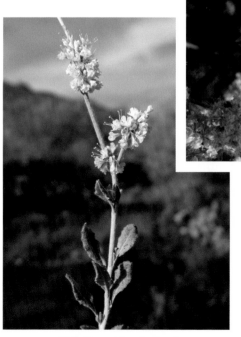

106. Flat-top buckwheat
(*Eriogonum fasciculatum*), flowers

107. Desert buckwheat
(*Eriogonum wrightii*)

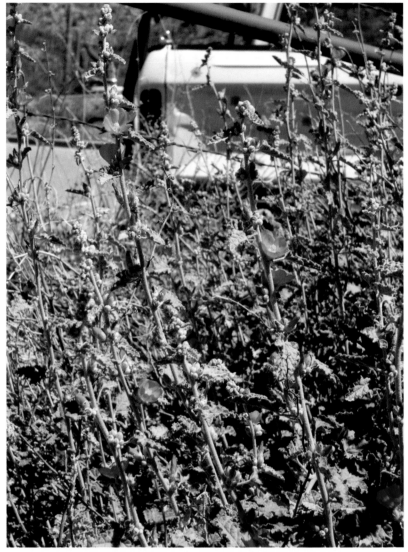

108. Globemallow (*Sphaeralcea spp.*)

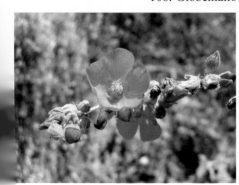 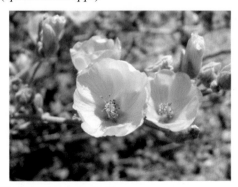

109. and 110. Globemallow (*Sphaeralcea spp.*), flowers

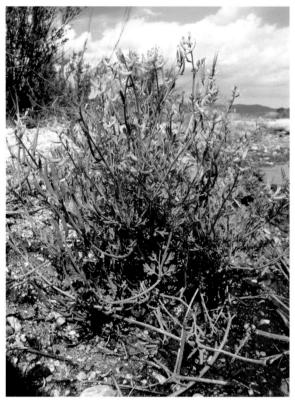

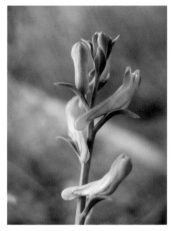

112. Golden smoke
(*Corydalis aurea*), flowers

111. Golden smoke (*Corydalis aurea*)

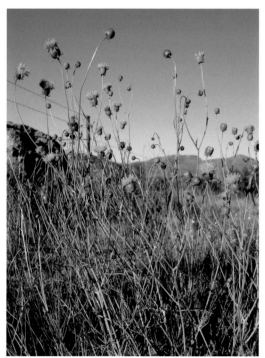

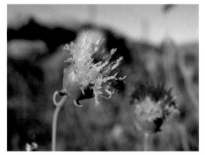

114. Greenthread
(*Thelesperma megapotamicum*),
flowers

113. Greenthread
(*Thelesperma megapotamicum*)

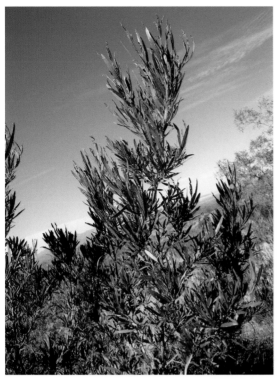

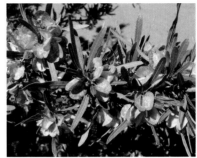

116. Hopbush
(*Dodonaea viscosa*), fruit

115. Hopbush (*Dodonaea viscosa*)

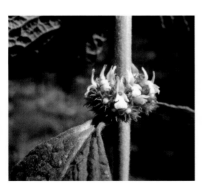

117. Horehound
(*Marrubium vulgare*), flowers

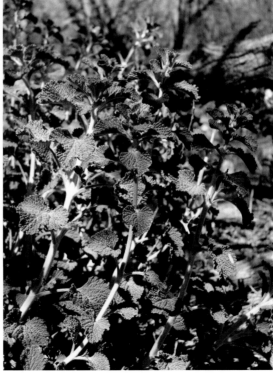

118. Horehound (*Marrubium vulgare*)

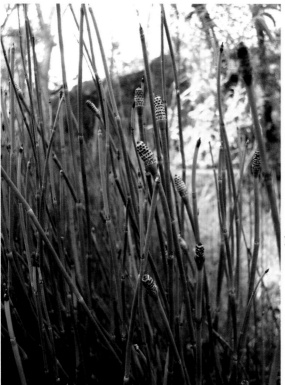

119. Scouring rush (*Equisetum hiemale*)

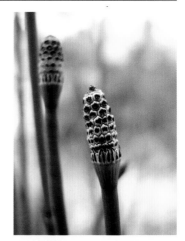

120. Scouring rush (*Equisetum hiema.*

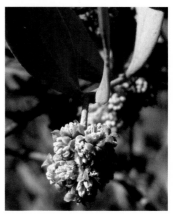

122. Jojoba (*Simmondsia chinensis*
male flowers

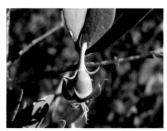

123. Jojoba (*Simmondsia chinensis*),
female flower

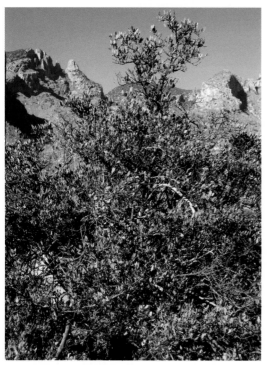

121. Jojoba (*Simmondsia chinensis*)

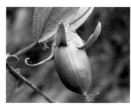

124. Jojoba (*Simmondsia chinensis*),
fruit

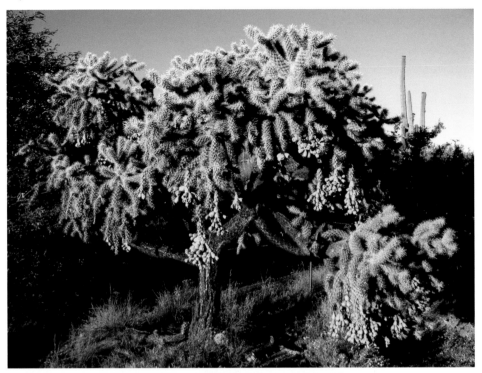

125. Jumping cholla (*Opuntia fulgida*)

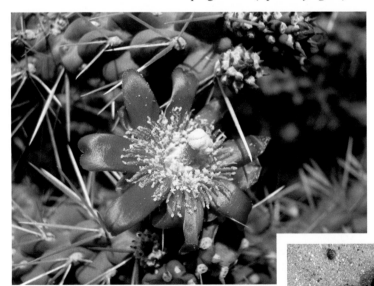

126. Jumping cholla (*Opuntia fulgida*), flower

127. Jumping cholla
(*Opuntia fulgida*), hardened sap

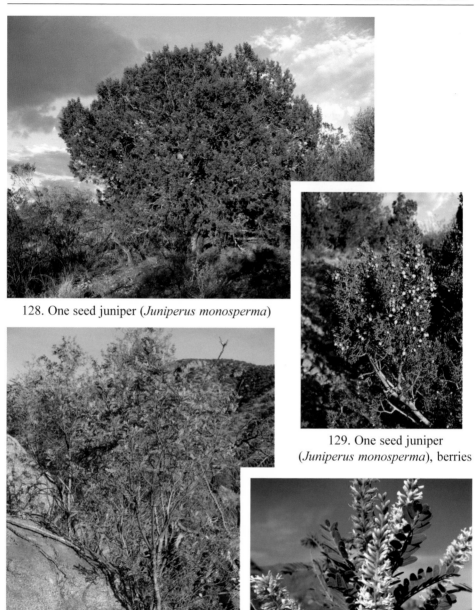

128. One seed juniper (*Juniperus monosperma*)

129. One seed juniper
(*Juniperus monosperma*), berries

130. Kidneywood
(*Eysenhardtia polystachya*)

131. Kidneywood
(*Eysenhardtia polystachya*), flowers

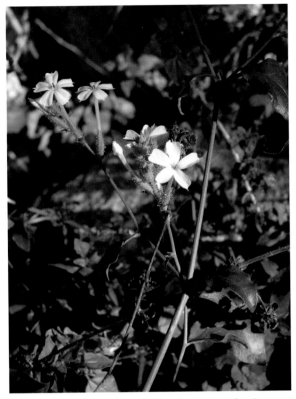

132. Leadwort (*Plumbago scandens*)

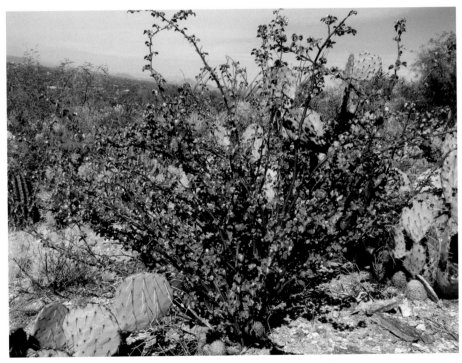

133. Limberbush (*Jatropha cardiophylla*)

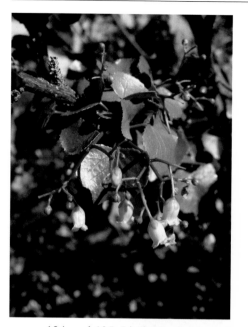 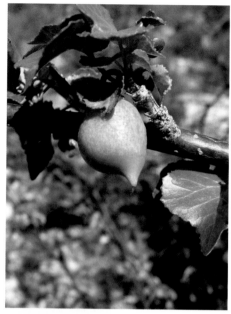

134. and 135. Limberbush (*Jatropha cardiophylla*), flowers left, fruit right

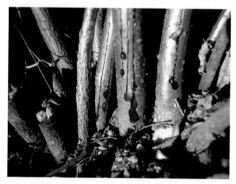

136. Limberbush (*Jatropha cardiophylla*), sap

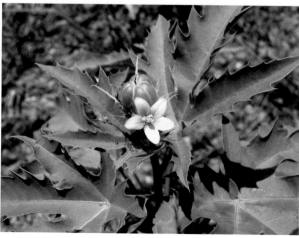

137. Nettlespruge (*Jatropha macrorhiza*)

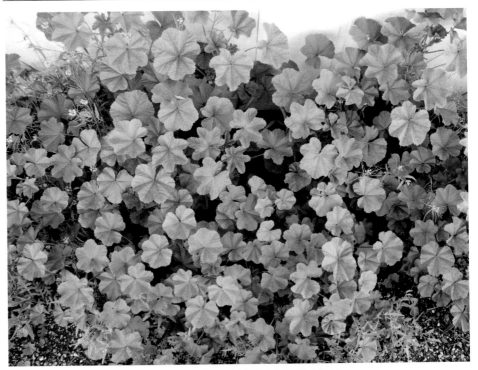

138. Mallow (*Malva parviflora*)

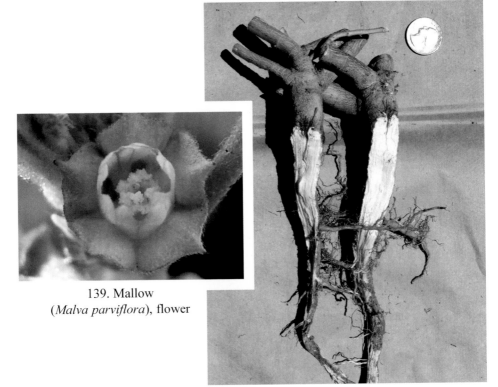

139. Mallow
(*Malva parviflora*), flower

140. Mallow (*Malva parviflora*), roots

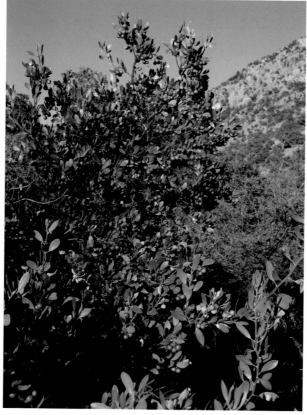

141. Manzanita (*Arctostaphylos pungens*)

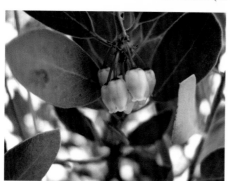
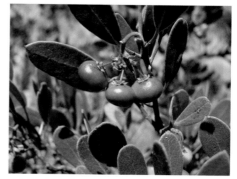

142. and 143. Manzanita (*Arctostaphylos pungens*), flowers left, fruits right

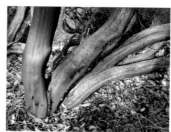

144. Manzanita (*Arctostaphylos pungens*), bark

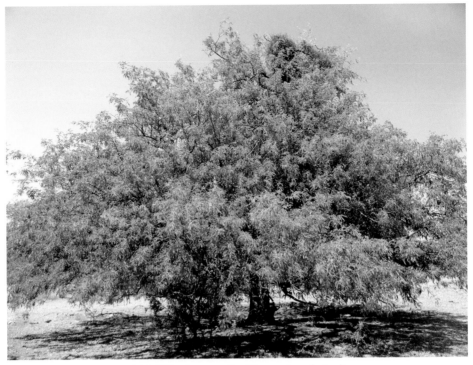

145. Velvet mesquite (*Prosopis velutina*)

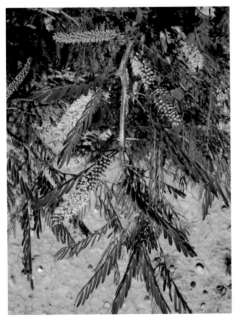

147. Western honey mesquite
(*Prosopis glandulosa var. torreyana*)

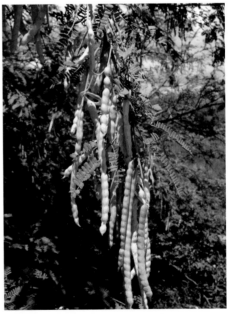

146. Velvet mesquite
(*Prosopis velutina*), pods

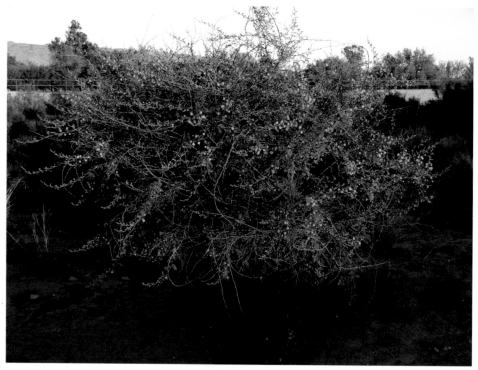

148. Wait-a-minute bush (*Mimosa biuncifera*)

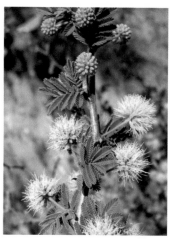

149. Wait-a-minute bush
(*Mimosa biuncifera*), flowers

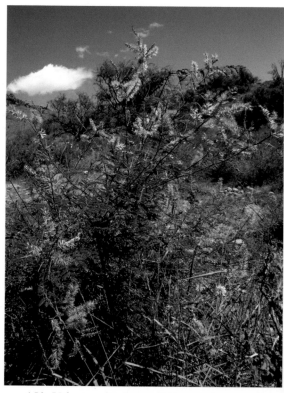

150. Velvet pod mimosa (*Mimosa dysocarpa*)

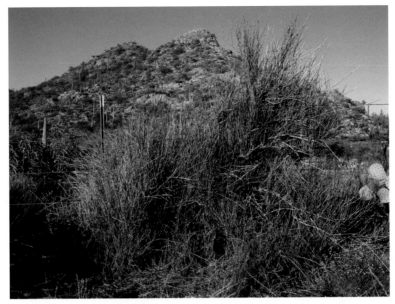

151. Mormon tea (*Ephedra trifurca*)

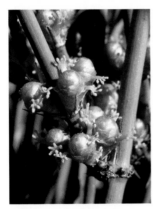
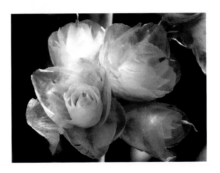

152. and 153. Mormon tea (*Ephedra trifurca*), male flowers left, female flowers right

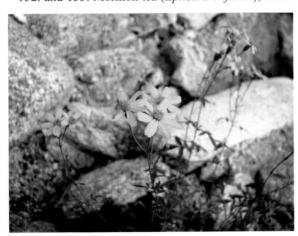
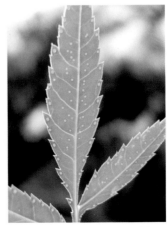

154. Mountain marigold (*Tagetes lemmoni*)

155. Mountain marigold (*Tagetes lemmoni*), leaf glands

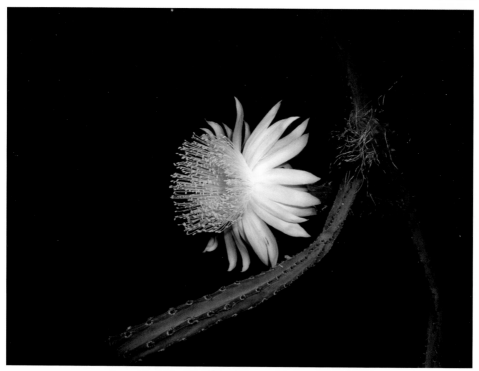

156. Night blooming cereus (*Peniocereus greggii*)

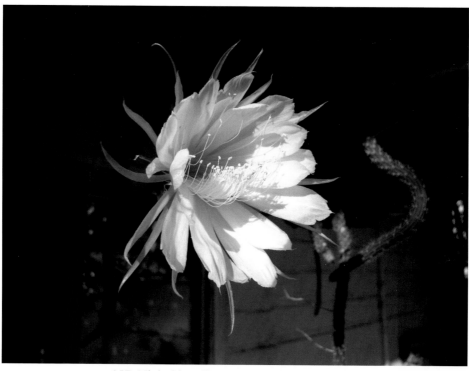

157. Night blooming cereus (*Selenicereus sp.*)

OCOTILLO

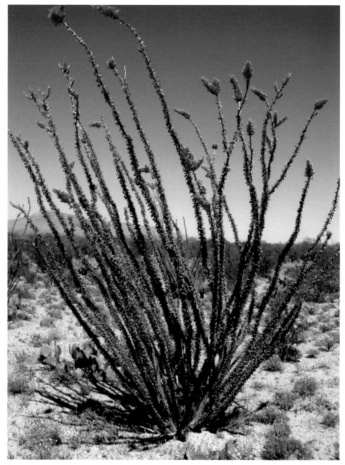

158. Ocotillo (*Fouquieria splendens*)

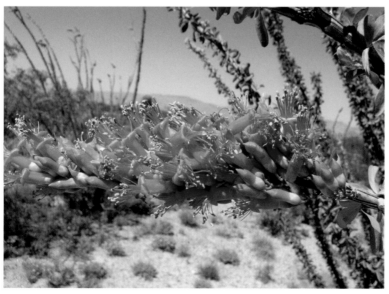

159. Ocotillo (*Fouquieria splendens*), flowers

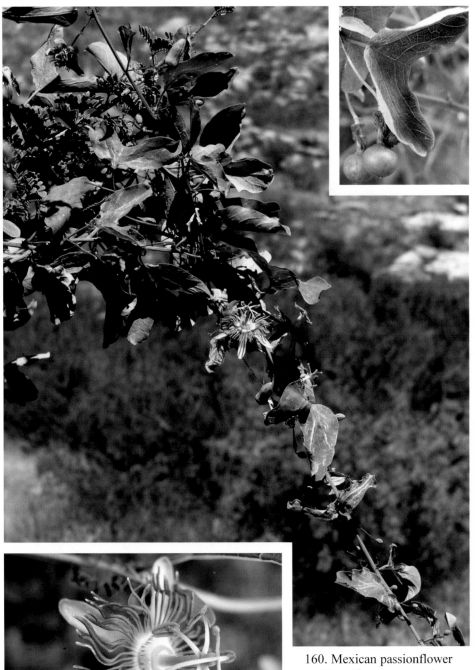

160. Mexican passionflower
(*Passiflora mexicana*)

161. Mexican passionflower
(*Passionflower mexicana*),
leaf and fruit (insert)

162. Mexican passionflower
(*Passiflora mexicana*), flower

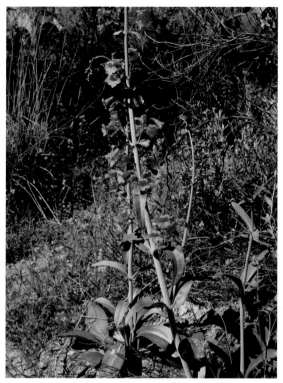

163. Penstemon (*Penstemon parryi*)

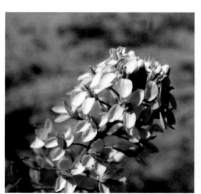

164. Peppergrass
(*Lepidium thurberi*), flowers

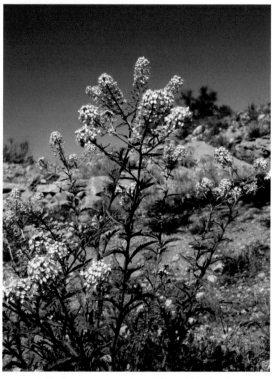

165. Peppergrass (*Lepidium thurberi*)

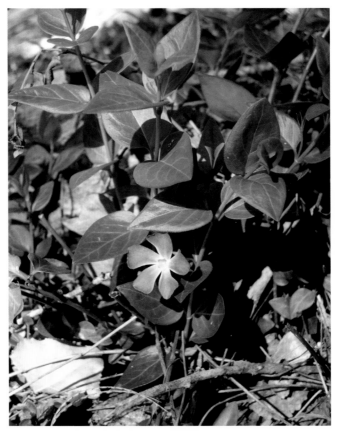

166. Periwinkle (*Vinca major*)

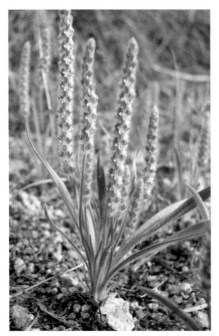

167. Wooly plantain
(*Plantago purshii*)

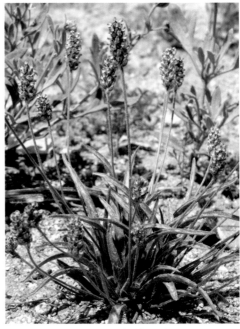

168. Desert indianwheat
(*Plantago insularis*)

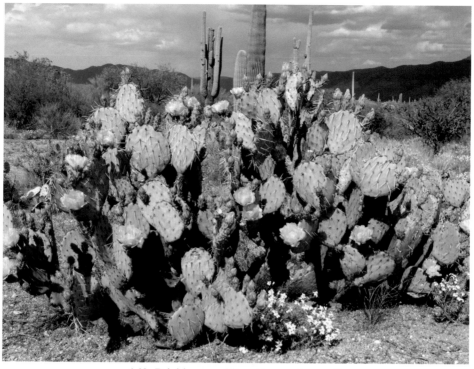

169. Prickly pear (*Opuntia engelmannii*)

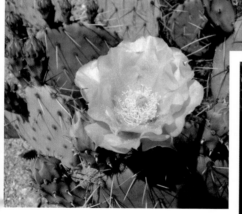

170. Prickly pear
(*Opuntia engelmannii*), flower

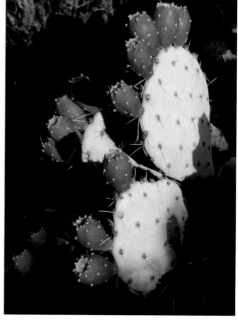

171. Prickly pear
(*Opuntia engelmannii*), fruit

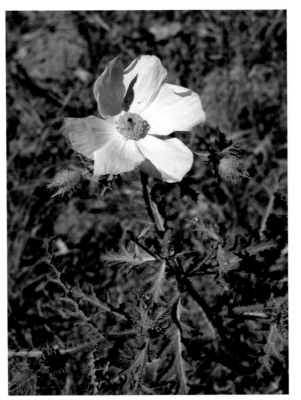

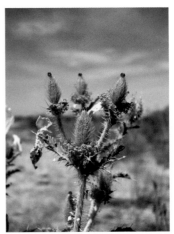

173. Prickly poppy
(*Argemone pleiacantha*),
seedpods

172. Prickly poppy (*Argemone pleiacantha*)

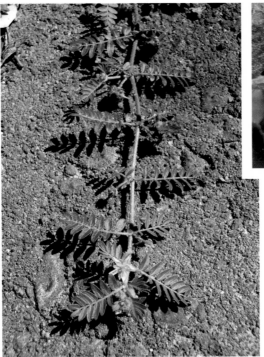

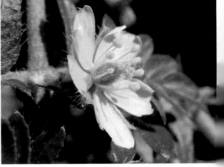

175. Puncturevine
(*Tribulus terrestris*), flower

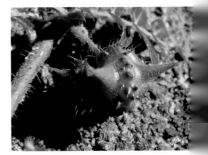

174. Puncturevine (*Tribulus terrestris*)

176. Puncturevine
(*Tribulus terrestris*), seedpod

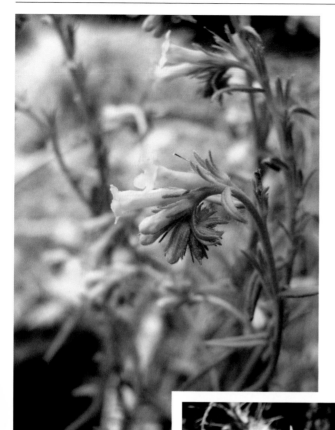

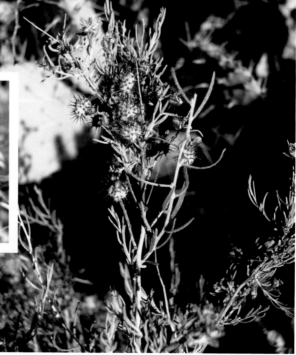

177. Purple gromwell
(*Lithospermum multiflorum*)

180. Ratany
(*Krameria parvifolia*),
seedpod

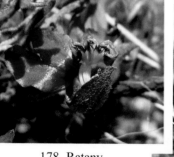

178. Ratany
(*Krameria parvifolia*),
flower

179. Ratany (*Krameria parvifolia*)

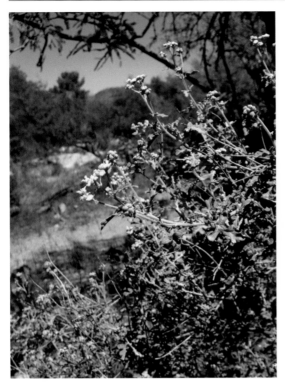

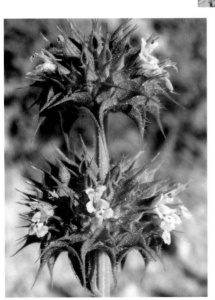

182. Rayweed
(*Parthenium incanum*), flowers

181. Rayweed (*Parthenium incanum*)

183. Chia
(*Salvia columbariae*), flowers

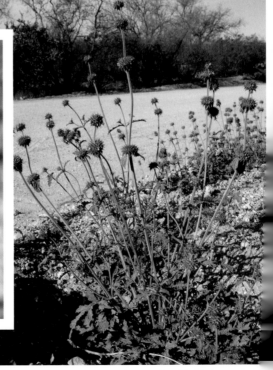

184. Chia (*Salvia columbariae*)

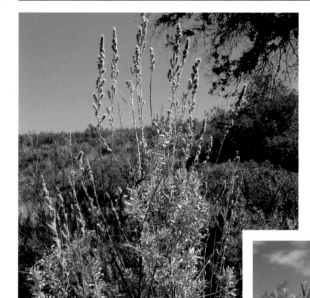

185. Sagebrush (*Artemisia tridentata*)

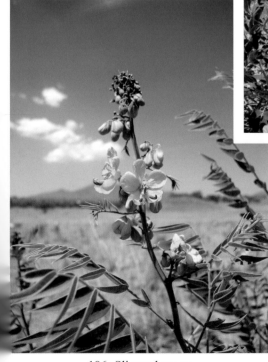

186. Slimpod senna
(*Cassia leptocarpa var. glaberrima*)

187. Desert senna (*Cassia covesii*)

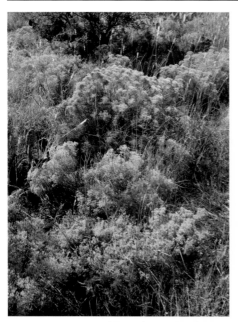
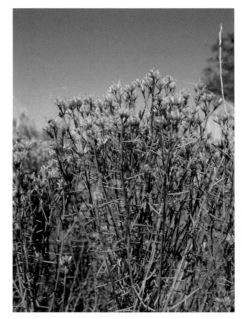

188. and 189. Snakeweed (*Gutierrezia microcephala*)

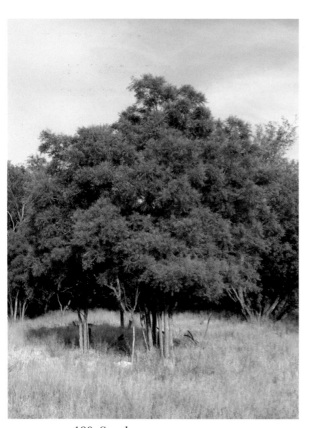
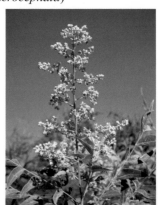
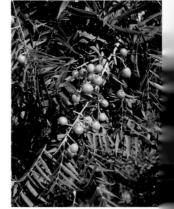

190. Soapberry
(*Sapindus saponaria var. drummondii*)

191. and 192. Soapberry (*Sapindus sapona
drummondii*), flowers above, fruits be

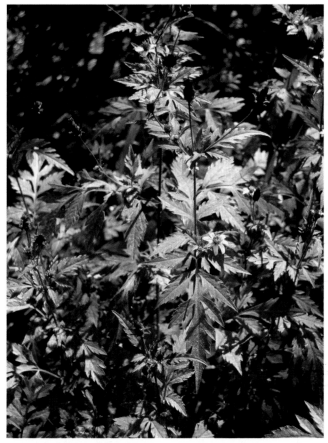

193. Spanish needles (*Bidens pilosa*)

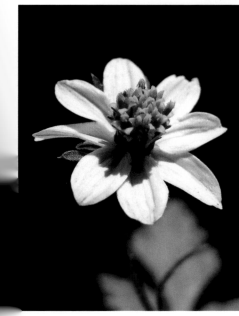

194. Spanish needles (*Bidens pilosa*),
flowers

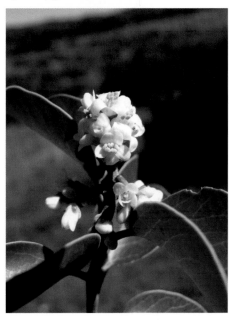

195. Sugar bush (*Rhus ovata*),
flowers

SUMAC

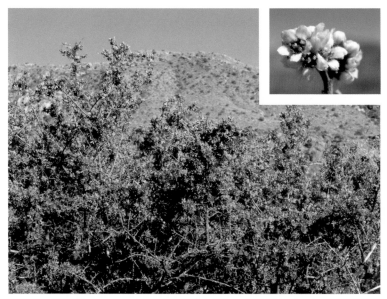

196. and 197. Little leaf sumac (*Rhus microphylla*), flowers (insert)

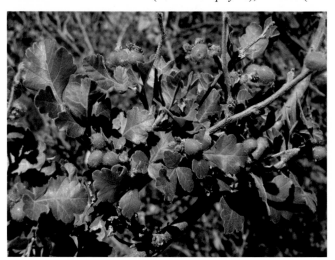

198. Squaw bush (*Rhus trilobata*)

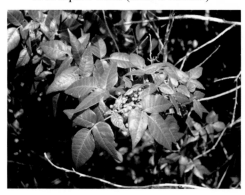

199. Western poison ivy (*Rhus radicans var. rydbergii*)

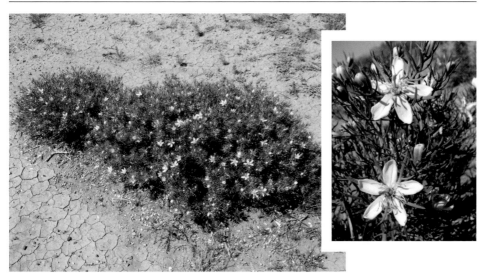

200. and 201. Syrian rue (*Peganum harmala*), flowers right

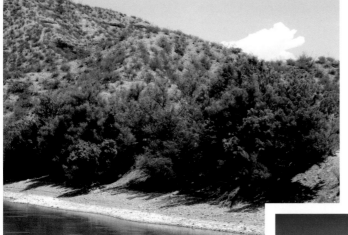

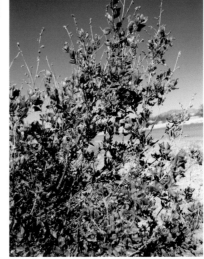

204. Tamarisk (*Tamarix pentandra*), flowers

202. Tamarisk (*Tamarix pentandra*)

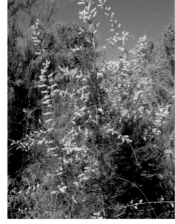

203. Tamarisk (*Tamarix pentandra*)

205. Tarbush (*Flourensia cernua*)

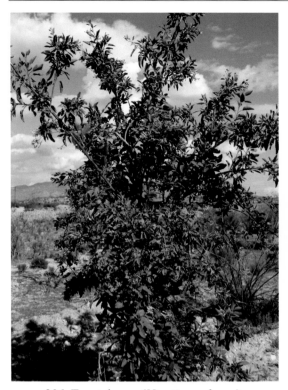

206. Tree tobacco (*Nicotiana glauca*)

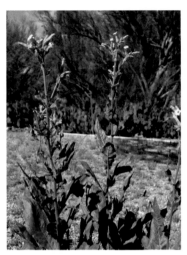

209. Desert tobacco
(*Nicotiana trigonophylla*)

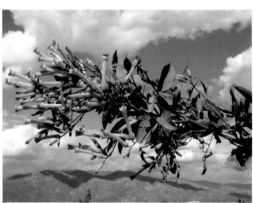

207. Tree tobacco (*Nicotiana glauca*), flowers

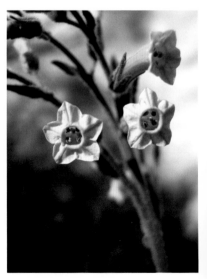

210. Desert tobacco
(*Nicotiana trigonophylla*), flowers

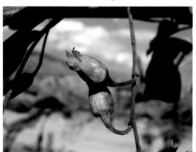

208. Tree tobacco
(*Nicotiana glauca*), seedpods

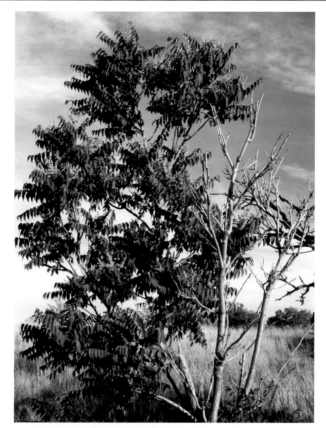

211. Tree of heaven (*Ailanthus altissima*)

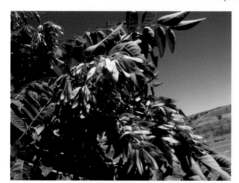

212. Tree of heaven (*Ailanthus altissima*), fruit

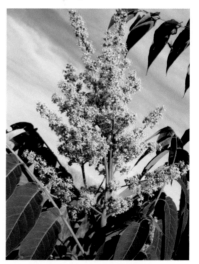

213. Tree of heaven
(*Ailanthus altissima*), flowers

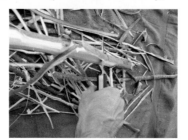

214. Tree of heaven
(*Ailanthus altissima*), collected bark

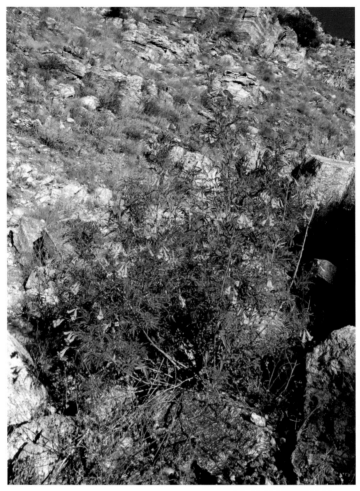

216. Trumpet flower (*Tecoma stans var. angustata*)

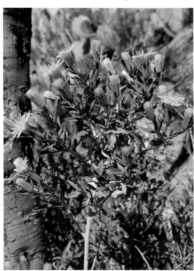

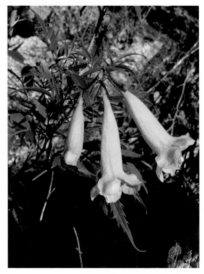

215. Trixis (*Trixis californica*)   217. Trumpet flower
(*Tecoma stans var. angustata*), flowers

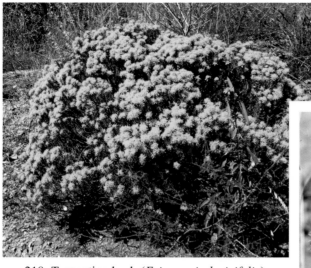

218. Turpentine bush (*Ericameria laricifolia*)

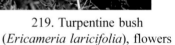

219. Turpentine bush
(*Ericameria laricifolia*), flowers

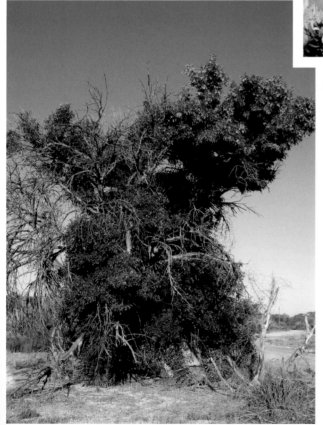

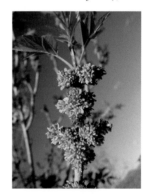

220. Velvet ash (*Fraxinus velutina*)

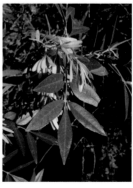

221. and 222. Velvet ash (*Fraxinus velutina*),
male flowers above, keys below

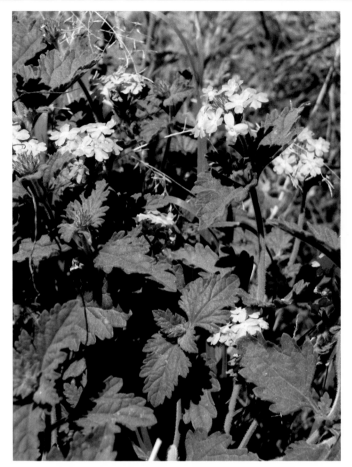

223. Desert verbena (*Verbena gooddingii*)

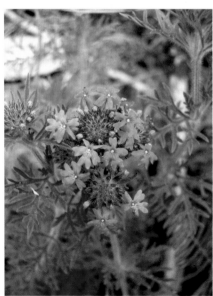

224. Mountain verbena
(*Verbena bipinnatifidia*)

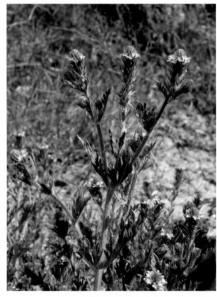

225. Bigbract verbena
(*Verbena bracteata*)

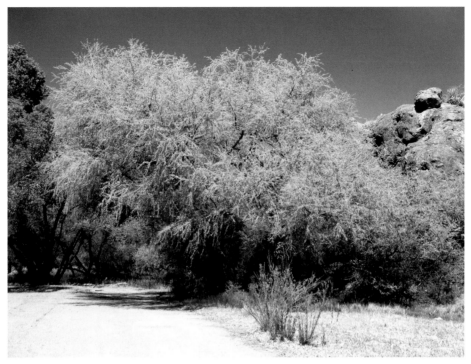

226. Western black willow (*Salix nigra var. vallicola*)

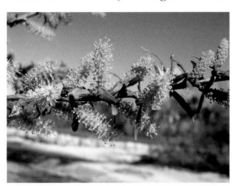

227. Western black willow (*Salix nigra var. vallicola*), male catkins

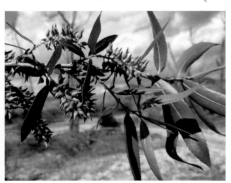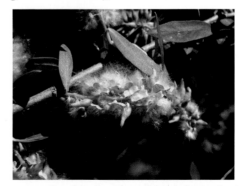

8. and 229. Western black willow (*Salix nigra var. vallicola*), female catkins left, seeds right

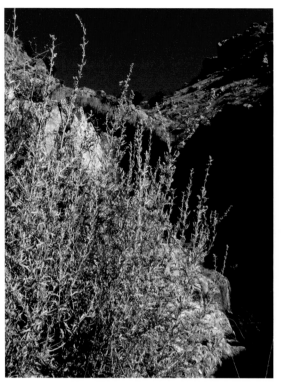

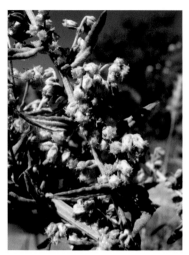

231. Western mugwort
(*Artemisia ludoviciana*), flowers

230. Western mugwort (*Artemisia ludoviciana*)

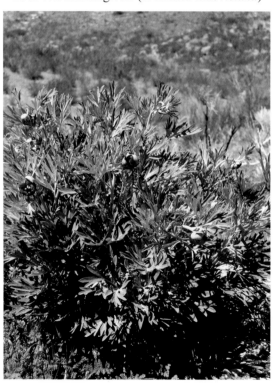

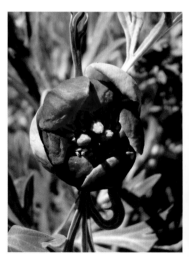

233. Western peony
(*Paeonia brownii*), flower

232. Western peony (*Paeonia brownii*)

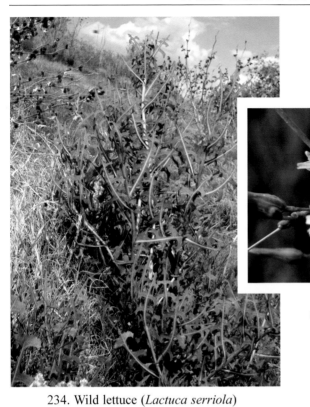

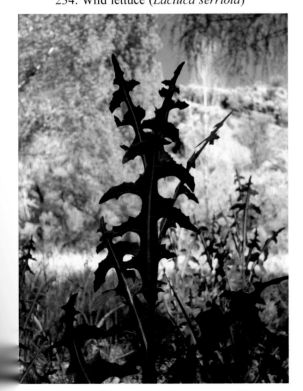

235. Wild lettuce
(*Lactuca serriola*), flowers

234. Wild lettuce (*Lactuca serriola*)

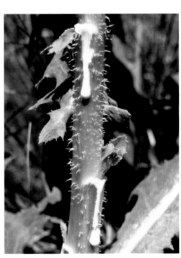

237. Wild lettuce
(*Lactuca serriola*), latex

236. Wild lettuce (*Lactuca serriola*)

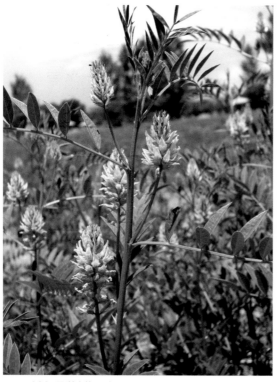

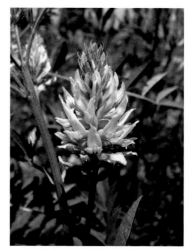

239. Wild licorice
(*Glycyrrhiza lepidota*), flowers

238. Wild licorice (*Glycyrrhiza lepidota*)

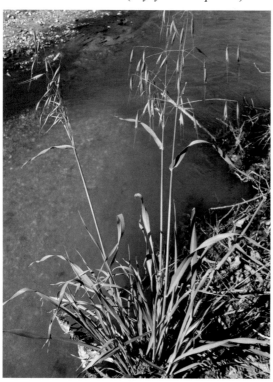

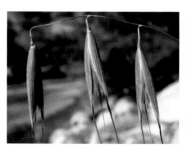

241. Wild oats
(*Avena fatua*), spikelets

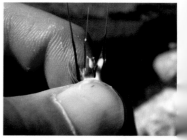

242. Wild oats (*Avena fatua*),
preformed seed

240. Wild oats (*Avena fatua*)

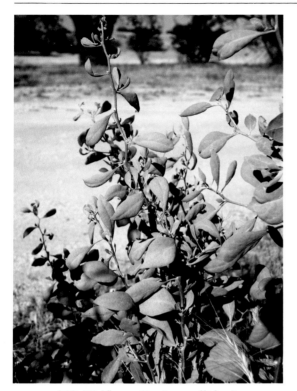

243. Wolfberry (*Lycium pallidum*)

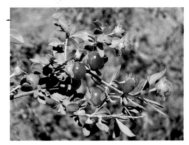

244. Wolfberry
(*Lycium pallidum*), fruit

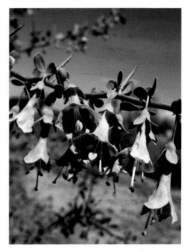

245. Wolfberry
(*Lycium pallidum*), flowers

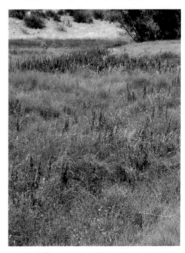

247. Yellowdock (*Rumex crispus*)

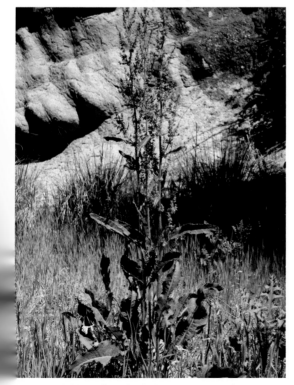

246. Yellowdock (*Rumex crispus*)

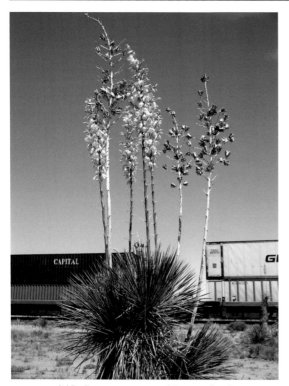

248. Soaptree yucca (*Yucca elata*)

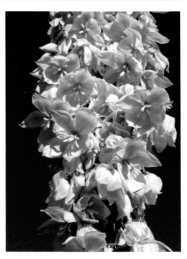

249. Soaptree yucca
(*Yucca elata*), flowers

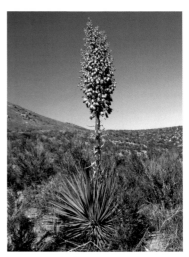

250. *Yucca sp.*

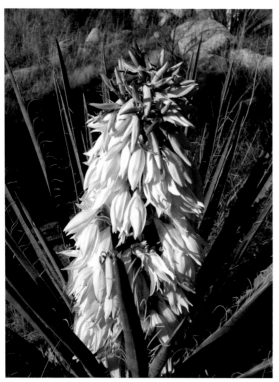

251. Banana yucca (*Yucca baccata*)

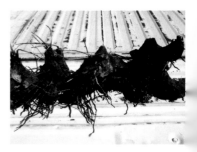

252. Banana yucca
(*Yucca baccata*), roots

seedpods have small amounts of anthraquinones; the mature seeds practically none. As previously mentioned the green, immature seedpods are the choice article. Collect and dry.

Preparations and Dosage:
♦ Cold infusion: 1-2 grams of whole pods to 1 cup of water; taken before bed

Cautions: Do not use during pregnancy due to the plant's potential sympathetic stimulation of uterine contractions. Senna will have a laxative effect in nursing infants through mothers drinking the tea. Senna is not recommended in constipation from dehydration, as the plant's effect on intestinal electrolyte absorption will exacerbate the situation, also muscular tetany has been observed with excess consumption – electrolyte balance, particularly of potassium, is disorganized by Senna. Excess consumption of the tea or over-the-counter preparations will cause dependence and habituation. Senna is best used for 1-2 weeks at a time, or longer in combination with supporting herbs.

SNAKEWEED   *Compositae* – Sunflower family

Gutierrezia sarothrae, G. microcephala
Snakebroom, Matchweed, Resinweed, Escoba de la víbora, Yerba de la víbora, Collálle

Description: Snakeweed is a low-growing small bush. This clump-forming deciduous perennial has somewhat of a woody base. The small, linear, green leaves are apparent from mid-spring though early to mid-fall when the plant flowers. The leaves are resinous and when crushed are sticky and aromatic. When in flower the small yellow blooms cover the upper portion of the plant giving it a frosted appearance. The two most abundant species in the west are Gutierrezia sarothrae and G. microcephala. They differ mainly in floral characteristics. G. microcephala's flowers are cylindrical and have 1 or 2 ray and disk flowers per head. G. sarothrae's flower heads are shaped more or less like a slender top, each flower having 3-8 ray and disk flowers.

Distribution: Snakeweed is a common plant widely distributed throughout the west. It can be found practically from almost sea level to almost 10,000 feet.

It is found in great abundance on over grazed rangelands. Gutierrezia microcephala is found from southern Colorado west to the White Mountains of California, east through much of Arizona, New Mexico, and southwest Texas. From 2,000-6,000 feet the plant inhabits several different vegetation zones: Oak-Juniper Woodlands, Desert Grasslands, and the Mojave Desert. Look for the plant on slopes, flats, and hillsides. G. sarothrae has the widest range of the two. Throughout the western interior, the plant is found on flats and plains from 3,000-6,000 feet.

Chemistry: terpenes: geraniol, γ-humulene, trans-verbenol, verbenone, α-pinene, β-pinene, limonene, nopinone, myrentol, polyalthic acid, and daniellic acid; flavonoids: sarothrin, calycopterin, jaceidin, and sudachitin

Medicinal Uses: Snakeweed is mainly used externally to reduce joint soreness, particularly from rheumatoid arthritis. The plant, being broadly antiinflammatory and especially sedative to muscular-skeletal pain, may be found particularly helpful to sufferers of "fibromyalgia". Not only is soaking in a bath of Snakeweed tea before bed the preferred method of application, it is also generally relaxing and therefore assisting to deeper sleep states, making it doubly beneficial for these individuals. A small amount of the tea can be sipped while soaking for added benefit. The liniment, oil, or salve can be applied for similar relief of painful areas. Like its close relative Turpentine bush, Snakeweed is antimicrobial. Applied to cuts and scrapes it will facilitate healing by retarding bacterial growth.

Indications:
♦ Rheumatoid arthritis/osteoarthritis (internal and external)
♦ Chronic muscular pain (internal and external)
♦ Cuts/scrapes (external)

Collection: Collect Snakeweed from late summer to early fall in bloom or not. Allergy sufferers may prefer to gather the plant without flowers. Prune the upper new growth. This can either be bundled with rubber bands or string, or collected loosely and then dried.

Preparations: Several ounces of herb are used to make a gallon of tea. This then is added to bath water. It is best to infuse the herb owing to its volatile oil content.

Dosage:
- ◆ Leaf infusion: add to bath water; internally, 1 cup daily
- ◆ Oil/salve/liniment: as needed

Cautions: Do not use during pregnancy due to the plant's potential stimulatory effect on uterine musculature. Large amounts are not recommended internally due to the plants remote possibility of causing liver toxicity.

SOAPBERRY   *Sapindaceae – Soapberry family*

Sapindus saponaria var. drummondii
Jaboncillo, Palo blanco

Description: Soapberry is a large bush or small tree capable of reaching 30 feet in height, but typically, it stands 10-15 feet tall. With age the tree's bark becomes gray and fissured. At first glance Soapberry looks to be some sort of stunted Walnut but upon closer examination the deciduous, pinnate leaves are smaller and are not serrated, as are Walnut's. Soapberry has between 13-19 leaflets that are 2-4 inches long and ½-1 inch wide. The small, whitish flowers develop into pyramidal shaped panicles at branch ends. Upon maturation, the fruits are yellowish-green. When dry the translucent fruits are unusual. The outer amber portion of the fruit is partially see-through, enabling the viewer to peer through its crinkled outer coating to the seed inside. In sandy soils, in canyons and small drainages, Soapberry tends to grow in thickets where the tree sprouts from laterally growing roots.

Distribution: From 2,500-6,000 feet Soapberry is found along canyon sides and drainages particularly where soils are sandy. Look for the plant from central Arizona, east to the Gila River and Rio Grande Drainages in New Mexico, to Texas, and east to Louisiana.

Chemistry: triterpenes: α-amyrin, β-amyrin, and hederagenin; flavonoids: luteolin and rutin; various saponins; lipids, mostly found within the seed: arachidic, linoleic, oleic, palmitic, and stearic acids

Medicinal Uses: Much like Yucca, Soapberry's medicinal effect is derived from the plant's saponin content interacting with the gastrointestinal tract's walls and contents. Use Soapberry when arthritic conditions are dependent upon poor intestinal health, particularly when poor dietary habits and constipation are factors. The plant's saponins form complexes with harmful colonic flora by-products and inhibit their systemic absorption, therefore proving systemically antiinflammatory. Soapberry is also directly antimicrobial; unfortunately, the plant does not discriminate between good and bad enteric microbes, so Lactobacillus and other "friendly floras" tend also to diminish slightly with internal use. When using the plant, internal supplementation with Lactobacillus acidophilus may be necessary to keep functional levels of these good microorganisms intact. Soapberry is broadly anti-protozoal. Its use is warranted in traveler's diarrhea and other similar conditions.

Indications:
♦   Arthritis, dependent upon constipation and poor intestinal health
♦   Diarrhea from protozoal infection

Collection: Gather the leaves from late spring through mid-summer; the fruits early to mid-fall.

Preparation and Dosage:
♦   Leaf infusion: 2-4 ounces 3 times daily
♦   Fruit decoction: 1-2 ounces 3 times daily
♦   '00' capsules, powdered leaf: 2-4, 3 times daily
♦   '00' capsules, powdered fruit: 1-2, 3 times daily

Cautions: Traditionally Soapberry has been used to stupefy fish. In various studies, the plant has been shown to kill snails and mollusks, and even has spermicidal properties, so the plant is not completely benign. Dosed properly, like any plant, its use is therapeutic. That said, do not use Soapberry during pregnancy, while nursing or with children. In addition, diarrhea can result with over use. It is best to use Soapberry for two consecutive weeks or less, and then rotate to another non-saponin plant.

Other Uses: A soapy wash can be made with the dried fruits.

SPANISH NEEDLES   *Compositae* – Sunflower family

Bidens pilosa
Bur marigold, Pitchforks, Stick tight, Beggar's ticks

Description: Spanish needles is a 3-4 foot tall herbaceous annual. The pinnate leaves are composed of 3-5 leaflets and are oppositely arranged along the stem. These large leaflets are lance to oval shaped and have toothed margins. The flowers form at branch ends and arise from the leaf axils on long petioles. They are composed of mostly yellow disk flowers. Less uniform in appearance are the slightly larger white ray flowers. The seeds are linear, 4-sided and have 2-4 awns terminating one end. They stick to clothes and animal fur easily, and are typically transported this way – a rather successful method, considering the extent of Spanish needles' range.

Distribution: The plant is originally native to South America, but now is found throughout the tropical and subtropical world. In the United States, it ranges from southern California to southern Arizona and east to Florida. Look to disturbed lowlands, moist riverbanks, fields, and vacant lots.

Chemistry: coumarins: aesculetin; triterpenes: β-amyrin, friedelan, lupeol, and lupeol acetate; flavonoids: quercetin and others; monoterpenes: borneol and limonene; sesquiterpenes: β-caryophyllene, germacrene d and t-muurolol; phenylpropanoids; steroid: daucosterol; benzenoid: phenylheptatriyne; alkenynes; diterpene: phytylheptanoate

Medicinal Uses: Spanish needles tea augments the quantity and quality of gastric mucus. It does this by activating prostaglandin activity at cellular levels within the epithelial lining of the gut wall. This effect increases vascularity of the area and glycoprotein content of gastric mucus. Proper viscosity and quantity of gut mucus is important in maintaining stomach health and in healing gastric and duodenal ulcers. Incidentally, continual emotional anxiety and tension have a diminishing effect on the gut's protective mucus layer, thereby exposing the stomach's sensitive mucosal layer to the causticness of hydrochloric acid. This greatly increases the chances of ulcer formation. Spanish needles also has application in pre-ulcerous gastritis.
   Spanish needles is useful in lowering elevated blood pressure. Traditionally the plant is used in treating a variety of cardiac ailments by

healers in Central America. Research has shown that Spanish needles' hypotensive effect mainly comes from the plant's ability to diminish influxes of extracellular calcium within aortic smooth muscle, subsequently reducing tonicity of those muscle fibers, thus lowering blood pressure. Although Spanish needles has little effect on sodium excretion it has been shown to diminish both essential and sodium induced hypertension.

Spanish needles has some affinity with Canadian fleabane as to its effect on the large and small intestines. Both have flavonoid contents that are sedating to inflammatory processes, particularly if they are autoimmune mediated. Specifically, Spanish needles diminishes excessive lymphocyte proliferation, making it of value in ulcerative colitis or crone's disease. Moreover, the plant tends to lessen diarrhea through its mild astringency.

In some areas of the tropical world where malaria is problematic Spanish needles is used as a treatment. This plant as well as other species, such as Bidens frondosa, B. bipinnatus and B. ferulaefolia has been found to retard the growth of Plasmodium falciparum, one of the main parasites responsible for malaria. Spanish needles is used advantageously as a co-therapy with pharmaceuticals where drug resistance is an issue. Although no research to my knowledge has been conducted there is potential in Spanish needles being of similar use in retarding Babesia growth. The organism is responsible for babesiosis, or various "tick fevers", particularly of concern throughout the northeast and northwest parts of the country. Both Plasmodium falciparum and Babesia reproduce within red blood cells.

Topically Spanish needles is somewhat antimicrobial and is useful in retarding bacterial growth responsible for infections. Using the tea as a wash, or the oil or salve, tends to be soothing to redness and irritation. Likewise, an eyewash made of the herb is cooling to inflamed conjunctiva. As a urinary tract medicine the plant is mild but worthy of note. Although not a urinary tract disinfectant, the plant is soothing to bladder and urethra irritability, and lessening somewhat to haematuria.

Indications:
- Gastric, duodenal ulcers
- Gastritis
- Ulcerative colitis
- Hypertension, essential and sodium induced
- Malaria, as a co-therapy with conventional medications
- Wounds/cuts (external)

♦ Conjunctivitis (eyewash)
♦ Urinary tract irritability, with passive hemorrhaging

Collection: From late spring through summer, collect the herbaceous portions of the plant.

Preparations and Dosage:
♦ Herb infusion: 4-8 ounces 3 times daily
♦ FPT/DPT (50% alcohol): 30-60 drops 3 times daily
♦ Wash/oil/salve: as needed

Cautions: None known.

SUMAC   *Anacardiaceae* – Cashew family

Rhus microphylla
Little leaf sumac, Desert sumac

Rhus trilobata
Squaw bush, Lemonade berry, Skunk bush

Rhus ovata
Sugar bush, Sugar sumac

Description: As a moderate sized, deciduous shrub, Rhus microphylla grows to be 6 feet high by 6 feet wide. The branches are weakly spined and form in dense tangles. This shrub has 5-9 small pinnate leaflets comprising each leaf. The white, very small 5-petaled flowers appear before the leaves in the early spring. The leaves and then fruits develop shortly after. The small, hair covered red fruits, are sticky, edible, and form in clusters at the branch ends. If particularly abundant they can cause the branches to droop.

Rhus trilobata is a slightly larger shrub. The leaves are comprised of 3 leaflets. They are lobed and non-leathery. The plant also develops edible-tart fruits. R. ovata is a large evergreen shrub occasionally reaching 12 feet in height. The oval leaves are leathery, entire, and are slightly longer than wide. The dense fruit clusters follow the small cream-colored flowers. The plant is adapted to brush fires, particularly in Chaparral Scrub of southern California where seeds germinate more successfully and root crowns sprout prolifically after burns.

Numerous species of Rhus not discussed here can also be used medicinally. It is important to be aware of the differences between Western poison oak (R. diversiloba) and Western poison ivy (R. radicans var. rydbergii) and non-toxic Rhuses. Poison oak's form is variable and can be shrub to vine-like. The leaves are divided into 3 leaflets, are usually shiny, and can be entire or present small serrations or lobes. Western poison ivy is typically a shrub with non-aerial roots. The fruits at maturity, for both plants, are white as opposed to the red-sticky fruits of non-toxic Rhuses. When a stem or leaf is broken, a white, milky, urushiol-containing sap is noticeable. This does not occur in non-toxic Rhuses.

Distribution: Rhus microphylla is found on rocky slopes and mesas from 3,500-6,000 feet. In Arizona from the Rincon and Santa Rita Mountains, the plant is found east to New Mexico and Texas along the Rio Grande and Pecos River Drainages. From Oklahoma, it ranges south. It is a typical Chihuahuan Desert plant. R. trilobata, an extremely variable species, is found at numerous elevations and can grow as high as 7,000 feet. It is extensively found throughout the west. R. ovata frequents Chaparral Scrub areas of southern California. In central Arizona the plant is found below the Mogollon Rim, although it does not reach into lower elevations where water scarcity and higher temperatures are limiting factors.

Chemistry: condensed and hydrolyzable tannins

Medicinal Uses: All tannin-bearing plants applied topically are tightening to tissue structure. Sumac leaves are astringent from their array of tannins. Use a fresh leaf poultice or the externally applied tea for stings, bites, rashes, and sunburn. The plant is decidedly soothing to skin irritations and superficial inflammations. The leaf powder applied topically will quickly astringe mild bleeding from cuts and scrapes. As a gargle for sore throats, mouth sores, and receding and bleeding gums, it is useful. A strong cup of tea will also prove lessening to episodic diarrhea.

Indications:
♦ Burns/cuts/scrapes (external)
♦ Sore throats/bleeding gums (gargle)

♦   Diarrhea

Collection: When fully leafed-out, from mid-spring to summer, clip the leaves from the upper portion of the plant. Use fresh or dry normally.

Preparations and Dosage:
♦   Leaf infusion: 2-4 ounces 3 times daily
♦   Leaf wash/powder/poultice/oil/salve: as needed

Cautions: Keep consecutive, internal use of the leaf to short term (2-3 weeks). Longer-term use, as with most other tannin bearing plants, may inhibit gastric function, irritate the kidneys and be mildly vasoconstricting to uterine lining. It is not recommended during pregnancy.

Other Uses: The red sticky fruits of Sumac make a refreshing, lemon-like beverage. Add 4 ounces of fresh fruits to 1 gallon of water. Let this stand for 24 hours, strain, and sweeten to taste. The fruits can also be dried for later use.

SYRIAN RUE   *Zygophyllaceae* – Caltrop family

Peganum harmala
Harmal, Wild rue

Description: Syrian rue is a small perennial bush. It typically stands 2 feet tall by about the same wide. The plant is somewhat dense due to its many-branched stems and finely divided leaves. They form alternately along the stem, are smooth, green, semi-succulent, and linear. The flowers form at branch ends, are white and have 5 petals. Syrian rue's capsules are 2-4 celled and contain many seeds.

Distribution: Syrian rue has a wide Central Asian and Middle Eastern distribution. The plant in this country, as an escapee, is most concentrated around the southern most part of the border between Arizona and New Mexico. From there it is found along primary and secondary roadsides to the El Paso area. An isolated grouping now exists in central Nevada.

Chemistry: indole alkaloids: harmol, harmalol, harmine, harmaline, harmalidine, and isoharmine; a non-indole alkaloid: vasicine; anthraquinones

Medicinal Uses: Syrian rue is a broadly acting medicinal plant, mainly due to its indole group of alkaloids, which have been extensively researched given their pharmacological activity. Seed preparations tend to be mildly mood elevating due to their monoamine oxidase inhibition. The plant reduces serotonin re-uptake in neuronal synapses. Although Syrian rue's immediate mood-altering effects are more pronounced than St. Johns wort's, after time its effect tends to lose potency. Syrian rue is better used in formula with other emotionally uplifting herbs, as alone it may impede coherent thought processes, usher in feelings of giddiness, and cause some gastro-intestinal upset.

Coincident with Syrian rue's traditional use as an antipyretic, research suggests the plant's indole alkaloid group reduces body temperature slightly. This is due to the plant's effect on the hypothalamus and other cerebral centers responsible for body temperature regulation. This activity suggests the plant is of use lowering a high fever. Being inhibiting to various bacterial and fungal strains, the tincture or seed poultice applied topically is broadly antimicrobial. Use on infected cuts and scrapes and on skin funguses.

Indications:
- Mild depression
- Fever
- Infection, bacterial and fungal (external)

Collection: Just before the seedpods split and open, clip them from the plant. Place loosely in a paper bag and dry. Crush the papery seedpods with your hands in the bag. Discard the seedpods. Keep the seeds for medicine.

Preparations: The seed tincture's dark red-burgundy color is quite striking.

Dosage:
- DPT (60% alcohol): 30-60 drops 3 times daily
- Seed poultice/powder/oil/salve: topically as needed

Cautions: Do not use Syrian rue with other psychoactive pharmaceuticals, particularly MAO inhibitors. The plant should not be used during pregnancy (or nursing) due to its potential emmenagogue effect.

Other Uses: A dye from the seeds, called Turkish red, was used in textile coloring and in dying Turkish rugs.

TAMARISK   *Tamaricaceae* – Tamarisk family

Tamarix aphylla
Athel

Tamarix pentandra (Tamarix ramosissima)
Salt cedar

Description: Tamarix aphylla is a large, pyramidal, 30-50 foot tall tree, with thin but dense foliage. The tree's overall appearance is delicate yet robust. The trunk bark is reddish-brown to gray. The scale-like leaves make the tree's appearance deceivingly Cypress-like, which did cause some botanical confusion at the end of the nineteenth century when botanists were trying to classify the tree. The leaves are grayish blue or green and glaucous; the branches are numerous and thin. The small white to pink, 5-petaled flowers form in spike-like panicles on branch ends.

Tamarix pentandra is almost identical in appearance to T. aphylla with one notable exception. T. pentandra is a large bush or small tree; it never approaches the size and girth of T. aphylla. In addition, as described below, how and where this plant grows is another useful distinguishing characteristic.

Distribution: Tamarix aphylla is non-native and originally from Eurasia. In this country it was originally planted as a windbreak, shade, or ornamental tree. The majority of trees throughout the southwest originate from approximately a ½-dozen cuttings from Algeria. Chances are, all clones here are from 1 or 2 trees abroad. Look for the tree throughout the hot and dry southwest. Old farms, homesteads, and ranches are good places to look. Rarely does the tree escape cultivation.

Tamarix pentandra is indigenous to the same regions as T. aphylla. Look for the tree along streams, wash sides, and irrigation ditches throughout the California deserts, east through Arizona, New Mexico, and to Texas. Up to nearly 6,000 feet, along waterways the plant can grow so densely it is known to choke out many native species. The plant is considered a noxious weed due to its aggressive nature. Its range expands yearly.

Chemistry: polyphenols: tamaridone, tamadone, gardenins, nevadensin, apigenin, tamarixellagic acid, dehydrotrigallic acid, isoferulic acid, gallic acid, isoquercitrin, and tamarixin

Medicinal Uses: Use Tamarisk externally on weepy rashes, bites, stings, and other problems that either Mesquite or Acacia remedy. Tamarisk is astringent from an array of bark and leaf tannins. The plant, also because of its tannin-derived astringency is moderately antibacterial and antifungal. There are stronger medicinal plants for either type of infection but if Tamarisk is the only plant on hand it can prove helpful in these situations.

Indications:
♦   Scrapes/cuts/skin abrasions/burns (external)
♦   Mouth sores/sore throats (gargle)

Collection: Gather the leaves and/or bark. The bark has a higher tannin yield and is subsequently the stronger part.

Preparations and Dosage:
♦   External preparations: as needed

Cautions: None for external use.

TARBUSH   *Compositae* – Sunflower family

Flourensia cernua
Varnishbush, Blackbrush, Hojase, Hojansen, Ojasé

Description: Tarbush is a 3-4 foot high, semi-deciduous long-lived shrub. For an arid desert plant, the leaves are large. They are an inch long and a ½-inch wide, green, generally oval shaped, and covered with a sticky-shiny resin. The older branches are dark gray, whereas newer stem growth is much lighter. The bell shaped inflorescences lack ray flowers. They are nodding and situated in axillary and terminal groupings.

Distribution: Tarbush is a typical Chihuahuan Desert plant, serving as an indicator of this desert region. It is found from 3,500-5,000 feet throughout valleys, slopes, and mesas. It ranges from southeastern Arizona through New Mexico's Rio Grande and Pecos River Basins to western Texas.

Chemistry: mono and sesquiterpenoids: camphene, β-myrcene, 3-carene, limonene, 1,8-cineole, borneol, cisjasmone, β-caryophyllene, caryophyllene oxide, and globulol; lactones: tetracosan, pentacosan, hexacosan, heptacosan, octacosan, nonacosan, and triacontan; flavonoids: kaempferol, quercetagetin, kumatakenin, cirsimaritin, and hispidulin

Medicinal Uses: Traditional Mexican usage is relied upon here in describing how Tarbush is best used. Few herbs surpass Tarbush's bitterness. Internally it is a stimulating bitter tonic, similar in use to Bricklebush. Tarbush enhances upper digestive process by stimulating an array of gastric secretions enabling food to be more adequately digested. Use the tea before meals if chronic indigestion, gas, and stasis are common, particularly with protein rich and fatty foods. Tarbush also is stimulating to bile production and release, thereby assisting in small intestinal fat digestion. Topically the plant has been found to be antifungal and antimicrobial, so apply external preparations when needed to related complaints. These latter activities of Tarbush are common for resinous plants that must develop complex defense mechanisms to ward off predators and protect themselves from the elements.

Indications:
♦ Indigestion/deficient protein and fat digestion
♦ Liver sluggishness
♦ Wounds/cuts/scrapes/topical fungal infection (external)

Collection: Tarbush's leaves are most hydrated throughout the spring and summer. Collect the upper herbage at this time.

Dosage:
♦ Leaf infusion: 2-4 ounces before meals
♦ Oil/salve/wash: as needed

Cautions: Large doses of Tarbush can be nauseating and laxative; avoid long-term use of large doses. Do not use during pregnancy or while nursing. Avoid use of the plant if there is a biliary blockage.

TOBACCO

Solanaceae – Nightshade family

Nicotiana glauca
Tree tobacco, Punche

Nicotiana trigonophylla
Desert tobacco, Tobaco loco

Nicotiana attenuata
Coyote tobacco

Description: Nicotiana glauca is a short-lived bush or small tree. It is distinctive in appearance due to its evergreen, ovate, large bluish-green leaves. They are prominently veined, smooth, glaucous, and alternate along the stems on long petioles. Clusters of long, yellow tubular flowers develop on leafless branch ends. The flower tubes are 5-lobed and close during the evening. They are followed by an oval seed capsule containing numerous small brown seeds.

Nicotiana trigonophylla is an annual, biannual, or sometimes a short-lived perennial. It stands 1-3 feet in height. Large plants have numerous multi-branched stems arising from their bases. The large leaves are oblong, green, and clasp the stem. They become smaller as they near the end of the branches' flowering top. The small, tubular, cream-colored, greenish white flowers form at branch ends. Like N. trigonophylla, the capsules contain many small brown seeds. The entire plant is sticky and covered with small hairs. It is common for it to be dust and debris covered.

Nicotiana attenuata is an annual reaching several feet in height. Like N. trigonophylla, the whole plant is hairy and sticky. The leaves alternate along the stems, are lanceolate, and are 2-6 inches long. The lower leaves are petioled, whereas the upper leaves are small and sometimes sessile. The tubular, white flowers form in racemes. They are followed by typical Tobacco-type ovoid seed capsules with minuscule brown seeds inside.

Distribution: Nicotiana glauca is a native of Argentina and Chile. Since its accidental introduction from a California botanical garden approximately 100 years ago, it is quite prolific in some areas. From 5,000 feet and below look for this plant in disturbed soils, vacant lots, along roadsides, streams, and wash sides. The plant has colonized numerous waterways throughout the southwest. The Salt and Gila Rivers in Arizona have dense stands of the plant. From the Rio Grande Plain in Texas, N. glauca is found east through parts of New Mexico, Arizona, to central California.

From 6,900 feet and below, Nicotiana trigonophylla is found from western Texas to Nevada and Utah. It ends its westward expansion in the Creosote bush and Joshua tree country of southern California. It is commonly found in Arizona and parts of New Mexico. Look for this native plant in disturbed soils, vacant lots, trail and roadsides, flood plains, and along washes and drainages.

Nicotiana attenuata has the largest range of the Tobaccos profiled here. From Montana and British Columbia, the plant is found south to Arizona, New Mexico, and California. From 1,000-7,500 feet look to disturbed areas similar to where N. trigonophylla is found. On occasion, they are found side by side.

Chemistry: major alkaloid for Nicotiana glauca: anabasine; N. trigonophylla: nornicotine; N. attenuata: nicotine

Medicinal Uses: Tobacco's primary use is as a topical analgesic. External preparations are useful in relieving pain and sensitivity from contusions, sprains, and other sport-accident type injuries. Soaking in a bath made with Tobacco tea is limiting to joint soreness, aches, and pains from a hard day's work. Topical preparations are also well applied to muscular spasm be it from overwork or injury. All three species profiled either have substantial amounts of nicotine, such as in N. attenuata, or other alkaloids that are therapeutically active, such as nornicotine in N. trigonophylla and anabasine in N. gluaca. Tobacco's alkaloid content has well documented inhibitory activity on body-brain pain transmission. The oil or leaf bolus is soothing to hemorrhoids and with internal Ocotillo use, the combination will offer relief that is more substantial. I have found the fresh leaf poultice or warm fomentation one of the best topical analgesics for spider and insect bites.

Indications:
♦ Acute pain from accidents and injury (external)
♦ Hemorrhoids (external)
♦ Insect bites and stings (external)

Collection: Collect and dry normally.

Preparations and Dosage:
♦   Fresh plant liniment/poultice/salve/oil/bath: topically as needed

Cautions: Do not use topical applications, particularly full body baths with an existing heart irregularity, hypertension, or if pregnant. Even healthy individuals may feel some chest tightness with extended bath application. Tobacco is for external use only.

Other Uses: Tree tobacco's anabasine content makes the tea a useful insecticide, particularly against aphids.

TREE OF HEAVEN   *Simaroubaceae* – Simarouba family

Ailanthus altissima
Chinese sumac, Ailanto

Description: Tree of heaven is a small to moderately sized tree occasionally reaching 80 feet in height. If not regularly pruned the tree is colony-forming – if manicured it resembles a small walnut tree. Its dark green leaves are composed of 6-12 pinnately arranged, pointed leaflets. Although some flowers are perfect, male and female flowers generally occur on separate trees with the male flowers being the strongest smelling. The seeds are encased in oblong samaras.

Distribution: Tree of heaven's range is sporadic owing to the fact that it once was planted as an ornamental throughout the southwest and potentially wider. It is extensively naturalized among old mining towns throughout California, Arizona, and New Mexico.

Chemistry: quassinoids: ailantinol, ailanthone, shinjulactone, shinjudilactone, amaloride, and others; triterpenoids and tannins

Medicinal Uses: We owe Tree of heaven's presence here in the southwest to Chinese immigrants of the mid-nineteenth century. Tree of heaven served the Chinese as a transportable medicine that easily transplants and remedies illnesses of travel. It contains a group of compounds called quassinoids, which are also found in Quassia and in a lesser-known southwestern shrub that could easily succumb to over-harvesting pressures if widely used, namely Castela emoryi.

Tree of heaven is best suited to quell diarrhea and dysentery caused from protozoal infections. Like most Simarouba family plants, Tree of heaven is active against an array of gastrointestinal tact pathogens, particularly Entamoeba histolytica, the cause of traveler's diarrhea, and Giardia. Tree of heaven is doubly beneficial because the plant is also tonic and rebuilding to weakened or damaged intestinal wall mucosa, which can easily result from these types of intestinal infections. Use Tree of heaven when diarrhea has become chronic and has caused a general state of weakness.

In times of emotional strife when the nervous system is hypersensitive and small insults are interpreted as greater dangers, Tree of heaven can prove soothing. The plant quiets extraneous muscular contractions and is useful in reducing mild seizure activity, tremors and shakiness, particularly from shock and trauma.

Indications:
◆ Diarrhea and dysentery with accompanying blood and intestinal wall injury
◆ Amebic, protozoal infections
◆ Nervous system excitability/tremors/mild seizure activity

Collection and Preparations: Ideally, gather the trunk and branch bark in the spring, but it can be collected year round if necessary. Tree of heaven lends itself well to most preparations. A cold infusion extracts both quassinoids and tannins. If the tea is found nauseating use alcoholic preparations as they are more easily handled by the stomach.

Dosage:
◆ Cold infusion/decoction: 2-4 ounces 2-3 times daily
◆ FPT/DPT (50% alcohol): 20-30 drops 2-3 times daily
◆ Fluidextract: 10-20 drops 2-3 times daily

Cautions: Too much Tree of heaven, particularly the tea, can cause nausea, weakness, and a cold-sweaty parasympathetic-like state. Use of this plant it is not recommended during pregnancy.

TRIXIS

Compositae – Sunflower family

Trixis californica
Cachano

Description: This is a small, roundish, mound-like shrub with fragile, grayish-white, many-branched stems. With adequate rainfall, Trixis's foliage is dense, otherwise it tends mainly to form unevenly on branch tips. The bright green leaves are lanceolate and typically are 1-2 inches long. The margins are toothed or entire, and occasionally curl slightly under the leaf body. In addition, the leaves are deciduous in response to lack of rain and cold temperatures. Trixis can flower throughout the year in response to adequate rain, but normally it is a spring to summer bloomer. The yellow flowers appear in dense, flat clusters. After flowering, the dried involucral tubes remain and are notable.

Distribution: From 2,000-4,000 feet, Trixis is found from scattered locations around the Grand Canyon, west to southern California. Throughout much of southern Arizona the plant extends east to New Mexico, particularly along the Rio Grande Drainage, and finally to southwestern Texas. Normally Trixis is found under shrubs and trees, such as Palo verde and Mesquite, in rocky crevasses, or in canyons that provide some protection from constant sun exposure.

Chemistry: not known

Medicinal Uses: Like many of the plants presented in this book, Trixis is not widely used north of the border. So it is put forth here as a medicine deserving more experimentation. The plant is traditionally used externally on wounds, ulcers, and inflammations to expedite healing.

Indications:
♦ Wounds/ulcers (external)

Collection: Clip the hydrated herbage with or without flowers. Dry normally.

Preparations and Dosage:
♦ External preparations: topically as needed

Cautions: None known.

TRUMPET FLOWER   *Bignoniacea* – Bignonia family

Tecoma stans
Tronadora, Palo amarillo, Retana

Description: As a tropical holdout in the southwest, Trumpet flower stands out from late spring through summer with its verdant foliage and large, tubular yellow flowers. It is a deciduous shrub usually reaching 4-6 feet in height. The leaves are oppositely arranged along the branches. The leaflets are pinnately formed with 1 terminal leaflet ending the grouping. Like Desert willow, the seedpod is elongated. The seeds themselves are surrounded by a winged membrane making air travel more likely.

Distribution: Tecoma stans var. angustata is found in the Sonoran and Chihuahuan Desert regions of southern Arizona, New Mexico, and Texas. The northern most reaches of Trumpet flower are determined by low temperatures. Some plants in southeast Arizona are frozen back to the ground after precipitously low temperatures, after in the spring they quickly rebound. The plant makes its home on foothills, rocky slopes, and among boulders where some cold protection can be gained. T. stans var. stans, which primarily differs from var. angustata by its slightly broader leaves, extends from northern Mexico and Florida south to Tropical America.

Chemistry: monoterpenes, triterpenes, benzenoids, phenylpropanoids, and flavonoids

Medicinal Uses: The tea or tincture of Trumpet flower is very useful taken internally before meals to stimulate appetite and upper digestive process. It is specific in treating atonic stomach conditions where upon ingesting food or drink there is fullness, distention, and gastric burning. The plant has a reputation for treating gastritis caused from long-term alcohol use. Trumpet flower modestly reduces blood sugar levels. It is most useful for individuals with NIDDM (non-insulin dependent diabetes mellitus) who are almost able to control blood sugar elevations with exercise and diet therapies. Taken between meals Trumpet flower will give an extra push to blood sugar normalcy.

Like most other Bignonia family plants, Trumpet flower is inhibiting to Candida albicans. If a round of steroids or antibiotics has led to a Candida flare-up, Trumpet flower is of value both topically and internally. For vaginal Candida infections, soaking in a sitz bath made with the tea along with internal usage is an efficacious plan. Campsis radicans or Trumpet creeper, a plant native to the southeastern part of the country, is cultivated in warmer parts of the west and can be used similarly in regards to its Candida inhibition.

Indications:
♦ NIDDM
♦ Indigestion
♦ Gastritis from alcohol abuse
♦ Candida infections, localized and systemic (internal and external)

Collection: During the spring and summer, collect the branch ends with the leaves and/or the flowers, as they all are medicinally active.

Preparations and Dosage:
♦ Herb infusion: 4-8 ounces 3 times daily
♦ Sitz bath: 2-3 times daily

Cautions: Do not use in IDDM (insulin dependent diabetes mellitus).

TURPENTINE BUSH   *Compositae* – Sunflower family

Ericameria laricifolia (*Haplopappus laricifolius*)
Cancerweed, Hierba del pasmo

Description: Turpentine bush is a small rounded shrub typically reaching 2-3 feet in height and width. In full sun locations, the plant is distinctly mound-like. However, among other shrubbery or trees it reaches upwards becoming less uniform. Its small linear leaves are compact and form at the upper terminal branch ends often appressed and cloaking the stems. In the fall, yellow flower clusters appear at the branch ends and with the leaves give the plant a leveled, flattop appearance. The leaves are very resinous and when crushed are sticky and emit an oily, turpentine-like scent.

In stature and overall appearance, Burroweed (Haplopappus tenuisectus) closely resembles Turpentine bush. The most prominent differences between the two plants are that Burroweed is slightly smaller and its leaves are pinnatifid where as Turpentine bush's are entire.

Distribution: From 3,000-6,000 feet, Turpentine bush can be found on rocky slopes and hillsides usually among Scrub oak, Mesquite, and Palo verde. From eastern stretches of the Mojave Desert in California, Turpentine bush stretches across to south-central New Mexico.

Chemistry: flavonoids: apigenin, jaranol, isokaempferide, kaempferol, luteolin, nepetin, quercetin, isorhamnetin, and rhamnocitrin; diterpene: grindelic acid

Medicinal Uses: Topically use Turpentine bush to resolve slow to heal ulcers, wounds, bedsores, and other similar conditions. Turpentine bush is also broadly antimicrobial. A topical powder, salve, or poultice is useful in clearing infected cuts and other superficial skin injuries. A warm poultice or the salve facilitates the process of boils, abscesses, and pimples in coming to a head.

Turpentine bush has a sedating effect on smooth musculature and to some degree on the central nervous system. Traditionally, the plant has been used in treating convulsions and spasms, particularly if initiated from moving from a hot environment to a cooler one in a short time period. A warm poultice can be applied to local pain and spasm, such as over the abdomen for menstrual, intestinal, or stomach cramps. Internally the plant is decidedly stimulating to menses. It also works well to sedate the pain of menstrual cramps.

Indications:
♦ Slow to resolve wounds and other skin conditions (external)
♦ Spasm and central nervous system excitability (internal and external)
♦ Amenorrhea with uterine cramps (internal and external)

Collection: Before flowering when new stem and leaf growth is apparent, snip the upper 6-8 inches of growth. The herb can be dried normally or bundled much like Snakeweed. When collecting have rubber bands or twine on hand for bundling the upper herbage.

Preparations and Dosage:
♦ Leaf infusion: 4-6 ounces 3 times daily

- ◆ DPT (50% alcohol): 30-60 drops 3 times daily
- ◆ Oil/salve/poultice/powder: as needed

Cautions: Do not use during pregnancy or while nursing.

VELVET ASH   *Oleaceae* – Olive family

Fraxinus velutina (F. pennsylvanica ssp. velutina)
Fresno

Description: Velvet ash is a tree of substantial size particularly when growing in moistened soils. Older trees can reach 30-40 feet in height, but usually they are less. The tree's crown is dense, rounded, and somewhat symmetrical. The bark is gray, fissured, and relatively soft. The deciduous leaves are 4-6 inches long and are composed of 3-9 leaflets. Their characteristics can be highly variable: toothed or entire, hairy or glabrous, and leathery or thin. Male and female flowers are borne on separate trees. Male flowers form in dense clusters on branch ends and appear like strange gall formations. After being pollinated the female flowers form into "keys" or seeds surrounded by a single wing.

Distribution: Velvet ash can be found from western Texas, New Mexico along the Rio Grande and Gila River Drainages, throughout southeast and central Arizona to southwestern Utah, southern Nevada, and finally to southeastern California. Between 1,000-6,000 feet, the tree is encountered along streamsides, canyon bottoms, wash sides, and gullies.

Chemistry: coumarins, secoiridoid glucosides, phenylethanoid glycosides, lignans, flavonoids, and tannins

Medicinal Uses: With little modern update, therapeutic use of Velvet ash comes to us largely from a time of the past. The bark tea is considered a digestive tonic; before meals, it is used to stimulate digestive secretion and appetite. The plant is also to be used in corresponding liver sluggishness; likewise it is a bile stimulant. Larger doses are laxative. Topically bark preparations can be used in many types of slowly healing cutaneous conditions. Velvet ash's flavonoid content is greatly responsible for its therapeutic action on the skin.

Indications:
◆ Chronic indigestion with liver sluggishness and mild constipation
◆ Poorly healing skin conditions (external)

Collection: Gather the unfissured bark from younger branches. Lay out in strips to dry.

Preparations and Dosage:
◆ Bark decoction: 4-6 ounces 3 times daily
◆ Poultice/oil/salve: externally as needed

Cautions: Do not take large amounts during pregnancy due to the plant's laxative properties, which are remotely capable of sympathetically stimulating contractions. Moreover do not use if there is a biliary blockage.

VERBENA   *Verbenaceae* – Vervain family

Verbena bracteata
Prostrate verbena, Bigbract verbena

Verbena gooddingii (*Glandularia gooddingii*)
Desert verbena, Mock vervain, Southwestern mock vervain

Verbena macdougalii
New Mexican verbena, MacDougal verbena

Verbena tenuisecta
Moss verbena

Description: Verbena bracteata is a small, low-growing, spreading annual or short-lived perennial. The leaves of this plant are deeply lobed and form oppositely along ridged stems. The entire plant is hairy. The flower spikes are long and composed mostly of leaf-like bracts. The flowers are small and pinkish-purple. V. gooddingii is a low-growing, clump-forming, short-lived perennial. The leaves are arranged oppositely along conspicuously angled stems. They are triangular and deeply lobed or serrated. The stems and leaves are hairy. The light-purple flower clusters form at branch ends. Each flower, as with other Verbenas, is 5-lobed, 2-lipped, tubular, and held within a tubular 5-toothed calyx.

Verbena macdougalii is a 2-4 foot tall perennial. It is a stately plant compared to others in the genus. The oblong-ovate shaped leaves are serrated, hairy, and arranged oppositely on the plant's ridged stems. The small and purplish flowers are arranged in upright spikes on the upper stem ends. V. tenuisecta is a low-growing, mounding annual or short-lived perennial. The leaves are finely divided and small. The laterally shaped flower clusters, depending on variety, are pink, purple, red, and other colors. In warmer parts of the west, it is a popular garden and nursery plant.

Distribution: At varying elevations, Verbena bracteata is widely distributed nearly throughout the entire country. Look to disturbed, moist soils, around cattle tanks, sumps, and bottomlands. V. gooddingii is found from nearly sea level to 6,000 feet. It is common in disturbed land, along drainages, mesas and on rocky slopes. The plant ranges from California, to Nevada and Utah, south and east to Arizona, New Mexico and southern Texas. V. macdougalii is found from Wyoming to western Texas, Arizona and New Mexico. Throughout the arid southwest, the plant is found at higher elevations (5,000-8,500 feet), lower in elevation in more northerly locals. Look to open Ponderosa pine forests and grassy meadows. V. tenuisecta is a common cultivated ornamental, originally from South America. Occasionally it is an escape where some moisture is afforded.

Chemistry: anthocyanines; flavonoids: naringenin and eriodictyol; triterpenoids

Medicinal Uses: Verbena is a sedative of mild strength. Its calming effect is useful in reducing nervousness, anxiety, and tension. Moreover, Verbena can be effective in relieving stress headaches with associated neck and upper back related tension. It is a good herb for individuals whose digestive process is impaired through stressful work or other life related stresses. Through the plant's bitterness and its countering effect on sympathetic-adrenaline discharge, digestion and assimilation are enhanced, as are other parasympathetic functions.

Verbena is a reliable diaphoretic. A warming feeling in the stomach can be felt after taking a small amount of the fresh plant tincture. It then slowly radiates outward. If feverish and dry-skinned Verbena stimulates diaphoresis.

In addition, like most other diaphoretic herbs, if there is no fever then the plant is diuretic. The plant is also stimulating to lactation as are other Vervain family plants, particularly its relative Chaste tree. Verbena may have some modulating effect on the neurotransmitter dopamine and the hormone prolactin. This combined with the plant's sedative qualities will be of help to stressed mothers who cannot produce enough milk for their child.

Some Verbenas have small but inconsistent amounts of cardiac glycosides. Occasionally in sensitive individuals, this can cause the heartbeat to slow and strengthen. The effect is rare but has been observed.

Indications:
- Anxiety/tension
- Headache, stress related
- Indigestion with poor circulation
- Fevers, dry
- Insufficient lactation

Collection: Gather the upper herbaceous portions of Verbena. Snip the individual stems down to where several sets of leaves are remaining. Lay out to dry or tincture fresh.

Preparations and Dosage:
- FPT/DPT (60% alcohol): 30-60 drops 3 times daily
- Herb infusion: 4-6 ounces 3 time daily

Cautions: Sensitive individuals may develop contact dermatitis from collecting the plant. Do not use during pregnancy due to Verbena's potential effect on prolactin levels.

WESTERN BLACK WILLOW *Salicaceae* – Willow family

Salix nigra var. vallicola (*Salix gooddingii*)
Dudley willow

Description: Western black willow is very closely related to Black willow of the eastern United States, and can be considered practically identical in terms of botanical morphology. Usually Western black willow starts as a multi-trunked bush; only later in its growth does it become a tree, and this is largely dependent on available water. The drooping branches give the tree a wide and open crown. Generally, the trunks are bowed and leaning, 2-3 feet in diameter at maturity, with dark, blackish-brown, furrowed bark. The toothed leaves are lanceolate, shiny, and yellowish to light green. Like Cottonwood, Western black willow's male and female flowers develop on separate trees. They form in tubular catkins. Because the mature fruits have cottony fibers attached to them, they are easily carried by the wind.

Distribution: From Shasta County, California, the Four Corners area, and the Texas Panhandle, Western black willow ranges southward along most waterways. Look for this tree from 6,000 feet and lower along waterways, washes, springs, and larger bodies of water. Occasionally dense thickets are encountered on flood plains where water is not too far from the surface.

Chemistry: phenolic glycosides: salicin, fragilin, and salicortin

Medicinal Uses: Like White willow of the east the bark of Western black willow does have a substantial phenolic glycoside content, making its application in chronic/acute pain disturbances indicated if Cottonwood is not available.

Western black willow is principally a remedy for the urinary tract. I apply here to Western black willow what the Eclectic physicians used Black willow (Salix nigra) for over one hundred years ago. Internally the fresh plant tincture made with the buds is quieting to irritative conditions of the geno-urinary tract. It particularly excels at diminishing irritation that triggers spermatorrhea and in both men and women, heightened sexual appetite from genital sensitivity, and to a lesser degree, psychological fixation. As an anaphrodisiac for men, it combines well with Chaste tree. Like Cottonwood,

Western black willow buds soothe urethral and bladder irritation as well as mild prostatitis dependent upon chronic laxity of involved tissues.

Indications:
♦ Genital irritation resulting in excessive sexual activity and preoccupation
♦ Spermatorrhea
♦ Chronic urinary tract irritation
♦ Prostatitis

Collection: Gather young buds in the early spring by stripping them from the branch ends.

Preparations and Dosage:
♦ FPT: 30-60 drops 3-4 times daily

Cautions: Like other Willow family plants use caution when mixing Western black willow with blood thinning pharmaceuticals due to the possible synergistic effect of the tree's glycosides. The chances of Western black willow triggering reye's syndrome in feverish children is remote, but it is best to err on the side of caution and not use internally in these situations.

WESTERN MUGWORT   *Compositae* – Sunflower family

Artemisia ludoviciana
Prairie sagewort, White sagewort, Estafiate

Artemisia douglasiana (Artemisia vulgaris var. californica)
California mugwort, Douglas mugwort, Ajenjo

Artemisia filifolia
Sand sagebrush, Sandhill sage, Romerillo

Description: Artemisia ludoviciana, like most others in the genus, is notorious for its variable foliage. Spring growth looks decidedly different from summer growth. If only looking at leaf characteristics, the plant growing in low-elevation deserts appears differently from its north-country kin. The leaves are entire, occasionally lobed or serrated, and alternate along the stem. New foliage can be bluish green or silver-gray in hue. The plant is highly successful at reproduction, using both seed and rhizome/stem clones to propagate itself. Individually, A. ludoviciana's flowers are inconspicuous, but in numbers, they form noticeable terminal spikes inter-mixed with small leaves. When flowering, the plant is upright, reaching for the sun, though it is not uncommon for flowering branches to droop in response to stem weakness or weighty flower spikes. This plant, as are other Artemisias, is very fragrant; when the leaves are crushed, they put forth a characteristic Sage-like smell. One of Howie Brounstein's abilities, as an herbalist in Eugene, Oregon, is his skill in making sense out of the morass of taxonomic darkness that A. ludoviciana and all of its sub-species tend to inhabit.

Like Artemisia ludoviciana, A. douglasiana roots from stem nodes so it too is found in bunched colonies. This perennial is usually several feet in height, but if conditions are optimal, it can occasion 6-7 feet. The leaves are variable but tend to be entire towards the top of the plant; lower along the stem they are toothed, cleft, or lobed. Above, the leaves are dark green, below, they are silvery due to a dense coating of leaf hairs. The small, whitish, cream-colored flowers are clustered in small spikelets, originating from the leaf axils on the upper stem ends.

Artemisia filifolia is a perennial sub-shrub, 3 feet tall by the same wide. The aromatic leaves are pubescent and are light gray, bluish-green. On the upper stems, the leaves are entire and thread-like. The lower leaves are also very thin and narrow, but are usually longer and cleft. They alternate along brownish-grey stems. The small inconspicuous flowers form in clusters on the upper stems. Like most Artemisias of the west, A. filifolia is a late summer to fall bloomer.

Distribution: From Wisconsin and Illinois Artemisia ludoviciana ranges south and west to the east side of the Cascade Range. Truly a ubiquitous western plant, A. ludoviciana is found in many microclimates and bioregions. This highly adaptable plant can be found anywhere between the Mixed Conifer-Pine Belts to lower desert washes and foothills.

A. douglasiana is found through most of California, Oregon, and eastern Washington. It ranges east to the Rocky Mountains. Look to rocky hillsides, mountain drainages, and streamsides. Artemisia filifolia has a wide distribution throughout the interior west. From Nebraska and Wyoming, the plant is abundant on well-drained sandy soils and rangelands. From this area, the plant is also found south to Colorado, Nevada, western Texas, New Mexico, and Arizona.

Chemistry: for Artemisia ludoviciana: sesquiterpenes: achillin, anthemidin, artedouglasia oxide, douglanine, ludovicin, tanaparthin-α-peroxide, and tanapartholide b; monoterpenes: borneol, camphor, chrysanthemol, transchrysanthenol, and α-pinene; flavonoids: butein, isoliquiritigenin, isorhamnetin, and quercetin; coumarins: lacarol and scopoletin

Medicinal Uses: Artemisias of the west are some of the most multi-faceted herbal medicines we can employ. The plants described here differ from Sagebrush (Artemisia tridentata) mainly in their lack of thujone and related aromatics. Some secondary differences will become evident as you read further.

Firstly, Western mugwort is a medicine for the gastrointestinal tract. All three Artemisias tend to be mild to moderate gastric stimulants, Artemisia ludoviciana being the most energetic. Each plant's gastric stimulation can largely be determined by its bitterness. The more bitter the plant, the more stimulation it will provide. Underlying Western mugwort's bitter tonic activity is its seemingly paradoxical cytoprotective effect on gastric and intestinal tissue. Western mugwort, particularly Artemisia filifolia and A. douglasiana have the ability of stabilizing cellular membranes and ultimately protecting gastrointestinal tissues from an array of inflammatory conditions. These plants have been shown to provide cyclooxygenase inhibition, increased glycoprotein (mucus) synthesis, granulocyte degranulation inhibition, as well as transcription factor NF-KB inhibition. All of these activities protect gastrointestinal tract mucosa from the body's own inflammatory responses. Use Western mugwort as a daily tea for ulcerative colitis, gastritis, or other inflammatory conditions affecting the area.

Western mugwort has a number of effects on the liver. Overtly it is choleretic, increasing bile synthesis and release. If prone to gall stone formation Western mugwort will thin bile enough to diminish precipitants. Deeper, these plants have a cooling, antioxidant effect on hepatocyte function. These liver centered effects tend to reduce elevated liver enzyme levels – all stress markers evident in viral and general hepatitis. In addition, the plant inhibits glutathione depletion within hepatocytes. Western mugwort's hepatoprotective effect can also be of benefit to individuals who consume excess alcohol, rancid oils, and processed foods with their array of artificial ingredients. Use Western mugwort to buffer these nefarious effects on the liver, although making better dietary choices is paramount in liver health. Several ounces of the cool tea taken before bed is one of the best approaches if prone to, upon waking the next morning, frontal headaches, red-irritated eyes, bad breath, and general liver congestion.

Topically, Western mugwort is mildly antibacterial and antifungal. It is effective against a wide array of microorganisms; it does not provide a strong effect, but it is broad. Artemisia ludoviciana is distinctly inhibiting to HSV (herpes simplex virus), type I and II. For cold sore treatment, the oil or salve in combination with Creosote bush is effective. With clients, I have observed genital herpes outbreaks diminish under internal use of the plant. Added benefit is achieved by topical application. Like its larger cousin, Sagebrush, Western mugwort is effective against a number of intestinal parasites. Drink several cups of tea daily for treatment of traveler's diarrhea, pinworm infections, and other infestations effecting intestinal function. Do not underestimate Western mugwort, particularly A. ludoviciana in these situations. The plant contains a number of compounds that are broadly anthelmintic.

The tea drunk hot is a stimulating diaphoretic; drunken cold with no elevated temperature Western mugwort is diuretic. The plant tends also to stimulate menses, so is useful in delayed menstruation where the pelvic area feels cold and rigid.

Indications:
♦ Dyspepsia/gastritis
♦ Intestinal inflammation
♦ Liver inflammation, with no hepatic/biliary blockage
♦ Bacterial/fungal infections (external)
♦ HSV, type I and II (internal and external)
♦ Intestinal parasites
♦ Fever, low-moderate temperature
♦ Amenorrhea, with pelvic rigidity

Collection: Depending on variety, Western mugwort's foliage is collectable from spring through fall. Gather without the flowers as the pollen can occasionally trigger hayfever reactions in sensitive individuals. Dry well spaced.

Preparations and Dosage:
♦ Leaf infusion or cold infusion: 4-6 ounces 2-3 times daily
♦ FPT/DPT (50% alcohol): 20-40 drops 3 times daily

♦ Oil/salve/wash: as needed

Cautions: Do not use during pregnancy due to Western mugwort's dilating effect on uterine vasculature. Due to the plant's cholagogue properties do not use if there is a biliary blockage.

Other Uses: Artemisia annua, principally used in TCM (Traditional Chinese Medicine) contains artemisinin, a compound used in conventional medicine as an antimalarial drug. Even whole herb preparations of A. annua have traditional use in intermittent fevers – one hallmark of malaria (Plasmodium falciparum) infection. Even though A. ludoviciana does not contain artemisinin, the plant has related compounds that have potential in resolving Plasmodium infections as well.

WESTERN PEONY
Paeoniaceae – Peony family

Paeonia brownii (*Paeonia californica*)
California peony

Description: Western peony is a 1-1½ foot tall by 2-3 foot wide herbaceous perennial. Its leaves, which are vibrantly green and somewhat fleshy, are numerous and form from the base of the plant. Occasionally the leaves are scarlet tipped when they first emerge; later in the season after flowering, the leaves easily wilt from lack of rain or intense sun exposure. The solitary large flowers are dark red, and occasionally shade to black. Typically, the nodding flowers are composed of 5-6 petals, although sometimes more; they are somewhat fragrant. When mature they can easily be mistaken for not being fully developed since the petals still cup the reproductive center. As the seed capsules mature the stem droops, and even may contact the ground. The roots on mature plants are numerous, vertically oriented, slender tubers. Some botanists place the plant in the Buttercup family.

Distribution: Western peony is abundant throughout coastal and northern California. Also, look to south and western Oregon, western Washington, into Nevada, Utah, Idaho and Wyoming where there exists extensive stands. Sagebrush is a common companion plant throughout its range in the Great Basin Desert.

Chemistry: not known

Medicinal Uses: Western peony is largely antispasmodic to smooth muscle tissue. Its two primary spheres of influence are on uterus and bronchial tissue. The plant is distinctly sedative to uterine cramps. It can be used as needed on the first or second day of menses to ease spasmodic pain, although some women find it more effective started a week or two before the onset of menses. Some also experience the plant as a menstrual stimulant; so is useful if menses is slow to start, or stop and start. If adrenal-stress is present then Western peony is doubly indicated since the plant is a gentle sedative of use in nervous excitability and tension.

Western peony is of value in relieving a spasmodic cough. Its effect on bronchial irritation is serviceable. Systemically, Western peony tends to diminish muscular twitching and excess nervous system discharge resulting in pre-seizure activity.

Indications:
♦ Uterine cramps
♦ Spasmodic cough
♦ Muscular twitching/pre-seizure activity

Collection: Select larger robust plants with corresponding large root masses. Start digging to one side of the plant and work in. Take only peripheral tubers while leaving the inner ones. This will ensure the plant's survival in years to come. After splitting open a tuber, the coloration is normally pink-purple; the darker the coloration the stronger the root medicine. Gather when the new foliage first appears or after flowering.

Preparations: If using for tea split the tuber length-wise to ensure proper drying. As the root dries, it will darken considerably.

Dosage:
♦ FPT/DPT (60%): 30-60 drops 3 times daily
♦ Root decoction: 4-6 ounces 3 times daily

Cautions: Western peony may interfere with consistent blood coagulation if mixed with blood-thinning pharmaceuticals. Also, do not take during pregnancy due to the plant's stimulating effect on menses.

WILD LETTUCE

Compositae – Sunflower family

Lactuca serriola
Prickly lettuce

Description: This annual, or sometimes biannual, grows to be 2-6 feet high. The leaves are alternately spaced, point upward, and clasp the stem; they are deeply lobed and toothed but occasionally are entire and lanceolate. On the underside of each leaf are spines aligned on the midrib. The flower heads are small, yellow, and Dandelion-like. They are borne on branching flower stalks and close by mid-morning. The seeds, like many other composites, are small and have a swirl of whitish fibers attached to them making wind dispersal the method of choice. When cut or injured the entire plant exudes a white milky sap.

Distribution: The plant was introduced from Europe and now exists throughout most of the United States. Like other introduced species, Wild lettuce is found along roadsides, buildings, walkways, and other areas where it is allowed through neglect and soil-disruption to flourish. Throughout drier areas in the west, the plant prefers moister soils and semi-shade.

Chemistry: lactucin, lactucopicrin, lactucic acid, caoutchouc, lactucerin, and other secondary compounds

Medicinal Uses: Wild lettuce is sedative and is of value when used for mild insomnia and restlessness upon retiring. It is best used when these states derive from mental and emotional stress, lesser so from the pain of physical injury. It works particularly well if the agitation is connected to, or dependent upon a sensation, either imagined or real, of physical heat, such as core body temperature being slightly elevated from fever, dehydration, or working outside during a hot day. As a sedative Wild lettuce has some similarities to California poppy. Although the former is not in the Poppy family, by effect, it can be considered a "sub-opiate", hence the antiquated name, Opium lettuce, once applied to several species of Lactuca. Moreover, Wild Lettuce is used in allying spasmodic coughs dependent on bronchial irritation

Indications:
♦ Insomnia and restlessness from overwork and stress

♦ Spasmodic coughs from bronchial irritation

Collection: Lactucarium is the name applied to the concentrated milky juice of several species of Lactuca. It can be collected through several time consuming methods. The first approach: clip the tops off a good-sized stand of Wild lettuce. Wait until the milky juice hardens slightly, and then scrape the milky beads off with a knife or razor blade. Re-snip each plant ¼-½ inch below the original cut, and continue on and on. The second method is similar to the first. Strip the leaves from the plant, then with a razor blade make vertical cuts along the plant's stalk. The copious exudate can be collected after it dries slightly or can be sponged up and squeezed out using a small amount of water. Finally, the last method is to collect the whole plant, before flowering, and juice it. Although the resulting juice is not technically lactucarium, the effect of the preparation is practically identical. Whatever method has been chosen, dehydrate the milky liquid or juice. This hardened material, typically reddish-brown in color, is lactucarium or close to it.

Preparations: Although the fresh and dried whole plant tincture and leaf infusion are feebler in effect then lactucarium they still have value. When making the tincture of lactucarium the hardened milky material should dissolve completely.

Dosage:
♦ DPT of lactucarium (80% alcohol): 30-60 drops 3 times daily
♦ FPT/DPT (60% alcohol): ½-1 tsp 3 times daily
♦ Leaf infusion: 4-8 ounces 3 times daily

Cautions: None known.

WILD LICORICE

Leguminosae – Pea family

Glycyrrhiza lepidota
American licorice

Description: Wild Licorice is a colony-forming perennial bush, spreading either from underground rhizomes or through typical seed reproduction. This deciduous plant stands 1-3 feet tall and has erect stems rising from the ground. The leaves are comprised of 11-19 oblong, narrow leaflets. The arrangement is called odd-pinnate because one leaflet always terminates the group; also, the leaflets are gland dotted at maturity and are slightly sticky when rubbed. The flower spikes originate from the upper part of the plant, and arise between leaf and stem joints. The spikes are arranged of compact yellowish-white to greenish-white small pea flowers. The burred seedpods are ½-¾ of an inch long and resemble Cocklebur pods. The beans within are small and reddish-brown.

Distribution: Wild licorice covers a wide range of territory throughout the country. Although the plant is absent from low-elevation arid areas of the southwest, such as the Sonoran Desert, it can be found throughout the west in moist and sandy soils along streams, fields, and roadsides.

Chemistry: glabidin, glabranin, glepidotin, pinocembrin, and glycyrrhizin

Medicinal Uses: Use Wild licorice in inflammatory conditions of the stomach dependent upon insufficient gastric secretions, namely mucin and hydrochloric acid. The plant is significantly inhibiting to Helicobacter pylori, a bacterium often associated with gastric ulcers. Note though gastric ulcers are not solely caused by H. pylori. This is why after a round of conventional antibiotics, designed to eliminate the bacterium, H. pylori does diminish and the corresponding ulcer resolves but all too often, both reoccur. Typically, there is an underlying stress pattern predisposing the gastric lining to H. pylori colonization. It is only when the surrounding tissues become vulnerable to H. pylori does the bacterium wreak havoc. In fact, H. pylori can be present in the gastric environment and not cause a problem. While being directly inhibiting to H. pylori, Wild licorice supports gastric secretion and membranes through a number of avenues. Taken before meals, Wild licorice can also be used as a functional bitter to allay indigestion and increase appetite.

Use Wild licorice when there is mild constipation and uncomfortable intestinal movement. The plant shifts fluids to the intestines and hydrates the feces somewhat, normalizing bowel movements. Moreover, the bronchial environment tends to be moistened by the plant. Use when there is a dry cough and the lungs feel hot. Wild licorice will be of greatest benefit to individuals who exhibit the above tendencies and who are under low-grade adrenaline fight or flight stress.

Recent research suggests that Wild licorice as well as European and Chinese species, due to their glabidin content, are all useful in diminishing inflammation, oxidative stress, and tissue damage in glomerulonephritis. The plant tends to stabilize nephrons and reduce albumin in the urine.

Wild licorice contains insignificant amounts of glycyrrhizin, one of the main bioactive constituents of European and Chinese licorice. Wild licorice has virtually no effect on mineralocorticoids and the like, making it safe to use in hypertension. The plant can sometimes stimulate menses through its isoflavone content. Its effect is unpredictable so care should be taken if cycles are irregular.

Indications:
- Gastric ulcer, H. pylori involvement
- Gastritis
- Indigestion
- Mild constipation
- Dry cough
- Kidney inflammation, chronic

Collection: Gather sub-surface rhizomes and taproots. Some stands can develop impressive networks of roots. In moist sandy soils, the runners can sometimes be pulled up by hand. Chop into small pieces and dry normally.

Preparations and Dosage:
- DPT (50% alcohol): 40-60 drops 3 times daily
- Fluidextract: 10-20 drops 3 times daily
- Root decoction: 4-6 ounces 3 times daily

Cautions: Do not take during pregnancy due to the plants unpredictable effect on circulating estrogen levels.

WILD OATS

Poaceae – Grass family

Avena fatua
Oatstraw, Oatgrass

Description: Wild oats is a robust annual, 2-4 feet tall with jointed, hollow stems and corkscrewing leaf blades. The inflorescences form in wide panicles; the individual spikelets droop tassel-like, resembling green cockroaches with their rearward stretched awns appearing as spindly legs. The small oat seeds mature from late spring to early summer and can remain viable in the ground for nearly 10 years. Cultivated oats (Avena sativa) is another commonly found oat. Often it is difficult to tell the two apart, but upon close study the bracts of this variety are not hairy, unlike Wild oats.

Distribution: With exceptions pertaining to the southeastern part of the United States, Wild oats, a European native, is ubiquitous throughout North America. Look for the plant in disturbed, rich soils, and around drainage ditches and culverts; occasionally it can be found along streams and canyon sides.

Chemistry: vitexin, apigenin, d5-avenasterol, avenocosides a and b, and nuatigenin

Medicinal Uses: Wild oats primarily exerts its effect on distresses arising from nervous system debility. Think of Wild oats as a nervous system stabilizer; it counteracts agitation from over work and prolonged periods of stress. There is some difficultly in describing what Wild oats actually does; it is not an overt sedative, nor is the plant overtly stimulating, but this does not detract from the fact that if you are physically and emotionally "rode hard and put away wet" the plant imparts a sense of stability.

Depressive states arising out of pushing through workloads on the job or at home are lifted. The edginess and frayed-end feeling of kicking nicotine, opiate, or alcohol habits is also lessened. As Michael Moore succinctly puts it, "This is crispy critter medicine".

Indications:
♦ Depressive states, emotional-nervous system debility from overwork, prolonged stress, or nicotine, opiate, and alcohol withdrawal

Collection: It is important to establish a relationship with Wild oats. Starting in the spring visit a stand several times a month as to not miss the oat "in milk" stage. You have a window where this plant is pickable for 1-2 weeks. The oat seed matures quickly so keep a close eye on it. When the spikelets are green and suspended in panicles, pick several and squeeze them. While squeezing the spikelet, you should feel a "pop" between your thumb and forefinger; this is followed by the milky-preformed seed coming out of the opposite end. At this point, they are prime for tincturing. Strip the spikelets from the rising stalks. Leave at least half of the immature oats on the collective group, so next year they will be equally abundant.

Preparations and Dosage:
♦ FPT: 30-60 drops 3-4 times daily

Cautions: None known.

Other Uses: The whole dried plant, also know as Oatstraw, prepared as a tea is a good source of readily absorbable electrolytes, particularly calcium.

WOLFBERRY   *Solanaceae* – Nightshade family

Lycium pallidum
Pale wolfberry, Thornbush, Desert thorn, Tomatillo

Description: Wolfberry is a large, dense shrub typically 3-6 feet high; its branches are thorny, smooth and whitish, and are crowded with clusters of spatula shaped small leaves, approximately an inch in length. They are pale green and fleshy. The greenish, tubular flowers are often tinged with purple and hang downward bell-like from leaf clusters. The smooth red fruits are the size of small grapes; they are juicy, contain a number of seeds, are slightly sweet to bitter, and have a subtle nightshade taste. Throughout the west, Lycium is a moderately sized genus. Most Lycium's are similarly formed with the main noticeable differences being berry and leaf size and general stature.

Distribution: From 3,000-7,000 feet, Wolfberry can be found throughout the Sonoran, Mojave, and Chihuahuan Deserts. At higher elevations look for Wolfberry among Oak Woodlands and Chaparral Scrub areas. The plant tends to inhabit varying areas such as basins, hillsides, and arroyos. Wolfberry can be found from Texas to Colorado, west to Utah and California, and south to Arizona and New Mexico.

Chemistry: an array of Nightshade family alkaloids; specific constituents not known

Medicinal Uses: The medicinal use of this genius in modern times has only come about in recent years. It is reasonable to speculate that most species can medicinally be used alike, however, approach the use of each species of Lycium with prudence. In allergic situations use Wolfberry when there is excessive eye and nose discharge. In addition, when lower respiratory tract tissues are congested and there are accompanying feelings of bronchial tightness Wolfberry can prove opening to the area. The plant's moderate anticholinergic activity shifts nervous system activity away from constricting respiratory tissues. This effect is most useful in mild-moderate humid asthma or other allergic-immune mediated bronchial responses; Wolfberry shrinks tissues and allays hyper-secretion.

Wolfberry's effect is also noticeable in gut and intestinal centered distresses. Nausea, intestinal spasms, and general over-excitability of these areas respond well to Wolfberry. The plant acts well to quell chills, sweating, and nausea (much like drinking the juice of one or two raw potatoes) from over-exposure to chemical herbicides, fertilizers, and other conventional agricultural productions.

It is important to note that Wolfberry is a mild drug plant, meaning it suppresses symptoms and does not have much underlying value beyond temporally diminishing distresses, albeit in a limited way. In chronic conditions, Wolfberry works well in formula. Combined with other more supportive herbs, it diminishes surfaces distresses while deeper issues, possibly exaggerated immune responses or stress patterns, can be addressed.

Topically the freshly poulticed plant or liniment can be applied to acute stings, swellings, contusions, and other injuries. In this respect, applied externally, Wolfberry acts like other Nightshade family plants. It moderately reduces pain and inflammation similarly to, although weaker than, Datura or Tobacco.

Indications:
♦ Rhinitis
♦ Constricted breathing from humid asthma and allergic reaction

- Nausea
- Intestinal spasm, with or without accompanying diarrhea
- Pain and inflammation from acute injuries (external)

Collection: In the spring or summer when Wolfberry's foliage is hydrated and full, collect the leaves by either stripping them from the young branches or pick individual leaf groupings where they are clustered. Be attentive to the thorns as they can prove to be an inconvenience.

Preparations and Dosage:
- FPT/DPT (50% alcohol): 20-30 drops 3 times daily
- Leaf infusion: 2-4 ounces 3 times daily
- Poultice/liniment/other external preparations: as needed

Cautions: Too much Wolfberry is apt to cause dizziness, overly dry skin and respiratory/GI tract membranes. Do not use Wolfberry during pregnancy, while nursing, or if taking anticholinergic pharmaceuticals.

Other Uses: The fruits can be eaten raw in limited quantities. Beyond a small handful, the medicinal effect of the plant may become evident. Not being the most palatable fruits, they are best cooked with other foods.

YELLOWDOCK

Polygonaceae – Buckwheat family

Rumex crispus
Curly dock, Lengua de vaca, Yerba colorado

Description: When flowering, this robust perennial can stand 5 feet tall. Yellowdock's long, lance-shaped leaves have wavy margins; they are mostly basal and form in large rosettes. As the stalk is produced, some leaves are arranged alternately along its length. The small green flowers form in dense clustered spikes. Unlike many other Docks that exhibit hook-like appendages on the seed's margins, Yellowdock's are completely smooth. After flowering, the seeds and stalks become reddish-brown.

Distribution: Yellowdock is found throughout most of North America. The plant is abundant at a great array of elevations, with the exception of extremely high elevations where low temperatures are a limiting factor. Look for this European non-native along streamsides, fields, ponds, and moist disturbed soils.

Chemistry: condensed and hydrolyzable tannins; anthraquinone pigments: nepodin, chrysophanol, physcion, and emodin; quercetin

Medicinal Uses: Yellowdock is an old-school alterative. Its primary effect is as a tonic on small and large intestinal walls. The plant has the ability through its beneficial effect on this area, particularly on small intestinal fat absorption, to lessen many skin and lymph derangements. Yellowdock is well used if there is a tendency towards eruptive and scaly skin conditions that appear to be linked to intestinal discomfort and stasis, especially from rich food consumption and nervousness. In addition, lymph enlargements are typically reduced due to Yellowdock's lipid-lymph organizational ability. Moreover, the plant improves absorption of fat-soluble vitamins. Therefore through its tonic activity it is nutritional to individuals who are dealing with functional anemia or sub-anemic tendencies.

Externally a fresh poultice of the whole plant or other topical preparations is used on many of the same conditions Yellowdock treats internally. Topically the plant works well to heal an array of chronic and acute conditions. Poorly healing ulcers and migrating itchy rashes dependent upon "bad blood", stress, Poison ivy exposure, or chemical sensitivity are Yellowdock specifics.

Indications:
♦ Skin rashes (internal and external)
♦ Skin eruptions/acne with poor fat digestion (internal and external)
♦ Fat malabsorption/nutritional malabsorption

Collection: A general rule of thumb when digging Yellowdock is, if the roots are difficult to dig and they are pigmented deep yellow-orange, then they will be strong medicine. Stronger plants will be found in drier, clay-laden, and dense soils. Yellowdock found partially submerged on streamsides is inferior.

Preparations: After cleaning the roots well, either split the taproots in ¼-½ inch strips or chop crossways into ¼-inch pieces, then dry.

Dosage:
♦ FPT/DPT (50% alcohol): 30-60 drops 3 times daily

- ◆ Fluidextract: 10-20 drops 3 times daily
- ◆ Root decoction: 4-6 ounces 3 times daily

The dosing of Yellowdock is important. In small amounts, the plant is tonic to intestinal walls, in larger amounts it is more irritative and tends to be laxative.

Cautions: Large doses should not be used during pregnancy or while nursing due to Yellowdock's anthraquinone-laxative effect.

Other Uses: The young leaves can be added to salads or cooked as a green.

YUCCA

Agavaceae – Agave family

Yucca elata
Soaptree, Spanish bayonet

Yucca schottii
Mountain yucca, Hoary yucca

Yucca baccata
Banana yucca, Blue yucca, Datil

Description: Yuccas come in all shapes and sizes. Depending on variety, at maturity their height can vary anywhere from several to 25 feet. The leaves of most Yuccas are stiff and pointed. On the tall, slender trunked varieties the old leaves have a tendency to droop downward making a protective layer over the trunk, much like an un-trimmed palm tree. All Yuccas produce a flowering stalk, if enough water and nutrients are available, upon which are borne, depending on variety, either fleshy or hard capsule-like fruits. They contain small, black, circular flattened seeds stacked in several columns. Yuccas, in the West, are long-lived perennials that are well adapted to their arid environments.

Yucca elata is tall and slender-trunked. It occasionally reaches 15 feet in height. On mature plants, 2-3 side trunks are not uncommon, although younger plants tend to have 1 small trunk. The bluish-green leaves are 10-20 inches long and very narrow with separating margin fibers. The large, showy, white flowers form from stalks that sprout during the spring. The woody capsule-like fruits contain numerous small black seeds. Y. schottii in some respects is similar to Y. elata. The plant is stout, thick trunked, and has stiff-leaves. Y. schottii reaches 20-25 feet in height and may have 2-3 trunks arising from its base, though 1 trunk is common. The long stiff leaves are stout, pointed, and 1-2 inches thick. Fleshy fruits develop after the showy, cream-colored flowers are pollinated. Y. baccata is a multi-trunked, lower-growing plant. The lower stems occasionally creep just below the ground's surface. The stiff leaves are pointed and have fibrous margins. The typical cream-colored flowers are followed by fleshy fruits.

Distribution: Yucca elata ranges from west of the Pecos River through southern New Mexico, along the Rio Grande Drainage, southeast-central Arizona, and finally to an isolated grouping in southwestern Utah. As a plant of the Desert Grasslands, it is found from 2,000-6,000 feet. Y. schottii is isolated to southeastern Arizona and southwestern New Mexico. It is a hillside and canyon plant that is commonly found throughout Desert Grasslands and Oak Woodlands; look for it from 4,000-7,000 feet. Y. baccata has the widest range of the three Yuccas profiled here. From southern Nevada, Utah, Colorado, and southeastern California it ranges south through much of Arizona, New Mexico, and southwestern Texas. Y. baccata enjoys a large array of habitat and elevation ranges; it is a common plant.

Chemistry: sapogenins: diosgenin, gitogenin, neogitogenin, hecogenin, manogenin, sarsasapogenin, smilagenin, stigmasterol, tigogenin, and neotigogenin; steroidal compounds: β-sitosterol, stigmasterol, and campesterol

Medicinal Uses: Yucca produces several therapeutic effects mainly through its influence imparted upon intestinal tract membranes and flora by its saponin content. Yucca forms complexes with abnormal colonic flora by-products rendering these toxins, to some degree, inert. Since Yucca's saponins are indigestible, the formed complexes are removed with other waste matter from the colon. Therefore, bacterial end-products are unable to exert an inflammatory effect because they literally are stuck to Yucca's saponins, making absorption into systemic circulation impossible. It is also interesting to note that constipation is often a factor in many arthritic/inflammatory conditions. When abnormal microorganisms have more time to interact negatively with intestinal waste matter there is a tendency for our internal environment to become pro-inflammatory. This is certainly one reason why laxative and liver stimulant therapies have a place in these chronic pain syndromes. Also old Mexican and White cowboys alike are known to use the plant to lessen the full body pains of years of hard work and cowboyin'.

Yucca is useful in lowering bile salt and cholesterol re-uptake by the lower duodenum. As above, the binding effect of these saponins subsequently can lower blood triglyceride and cholesterol levels. High protein/high fat/low carbohydrate diet followers will benefit from Yucca's effective binding of ammonia in the colon, allowing it to pass out with the feces and not be reabsorbed through the portal circulation. Thus, liver stress in response to a high protein diet, will diminish. Ammonia, one of the end results of protein breakdown is converted from urea in the colon by colonic flora. If the liver is not able to reconvert ammonia back to urea, because of large protein qualities from diet or impaired renal or liver function, resulting ammonia toxicities can ensue.

Indications:
♦ Rheumatoid arthritis
♦ Chronic pain, dependent upon constipation
♦ Elevated LDL levels, triglycerides

Collection: Collect the roots and lower trunk in the fall. Yucca's saponin content varies in response to season and species. The highest yields are in the fall when the plant draws back in and again starts the cycle of accumulation for next years spring growth. The lower-growing, multi-trunked varieties, such as Yucca baccata, with more substantial trunk/root networks, not only are easier to collect but overall are less damaged by collection.

Preparations: Chop the gathered material into ¼-½ inch pieces. Lay out on a flat to dry if in an arid place or if in a more humid environment use a dehydrator. Either way the root will dry quickly given its porous nature.

Dosage:
♦ Root decoction: 4-6 ounces 2-3 times daily
♦ DPT (50% alcohol): 30-60 drops 2-3 times daily
♦ Fluidextract: 10-20 drops 2-3 times daily
♦ '00' capsules: 2-3, 2-3 times daily
It is best to approach Yucca as a short-term plant used concurrently for 3-4 weeks. If longer term use is needed try a rotation of Yucca for 3-4 weeks followed by 1 week of Creosote bush or Figwort.

Cautions: Used in excessive quantities Yucca can cause intestinal distress. Do not use during pregnancy, due to the plant's potential altering effect on reproductive hormones.

Other Uses: 1-2 ounces of the powdered root can be added to water making a useable soap/shampoo. The fruits from the fleshy varieties are sweet and edible. Collect and eat when small brown marks of sugar fermentation are just starting to appear on the outer light green surface of the fruit skin. According to Peter Bigfoot, a seasoned herbalist who lives in the Superstition Mountains of Arizona, the seeds will cause diarrhea.

FAMILY GROUPINGS

Agave family
Beargrass, Yucca

Barberry family
Desert barberry

Bignonia family
Desert willow, Trumpet flower

Borage family
Purple gromwell

Buckwheat family
Desert rhubarb, Flat-top buckwheat, Yellowdock

Buttercup family
Clematis, Desert anemone

Cactus family
Jumping cholla, Prickly pear, Night blooming cereus

Caltrop family
Caltrop, Creosote bush, Puncturevine, Syrian rue

Cashew family
Sumac

Cypress family
Cypress, Juniper

Dogbane family
Periwinkle

Figwort family
Penstemon
Honeysuckle family
Elder

Geranium family
Filaree

Grass family
Wild oats

Heath family
Manzanita

Horsetail family
Horsetail

Joint-fir family

Mormon tea

Jojoba family
Jojoba

Lily family
Aloe

Madder family
Buttonbush

Mallow family
Desert cotton, Globemallow, Mallow

Milkweed family
Antelope horns, Desert milkweed

Mint family
Desert lavender, Desert oregano,
Horehound, Sage

Mustard family
Peppergrass

Nightshade family
Datura, Tobacco, Wolfberry

Ocotillo family
Ocotillo

Olive family
Velvet ash

Pea family
Acacia, Bird of paradise,
Kidneywood, Mesquite, Mimosa,
Senna, Wild licorice

Passionflower family
Passionflower

Peony family
Western peony

Pink family
Chickweed

Plantain family
Plantain

Plumbago family
Leadwort

Poppy family
California poppy, Golden smoke,
Prickly poppy

Ratany family
Ratany

Simarouba family
Tree of heaven

Soapberry family
Hopbush, Soapberry

Spurge family
Copperleaf, Limberbush

Sunflower family
Baccharis, Bricklebush, Brittlebush,
Burrobrush, Camphorweed, Canadian
fleabane, Canyon bursage,
Chinchweed, Cocklebur, Crownbeard,
Cudweed, Dandelion, Deerweed,
Dogweed, Greenthread, Marsh

L3siIjoi

fleabane, Mountain Marigold,
Rayweed, Sagebrush, Snakeweed,
Spanish needles, Tarbush, Trixis,
Turpentine bush, Western Mugwort,
Wild lettuce

Tamarisk family
Tamarisk

Vervain family
Chaste tree, Verbena

Walnut family
Canyon walnut

Willow family
Cottonwood, Western black willow

THERAPEUTIC INDEX

Cardiovascular

Angina pectoris (Puncturevine)

Cardiac weakness, from age/tobacco heart (Antelope horns, Desert milkweed, Night blooming cereus)

Hypertension, essential (Puncturevine, Spanish needles)

Leg heaviness, fatigue, and fluid retention (Beargrass, Ocotillo)

Tachycardia with hypertension and forceful pulse (Passionflower)

Gastrointestinal

Amebiasis (Cypress, Desert barberry, Sagebrush, Soapberry, Tree of heaven, Western mugwort)

Constipation (Aloe, Buttonbush, Rayweed, Senna, Velvet ash, Wild licorice)

Cramps, intestinal (Baccharis, Burrobrush, Canyon bursage, Canyon walnut, Datura, Hopbush, Passionflower, Prickly poppy, Sage, Sagebrush, Wolfberry)

Diarrhea (Bird of paradise, Caltrop, Canadian fleabane, Cocklebur, Flat-top buckwheat, Jojoba, Jumping cholla, Limberbush, Ratany, Sumac, Tree of heaven)

Diarrhea with intestinal cramps (Bricklebush, Chinchweed, Marsh fleabane)

Dyspepsia (Desert anemone, Bricklebush, Buttonbush, Cottonwood, Dandelion, Desert barberry, Golden smoke, Horehound, Rayweed, Tarbush, Trumpet creeper, Verbena, Western mugwort, Wild licorice)

Dyspepsia with bloating (Chinchweed, Deerweed, Desert oregano, Dogweed, Juniper, Mountain marigold, Peppergrass, Sagebrush)

Food poisoning (Cypress, Desert barberry, Sagebrush)

Gastritis (Baccharis, Bird of paradise, Bricklebush, Caltrop, Crownbeard, Dogweed, Jumping cholla, Mallow, Mormon tea, Mountain marigold,

Prickly pear, Spanish needles, Trumpet flower, Western Mugwort, Wild licorice)
Giardiasis (Cypress, Desert barberry, Tree of heaven)
Hemorrhoids (Crownbeard, Datura, Ocotillo, Ratany, Tobacco)
Hemorrhoids, bleeding (Periwinkle, Ratany)
Hiccups (Chinchweed)
Inflammation, intestinal (Baccharis, Bird of paradise, Caltrop, Canadian fleabane, Canyon walnut, Chickweed, Horsetail, Marsh fleabane, Plantain, Spanish needles, Tree of heaven, Western mugwort)
Infection, Candida albicans (Canyon walnut, Desert willow, Trumpet flower)
Malabsorption, nutrient/lipid (Buttonbush, Canyon walnut, Dandelion, Yellowdock)
Ulcer, duodenal (Baccharis, Spanish needles)
Ulcer, gastric (Crownbeard, Prickly pear, Spanish needles, Wild licorice)
Ulcer, peptic (Aloe, Desert lavender, Horsetail, Jumping cholla)
Worms (Sagebrush, Western mugwort)

Liver-Gallbladder
Congestion, liver and gallbladder (Bricklebush, Buttonbush, Dandelion, Desert barberry, Rayweed, Sagebrush, Tarbush, Velvet ash)
Inflammation, liver (Dandelion, Desert barberry, Western mugwort)
Spasm, gall bladder (Hopbush)

Lymph-Immune
Skin conditions from allergy or autoimmune disturbances, chronic (Golden smoke)
Enlargements, lymph node (Golden smoke, Ocotillo)

Men
Debility, genital (Desert anemone)
Irritation, genital, resulting in excessive sexual activity and preoccupation (Western black willow)
Herpes simplex virus, type II (Creosote bush, Crownbeard, Western mugwort)
Libido, decreased (Desert anemone, Puncturevine)
Prostatitis (Cypress, Cottonwood, Ocotillo, Western black willow)
Sperm count, low and poor quality (Puncturevine)
Spermatorrhea (Western black willow)
Warts, genital (Creosote bush, Cypress)

Metabolic

Hyperglycemia-NIDDM (Aloe, Bricklebush, Prickly pear, Trumpet flower)

Gout (Dandelion, Prickly pear)

LDL levels, elevated (Prickly pear, Yucca)

Mouth and Throat

Gingivitis (Cypress)

Gums, spongy and bleeding (Limberbush, Ratany, Sumac)

Periodontitis (Ratany)

Sores, mouth (Desert rhubarb, Limberbush, Mesquite, Mimosa, Ratany, Tamarisk)

Strep throat (Cypress, Desert barberry, Sage)

Sore throat-general (Cypress, Desert barberry, Desert rhubarb, Filaree, Jojoba, Mesquite, Sage, Sumac, Tamarisk)

Nervous System

Depression (Desert anemone, Syrian rue, Wild oats)

Insomnia/anxiety (California poppy, Desert lavender, Passionflower, Prickly poppy, Verbena, Wild lettuce, Wild oats)

Memory loss/poor cognition/Alzheimer's (Sage)

Seizure activity/tremors/tics (Golden smoke, Passionflower, Tree of heaven, Turpentine bush, Western peony)

Pain

Arthritis, general (Desert anemone, Brittlebush, Clematis, Cottonwood, Peppergrass, Snakeweed, Soapberry)

Arthritis, rheumatoid (Beargrass, Clematis, Creosote bush, Soapberry, Yucca)

Injury, acute, with pain (California poppy, Prickly poppy, Camphorweed, Cottonwood, Wolfberry)

Injury, acute, with pain and unbroken skin (Datura, Tobacco)

Muscular pain, chronic (Snakeweed)

Headache, migraine, beginning stages (Clematis, Desert anemone)

Headache, migraine, acute pain (Periwinkle)

Headache, general (Peppergrass)

Headache, stress (Verbena)

Spasm, muscle, from injury (Datura, Passionflower)

Renal-Urinary

Debility, general (Desert anemone)

Fluid retention (Elder, Filaree, Horehound, Horsetail, Prickly pear)

Incontinence/bed wetting from lack of bladder tone (Cypress)

Inflammation/pain, lower urinary tract (Chickweed, Cocklebur, Filaree, Flat-top buckwheat, Globemallow, Horsetail, Jumping cholla, Kidneywood, Mallow, Mormon tea, Plantain)

Inflammation/pain, lower urinary tract, weakened tissues (Cypress, Juniper, Western black willow)

Inflammation with haematuria (Filaree, Horsetail, Periwinkle, Ratany, Spanish needles)

Infection, alkaline urine (Manzanita)

Infection, general (Cypress, Juniper)

Kidney stones, general (Kidneywood)

Kidney stones, preventative (Horsetail, Jumping cholla, Mallow, Puncturevine)

Kidney stones, uric acid (Dandelion, Jumping cholla, Kidneywood, Prickly pear)

Nephritis, acute (Globemallow, Mallow)

Nephritis, chronic (Cottonwood, Juniper, Kidneywood, Wild licorice)

Respiratory (Lower)

Asthma, copious phlegm (Horehound, Wolfberry)

Asthma, dry, non-spasmodic (Antelope horns, Desert milkweed)

Asthma, general (Creosote bush, Datura)

Bronchitis with copious phlegm and weak cough (Cypress)

Bronchitis with difficult expectoration (Antelope horns, Cudweed, Desert milkweed, Horehound, Ocotillo, Sagebrush)

Bronchitis with dry fever (Cudweed, Horehound, Sagebrush)

Cough, dry and painful (Cudweed, Globemallow, Mallow, Plantain, Wild licorice)

Cough, spasmodic (California poppy, Passionflower, Prickly poppy, Western peony, Wild lettuce)

Hemorrhaging, passive (Horsetail, Ratany)

Pleurisy (Antelope horns, Desert milkweed)

Respiratory (Upper) and Eyes

Conjunctivitis (Desert anemone, Caltrop, Mesquite, Prickly poppy, Spanish needles)

Glaucoma (Desert anemone)

Rhinitis (Brittlebush, Burrobrush, Canyon bursage, Cocklebur, Mormon tea, Wolfberry)
Sinusitis (Canyon bursage, Burrobrush, Cocklebur, Desert barberry)
Styes (Desert anemone, Prickly poppy)

Skin
Abscess (Globemallow, Copperleaf, Leadwort, Mallow)
Actinic keratosis (Creosote bush)
Bedsores (Copperleaf, Cypress, Leadwort)
Bites, insect, venomous (Creosote bush)
Bites, stings (Bird of paradise, Chickweed, Creosote bush, Flat-top buckwheat, Hopbush, Penstemon, Plantain, Tobacco)
Boils (Mallow)
Burns form heat and sunburn (Aloe, Chickweed, Crownbeard, Datura, Jumping cholla, Prickly pear, Prickly poppy)
Candida infections (Cypress, Desert lavender, Desert willow, Hopbush, Trumpet flower)
Chicken pox (Crownbeard)
Contusions (Aloe, Prickly pear, Sagebrush, Wolfberry)
Dermatitis, dry scabby (Cypress)
Eczema (Creosote bush, Juniper, Puncturevine, Purple gromwell)
Herpes simplex virus, type I (Creosote bush, Crownbeard, Western mugwort)
Hives, Rashes (Bird of paradise, Burrobrush, Caltrop, Canyon bursage, Chickweed, Desert rhubarb, Filaree, Flat-top buckwheat, Golden smoke, Hopbush, Jojoba, Penstemon, Puncturevine, Yellowdock)
Infections, bacterial – Aloe, Creosote bush, California poppy, Cypress, Desert barberry, Desert lavender, Hopbush, Prickly poppy, Purple gromwell, Sagebrush, Syrian rue, Western mugwort)
Infections, fungal (Aloe, Antelope horns, California poppy, Creosote bush, Cypress, Desert barberry, Desert milkweed, Purple gromwell, Sagebrush, Syrian rue, Tarbush, Western mugwort)
Poison ivy reactions, systemic (Brittlebush)
Poorly healing tissue with tendency towards ulceration (Golden smoke)
Psoriasis (Creosote bush, Desert barberry, Juniper, Puncturevine, Purple gromwell)
Shingles (Crownbeard)
Scrapes, abrasions, cuts – Acacia, Aloe, Baccharis, Bird of paradise, California poppy, Cocklebur, Cottonwood, Crownbeard, Desert lavender, Desert

rhubarb, Flat-top buckwheat, Hopbush, Limberbush, Marsh fleabane, Mesquite, Mimosa, Mountain marigold, Penstemon, Plantain, Prickly pear, Prickly poppy, Snakeweed, Spanish needles, Sumac, Tamarisk, Tarbush)

Splinters (Globemallow, Copperleaf, Leadwort, Mallow)

Ulcers, poorly healing (Copperleaf, Cypress, Leadwort)

Varicosities/spider veins (Beargrass, Prickly pear)

Vitiligo (Puncturevine)

Warts, common (Antelope horns, Cypress, Creosote bush, Desert milkweed)

Wounds (Aloe, Horsetail, Marsh fleabane, Penstemon, Plantain, Purple gromwell, Sagebrush, Spanish needles, Tarbush, Trixis)

Wounds, poorly healing (Copperleaf, Cypress, Elder, Leadwort, Mountain marigold, Prickly pear, Turpentine bush, Velvet ash)

Women

Anovulatory cycles (Chaste tree)

Cramps, uterine (Desert anemone, Datura, Hopbush, Western peony)

Cramps, uterine with pelvic congestion (Canyon bursage, Burrobrush, Sagebrush, Turpentine bush)

Fibroids, breast and uterine (Desert cotton)

Fibroids, uterine, subserous (Chaste tree)

Herpes simplex virus, type II (Creosote bush, Crownbeard, Western mugwort)

Irritation, genital, resulting in excessive sexual activity and preoccupation (Western black willow)

Inflammation, vaginal and cervical (Filaree, Manzanita)

Lactation, insufficient (Chaste tree, Verbena)

Lactation, to lessen (Sage)

Labor, slowed (Antelope horns, Desert milkweed)

Libido, decreased (Desert anemone)

Menstruation, heavy (Chaste tree, Caltrop, Filaree, Periwinkle, Ratany)

Menstruation, slowed (Desert anemone, Antelope horns, Desert cotton, Desert milkweed, Peppergrass, Sagebrush, Turpentine bush, Western mugwort)

Perimenopause (Chaste tree)

Premenstrual discomfort with breast tenderness, agitation, and anxiety (Chaste tree)

Post-partum tonic (Manzanita)

Warts, genital (Creosote bush, Cypress)

Miscellaneous

Connective tissues, hair, nails, skin, and bones, weakened (Horsetail)

Fever, dry, low-moderate temperature (Desert lavender, Elder, Marsh fleabane, Mountain marigold, Sage, Verbena, Western mugwort)

Fever with autoimmune inflammation (Desert barberry)

Fevers with moderately high temperature, dry skin, strong determination of blood (Cottonwood, Sagebrush, Syrian rue)

Sweating, colliquative (Cocklebur, Sage)

Valley fever (Cypress Desert willow)

GLOSSARY

Abscess: an accumulation of pus (defunct leucocytes, damaged tissue cells, and cellular wastes) within tissues or organs either resolving by coming to "a head" or diminishing internally.

Acetylcholinesterase (AchE): an enzyme of the central nervous system that breaks down acetylcholine into choline and acetate.

Achene: a term used to describe a seed common to the Sunflower family.

Adrenaline: (Epinephrine) both a catecholamine hormone and a neurotransmitter. It is secreted by the adrenal medulla and is used by the sympathetic branch of the central nervous system. It is a prominent physiologic agent in flight or flight reactions and low-grade stress states.

Albumin: a plasma protein crucial in transporting many organic substances – bile acids, hormones, and fatty acids. It is also important in maintaining proper plasma osmotic pressure. Plasma albumin levels diminish in certain renal and hepatic diseases, as well as if dietary levels of protein are insufficient.

Allopathic: pertaining to present day conventional medicine when solely used to suppress or oppose symptoms, such as steroids for inflammation, analgesics for pain, etc.

Alterative: pertaining to the quality, or a substance (usually an herbal medicine) that positively alters organs or functions of elimination, detoxification, or immunity.

Alveoli: (pulmonary alveoli) small sacs within the lungs where carbon dioxide and oxygen exchange takes place.

Alzheimer's disease: a progressive brain disease with a number of potential causative factors. Senile plaques, neurofibrillary tangles, and loss of acetyltransferase activity are common. Progressed effects are dementia and personality change.

Amebiasis: (montezuma's revenge or traveler's diarrhea) an intestinal infection involving Entamoeba histolytica from contaminated food or water. Usually the large intestine is affected but in severe cases infection can migrate to the liver, spleen, brain, lungs, and other areas.

Amenorrhea: the abnormal cessation of menses, often due to extreme weight loss, physical-emotional stress or the alteration of ovarian hormones.

Anaphrodisiac: that which curbs libido.

Angina pectoris: a particular spasmodic, suffocative pain due to heart tissue ischemia; radiating left arm pain is common as well. It may be precipitated by physical exertion and is caused by coronary artery obstruction from plaque buildup.

Annual: any plant that germinates, then sets seed and dies in one year.

Anovulatory cycle: a menstrual cycle without ovulation.

Anticholinergic: inhibiting to the parasympathetic nervous system; pertaining to any substance whether pharmaceutical, herbal, or otherwise that lessens gastrointestinal tract, mucosal, and skin secretion and excretion.

Antiviral: inhibiting to virus reproduction or cellular attachment.

Aphthous stomatitis: (Canker sores) a small white ulcer of the oral mucosa. Stress, immune deficiency, and allergic reaction are common underlying factors.

Asthma: a condition of bronchial constriction due to spasm or autoimmune inflammation.

Asthma, humid: Asthma with copious expectoration.

Ayurveda: traditional Indian medicine, thought to predate Traditional Chinese Medicine; the system also describes herbs as having energetic qualities and people being of three different constitutional types.

Bifidobacteria: one of a number of gram-positive, anaerobic bacteria belonging to the Bifidobacterium genus. Common species found in the large bowel are B. adolescentis, B. erikosnii, and B. infantis.

Bile: an alkaline liquid secreted by the liver composed of cholesterol, bile salts, phospholipids, bilirubin diglucuronide, and electrolytes necessary in fat digestion.

Boil: (furuncle) a painful, subcutaneous nodule with an enclosed core. Usually caused by Staphylococci entering through hair follicles. Liver and immune deficiencies are common constitutional factors.

Bract: a modified leaf situated at the base of a flower.

Bronchitis: mechanical, bacterial, viral, or allergy induced inflammation of one or more bronchi.

Canker sores: see Aphthous stomatitis

Cardiac glycoside: glycosides found in some Cactus, Figwort, Dogbane, and Lily family plants. In therapeutic doses, they are slowing and strengthening to the heart.

Carminative: a term used to describe a medicine that relieves gas pains and bloating.

Catkin: (ament) a compact male or female, spike-like inflorescence, typically found in Willow or Birch family plants.

Chicken pox: (varicella-zoster) a contagious herpes virus causing reddened and itching vesicles, normally affecting children.

Cholecystokinin (CCK): both a hormone secreted by the upper small intestine and by the hypothalamus as a neurotransmitter. It stimulates gallbladder contractions, secretion of pancreatic enzymes and is involved in feelings of satiety and fullness in response to food.

Cholesterol: a common sterol produced by the liver and obtained from the diet; it is involved in cell-membrane structure, and is also a base for steroidal hormones and the precursor in bile formation. It is a contributing factor in arterial plaques and in some gallstones.

Cholagogue: any substance that stimulates bile release from the gallbladder; many of these herbs are choleretics as well, stimulating bile synthesis in the liver.

Coccidioides immitis: the fungus responsible for Coccidioidomycosis or Valley fever.

Coccidioidomycosis: (Valley fever) the disease caused by Coccidioides immitis. Primary manifestations are cough, fever, and joint pain. The infection is usually self-resolving but can be serious in some racial groups and immune compromised individuals.

Collagenation: the process of collagen formation in cartilage or other tissues.

Colonic flora: bacterial strains existing in the large intestine, many of which are necessary for gastrointestinal and systemic health.

Condyloma acuminatum: (venereal or genital warts) caused from Human papillomavirus (HPV). It is infectious, sexually transmitted and predisposes women to cervical dysplasia. Infections are on the rise, as with most other STD's, mainly through relaxed mores.

Conjunctivitis: an inflammation of the conjunctiva, typically involving redness, swelling, and discharge. There can be bacterial, viral, mechanical, or allergic involvement.

Cyclooxygenase: an enzyme or activity involved in prostaglandin synthesis, particularly inflammatory processes.

Cystitis: inflammation of the urinary bladder.

Deciduous: describing a plant that is not evergreen; herbage falling from the plant seasonally.

Dehydroepiandrosterone (DHEA): An adrenal cortex steroid hormone. It plays a large role as an androgen precursor in premenopausal women and as a major androgen in postmenopausal women. Supplementation in women can often cause masculine tendencies.

Diaphoresis: perspiration or sweating.

Diaphoretic: a substance that promotes sweating (diaphoresis) or the activity of something that promotes sweating.

Dioecious: imperfect male and female flowers borne on different plants.

Diuretic: a substance that promotes urine excretion or the activity of increasing urine excretion.

Duodenal ulcer: an ulcer of the upper small intestine or duodenum.

Dust cells: (Alveolar macrophage or Alveolar phagocyte) a phagocyte that resides within the lung's alveoli; they ingest inhaled particulate matter and are important in pulmonary immunity.

Dyspepsia: faulty digestion, resulting in discomfort, gas, and sometimes, gastrointestinal tract stasis.

Edema: increased intercellular fluid buildup from numerous causes, but typically from kidney or heart dysfunction, or venous or lymphatic obstruction.

Emmenagogue: something that induces menstruation.

Endometrium: inner mucus membrane layer of the uterus.

Entamoeba histolytica: a common ameboid protozoa; the cause of amebiasis. Severe infections may affect the lungs, liver, spleen, and other organs.

Entire: referring to the margin of a leaf; not toothed, lobed, or divided, but continuous.

Escherichia coli: a gram negative, anaerobic bacterium normally found in the large intestine. The organism typically causes urinary tract infections. Colonization often takes place through poor hygiene and alkaline urine.

Essential hypertension: (idiopathic or primary hypertension) elevated blood pressure without organic causes. It is largely a functional problem with sodium intake, weight, and stress being primary causative agents.

Essential oil: non-polar, volatile oil content of an aromatic plant. Commonly extracted through distillation. Mint family plants are typical subjects.

Eupatory tribe: a division of the Sunflower family. Plants in this division are apt to contain either toxic or non-toxic pyrrolizidine alkaloids. Brickellia and Eupatorium geneses are both in this tribe.

Extracellular fluid: pertaining to fluid outside of a cell, such as lymphatic fluid.

Flavonoids: a group of phenolic compounds closely related to tannins; many have therapeutic effects on cell/tissue structure.

Follicle stimulating hormone (FSH): a pituitary hormone necessary for women's follicle maturation and in men, proper spermatogenesis.

Gastritis: simply inflammation of the stomach often caused from stress, poor diet, mechanical insults, or pharmaceutical side effects.

Gastroenteritis: inflammation of the stomach and intestinal lining. It can be viral or bacterial initiated, and in some cases, is triggered by intense adrenergic reactions. It is most commonly the result of food poisoning.

Genital warts: See Condyloma acuminatum

Giardia: a parasite in humans and in other invertebrates, commonly spread by contaminated food, water, and direct human/animal contact. Giardia lamblia is the most notorious species. The organism attaches itself to the microvilli of the intestinal walls causing diarrhea, nausea, weight loss, and fatigue among other symptoms.

Gingivitis: An acute or chronic inflammation of the gingivae or gums, caused through a number of factors.

Glomerulonephritis: autoimmune mediated or from a residual hemolytic infection causing kidney inflammation with accompanying inflammation of the capillary structures in the glomeruli of the kidney.

Glucose-6-phosphate-dehydrogenase deficiency (G6PD): a genetic deficiency causing, to varying degrees, hemolytic anemia.

Glycogen: The primary storage carbohydrate found in liver and muscle tissue. It is broken down into glucose.

Granulocyte: typically a neutrophil, basophil, or eosinophil (all white blood cells) that contain immuniologic granules that when released heighten inflammatory-defense processes.

Helicobacter pylori: (Campylobacter pylori) a gram-negative bacterium involved in gastric ulcer formation and gastritis.

Hemolysis: the break down of red blood cell membranes resulting in the liberation of hemoglobin. This can be caused from a myriad of factors but most predominantly, it is triggered by an autoimmune reaction, exposures to certain snake venoms, microorganisms, and other substances such as saponins from some Agaves. **Intravascular:** severe red blood cell breakdown within blood vessels.

Hemostatic: an activity or something that slows or stops blood flow; typically astringents or other substances that have a localized or systemic vasoconstrictive effect.

Herpes zoster: (see Shingles)

Hydrochloric acid (HCl): solutions of hydrogen chloride secreted by gastric parietal cells in response to hormonal, local, or nervous system stimulation; necessary for initial protein breakdown in the stomach.

Hypertension: (see Essential hypertension)

Immunoglobulin E (IgE): An antibody that has a significant role in allergic process.

Insulin dependent diabetes mellitus (IDDM): (Juvenile onset or Type I) onset usually occurs in late childhood or in the early teens and is characterized by the destruction of the pancreatic beta cells by viral infection or autoimmune reactions; there is some genetic predisposition as well. Lack of endogenous insulin is the hallmark of IDDM. Reliance upon exogenous insulin is necessary, otherwise hyperglycemia and corresponding problems result. IDDM is difficult, if not nearly impossible to treat solely with natural therapies.

Interleukin: a broad group of immunologic compounds (cytokines); many are produced by T-cells and macrophages. They are involved in an array of immunologic activities, including inflammatory responses.

Interstitial fluid: fluid of lymph between cells or tissue; as opposed to intracellular fluid.

Intraocular pressure: pressure within the eye; when elevated it is associated with glaucoma.

Involucre: a whorl of bracts at the base of a flower.

Isotonic: a solution that has the same tonicity as the tissues that are exposed to it. Most notable are eyewash solutions that have roughly the same tonicity/salinity as ocular membranes or tears.

Lactobacillus: a genus of naturally occurring bacteria found in the mouth, intestine, and vagina. In proper concentrations the bacteria plays a role in surrounding tissue health.

Latex: a milky sap from a plant.

Leukocyte: (white blood cell) a granular or nongranular type cell, largely involved in immunologic processes.

Lutenizing hormone (LH): a pituitary hormone that promotes ovulation and progesterone secretion. In men, it is important in the formation of the Leydig cells of the testes.

Macrophage: a mononuclear phagocyte widely distributed throughout varying tissues. It comprises one of the first lines of defense in response to pathogens; part of the body's innate cellular immunity.

Malaria: an infectious disease caused by the protozoa genus Plasmodium. It is transmitted through mosquito bites.

Melanocyte: surface skin cells that synthesize the pigment melanin.

Menorrhagia: painful menstruation.

Menorrhea: excess menstruation.

Mineralocorticoids: mainly aldosterone secreted by the adrenal cortex necessary in proper water and electrolyte balance. This group of adrenal hormones causes water and sodium retention and potassium loss.

Monoecious: Separate male and female flowers borne on the same plant.

Montezuma's revenge: see Amebiasis.

Mucin: the main component of mucus; composed of glycoproteins, glycolipids, and polysaccharides.

Mucus: composed of mucin, inorganic salts, and leucocytes. It is secreted by mucus membranes and is necessary for proper functioning of many organs and tissue groups.

Nephron: a functional unit of the kidney. The majority of renal activities are carried out by nephrons.

Nightshade alkaloids: alkaloids found in the Nightshade family. Many of these compounds have profound anticholinergic effects. Atropine and scopolamine are two of these compounds that are still used in conventional medicine.

Nocturnal emissions: (See Spermatorrhea)

Non-insulin dependent diabetes mellitus (NIDDM): (Adult onset or Type II) mostly a result of a sedentary lifestyle and poor dietary choices, although there is some genetic predisposition. Typically, insulin levels are normal or even elevated. The situation is closely related to the notorious "Syndrome X". If insulin sensitivity is left impaired, cardiovascular and peripheral nervous system disturbances can ensue. With adherence to diet, lifestyle, and other natural therapies, reversing the situation is likely.

Norepinephrine: (Noradrenaline) a catecholamine acting as a hormone and as a neurotransmitter. Secreted by the adrenal medulla and the sympathetic nervous system; it is largely involved in stress (fight or flight) reactions.

Also it is one of the most likely catecholamines to be involved in functional imbalances that can be influenced with herbal medicines.

Oblanceolate: being generally lance shaped, but slightly rounded towards the end of the leaf and narrower towards the leaf stem.

Panicles: flowers maturing in branched groupings from the bottom of the cluster, up.

Parasympathetic: the cholinergic branch of the autonomic nervous system involved in rest, repair, and nutritive functions of the body.

Parenchymal cells: functional cells of an organ or group of tissues, as opposed to structural cells.

Pepsin: a proteolytic enzyme derived from pepsinogen by hydrochloric acid. It is responsible for the bulk of gastric protein breakdown into smaller peptides.

Perennial: a plant that lives three years or more.

Perimenopause: the period before menopause when reproductive hormones and their effects within the body become irregular.

Periodontitis: inflammation of the tissues surrounding the teeth, often a progression of chronic gingivitis. It can ultimately cause tooth and bone loss.

Petiole: a leaf stalk.

Phagocytosis: a process by which white blood cells – macrophages and neutrophils – engulf and eliminate particulate material or microorganisms deemed harmful to the internal environment.

Pimples: a pustule usually on the upper parts of the body, commonly a result of Acne vulgaris.

Pinnae: (Pinna) a leaflet of a pinnate leaf.

Pinnatifid: pinnately cleft, narrow lobes of a leaf not reaching the mid-vein.

Pinworms: (Enterobius vermicularis, formally called Ascaris vermicularis or Oxyuris vermicularis) Nematode type worms that can colonize the upper large intestine; common in children and causes anal itching. Infection can occasionally spread to female genitals and bladder.

Pistillate: used to describe a female flower. A flower lacking stamens.

Placenta: a temporary organ that forms between the mother and fetus. It provides blood borne nutrients, hormones, and other necessary substances for the fetus's development.

Plasmodium falciparum: the main protozoa that causes malaria.

Pleurisy: an acute or chronic inflammation of the lung and thoracic cavity's serous membrane or pleura. Fever, dry cough, and stitch in the side are common symptoms.

Progesterone: a reproductive hormone secreted by the corpus luteum, placenta, and in small quantities, by the adrenal cortex. Aside from uterine preparatory and pregnancy sustaining effects, altered circulating levels of the hormone is a factor in premenstrual discomforts and menstrual cycle irregularities.

Prolactin: traditionally defined as a hormone secreted by the anterior pituitary responsible for lactation. Recent research suggests the hormone has a broader role in chronic stress states.

Prostaglandin: a diverse group of naturally occurring compounds involved in a wide array of physiological responses. Many are pro-inflammatory, cellular excitants.

Prostatitis: inflammation of the prostate.

Proteolytic enzymes: enzymes that breaks down proteins into smaller polypeptides by splitting peptide bonds. In supplement form they are used as digestive aids and as antiinflammatories.

Protozoa: simple, single celled organisms; many are parasitic.

Pyrrolizidine alkaloids: a group of compounds common in the Sunflower and Borage families responsible for liver inflammation and subsequent hepatocyte breakdown.

Reye's syndrome: usually occurring as a result of an acute viral infection (often respiratory centered or associated with chicken pox). Fever, vomiting, elevated liver enzyme levels, and brain swelling are common. This childhood syndrome is rare, but can result in seizures and death. Aspirin use in febrile conditions has been linked as a causative factor.

Rheumatoid arthritis: chronic joint inflammation usually affecting the hands and feet. It is autoimmune mediated and if left untreated leads to lack of mobility and joint deformation.

Rhinitis: inflammation of nasal mucus membranes; a typical hayfever response.

Roundworm: (nematode) an organism from the nematode class; many are intestinal parasites.

Rubefacient: something that reddens the skin by causing blood movement to that area, commonly through vasodilation; a reddening of the skin.

Salmonella: a genus of gram-negative bacteria. Many species cause gastroenteritis and fever, better known as food poisoning.

Samara: a winged fruit, common in the Fraxinus and the Ailanthus genuses.

Seborrheic dermatitis: (cradle cap, seborrheic eczema, or seborrhea) a chronic skin condition characterized by redness and yellow scaly patches on the trunk, groin, face, and/or scalp. Allergic and constitutional factors are involved.

Serrate: designating a toothed margin; saw-like.

Shigella: a gram-negative genus in the Enterobacteria family. Many cause severe diarrhea/dysentery.

Shingles: (Herpes zoster) more common in the elderly and in immune compromised individuals, shingles manifests as nerve pain and corresponding vesicles over affected dermatomes. Occurrence is normally on only one side of the body and is thought to involve expression of latent varicella-zoster virus – called H. opthalmicus when the virus affects the trigeminal nerve.

Simple: an undivided leaf that is not separated into leaflets. Describing an herb used singly, not in formula.

Sinusitis: inflammation of the sinuses. Typical causes are allergic reaction or bacterial, viral, or fungal infections. Poor tissue health and local immunity are predisposing factors to reoccurring infections.

Spermatorrhea: involuntary and excessive discharge of semen without copulation; excessive wet dreams or nocturnal emission.

Spikelet: the flower cluster of grasses and sedges, or a secondary spike.

Staminate: used to describe a male flower bearing only stamens, not pistils.

Staphylococcus: a genus of gram-positive, anaerobic bacteria; many are pathogenic.

Strep throat: Streptococcus infection affecting the throat.

Streptococcus: a gram-positive genus of bacteria. To varying degrees most species are pathogenic, notably S. pyogenes.

Sudorific: diaphoretic; an agent that causing sweating.

Tepals: a specialized sepal or petal; common in the Passionflower family.

Testosterone: a major male sex hormone produced in the testes. It is crucial for bone and muscle growth in the male as it is for sperm formation.

Thyroid stimulating hormone (TSH): (Thytotropin) a pituitary hormone that is necessary in the thyroid's normal functioning. Low levels can be an indicator of hyperthyroidism.

Tobacco heart: cardiovascular weakness caused from years of smoking.

Tonsillitis: inflammation of the small rounded masses of lymph tissue (palatine tonsils) located near the back of the tongue. This normally occurs through heightened leukocyte activity.

Traveler's diarrhea: See Amebiasis

Ulcerative colitis: (crone's disease) chronic inflammation effecting the mucosa and submucosa of the colon wall. Symptoms of abdominal pain, diarrhea, stool with blood, and mucus are common. Autoimmune involvement is typical. It is unrelated to irritable bowel syndrome, which is a functional problem.

Urethritis: inflammation of the urethra (a urinary tract tube leading from the bladder to the body's exterior).

Vagus nerve: a key parasympathetic cranial nerve involved in viscera innervation. It affects the digestive tract, lungs, heart, liver, and other areas. Certain herbs (Asclepias spp.) stimulate vagus nerve function, particularly when digestive function is depressed by adrenaline stress.

Vermifuge: an agent that kills or expels parasites.

Verruca vulgaris: common wart.

Vitiligo: a chronic pigmentary disorder resulting in depigmented skin. A hyperpigmented border may surround these white patches. It is possibly autoimmune mediated with some genetic predisposition.

Volatile oil: non-polar aromatics that disperse easily through sun exposure or through other forms of heat such as boiling.

White blood cell: (See leukocyte)

BIBLIOGRAPHY

Botany

Benson, Lyman and Robert A. Darrow. *Trees and Shrubs of the Southwestern Deserts*, 3rd. ed. Tucson: The University of Arizona Press, 1945.

Harris, James G. and Melinda Woolf Harris. *Plant Identification Terminology an Illustrated Glossary*. Spring Lake: Spring Lake Publishing, 1994.

Hopkins, William G. *Introduction to Plant Physiology*. 2nd ed. New York: John Wiley and Sons Inc., 1995.

Jaeger, Edmund C. *Desert Wildflowers.* 2nd ed. Stanford University: Stanford University Press, 1940.

Kearney, Thomas H., and Robert H. Peebles. *Arizona Flora*, 2nd. ed. Berkeley and Los Angeles: University of California Press, 1951.

McDougall, W.B. *Seed Plants of Northern Arizona*. Flagstaff: The Museum of Northern Arizona, 1973.

Munz, Philip A. *A Flora of Southern California*. Berkeley, Los Angeles, and London: University of California Press, 1974.

Niehaus, Theodore F. *Peterson Field Guides, A Field Guide to Southwestern and Texas Wildflowers*. Boston: Houghton Mifflin Company, 1984.

Parker, Kittie F. *An Illustrated Guide to Arizona Weeds*. Tucson: The University of Arizona Press, 1972.

Parsons, Mary Elizabeth. *The Wild Flowers of California*. New York: Dover Publications, 1966.

Stubbendieck, James, Stephan L. Hatch, and Charles Butterfield. *North American Range Plants*. 4th.ed. Lincoln and London: University of Nebraska Press, 1981.

Sudworth, George B. *Forest Trees of the Pacific Slope*. Washington D.C.: United States Government Printing Office, 1908.

Thornber, John James and Frances Bonker. *The Fantastic Clan, The Cactus Family*. New York: The Macmillan Company, 1932.

Turner, Turner M., Janice E. Bowers, and Tony L. Burgess. *Sonoran Desert Plants*. Tucson: The University of Arizona Press, 1995.

Whitson, Tom D., Larry C. Burrill, Steven A. Dewey, David W. Cudney, B.E. Nelson, Richard D. Lee, and Robert Parker. *Weeds of the West.* 5th ed. Newark: The Western Society of Weed Science, 1996.

Physiology

Anderson, Douglas M. *Dorland's Illustrated Medical Dictionary.* 28th ed. Philadelphia: W.B. Saunders Company, 1996.
Fauci, Anthony S., Eugene Braunwald, Kurt J. Isselbacher, Jean D. Wilson, Joseph B. Martin, Dennis L. Kasper, Stephen L. Hauser, and Dan L. Longo. *Harrison's Principals of Internal Medicine.* 14th ed. New York: McGraw-Hill, 1998.
Guyton, Arthur C. and John E. Hall. *Textbook of Medical Physiology.* 9th ed. Philadelphia: W.B. Saunders Company, 1994.
Sheldon, W.H., S.S. Stevens, and W.B. Tucker. *The Varieties of Human Physique.* New York: Harper and Brothers Publisher, 1940.

Medicinal Uses, General

Boericke, William. *Homoeopathic Materia Medica.* 9th ed. Santa Rosa: Boericke and Tafel, Inc., 1927.
Brinker, Francis. *Complex Herbs-Complex Medicines.* Portland: Eclectic Medical Publications, 2004
_____. *Native Healing Gifts. Rediscovering Indigenous Plant Medicines of the Greater Southwest.* Portland: Eclectic Medical Publications, 1995.
Brown, E. Richard. *Rockefeller Medicine Men.* Berkeley: University of California Press, 1979.
Ellingwood, Finley. *American Materia Medica, Therapeutics and Pharmacognosy.* 1919. Reprint, Bisbee: Southwest School of Botanical Medicine, 2001.
Felger, Richard Stephen and Mary Beck Moser. *People of the Desert and Sea, Ethnobotany of the Seri Indians.* Tucson: The University of Arizona Press, 1985.
Felter, Harvey Wickes and John Uri Lloyd. *King's American Dispensatory.* 1898. Reprint, Bisbee: Southwest School of Botanical Medicine, 2001.
Felter, Harvey Wickes. *The Eclectic Materia Medica, Pharmacology and Therapeutics.* 1922. Reprint, Bisbee: Southwest School of Botanical Medicine, 2001.
Finkler, Kaja. *Spiritualist Healers in Mexico.* South Hadley: Bergin and Garvey Publications, Inc., 1985.
Ford, Karen Cowan. *Las Yerbas de la Gente: A Study of Hispano-American Medicinal Plants.* Ann Arbor: The University of Michigan, 1975.
Grieve, M. *A Modern Herbal.* 1931. Reprint, New York: Dover Publications, 1971.
Harrington, H.D. *Edible Native Plants of the Rocky Mountains.* Albuquerque: The University of New Mexico Press, 1967.
Jones, Eli G. *Reading the Eye, Pulse and Tongue for the Indicated Remedy.* Edited by Wade Boye. East Palestine: Buckeye Naturopathic Press, 1989.
Kay, Margarita Artschwager. *Healing with Plants in the American and Mexican West.* Tucson: The University of Arizona Press, 1996.

Kirk, Donald R. *Wild Edible Plants of the Western United States*. Healdsburg: Naturegraph Publishers, 1970.

Moore, Michael. *Herbal Materia Medica.* 5th ed. Bisbee: Southwest School of Botanical Medicine, 1995.

_____. *Medicinal Plants of the Desert and Canyon West*. Sante Fe: Museum of New Mexico Press, 1989.

_____. *Medicinal Plants of the Mountain West*. Sante Fe: Museum of New Mexico Press, 1979.

_____. *Medicinal Plants of the Pacific West*. Sante Fe: Red Crane Books, 1995.

_____. *Specific Indications for Herbs in General Use.* 2nd ed. Bisbee: Southwest School of Botanical Medicine, 1997.

Niethammer, Carolyn. *American Indian Food and Lore*. New York: Macmillan Publishing Co., Inc., 1974.

Pereira, Jonathan. *The Elements of Materia Medica and Therapeutics*. Philadelphia: Blanchard and Lea, 1854.

Scudder, John M. *Specific Diagnosis. A Study of Disease*. 1874. Reprint, Sandy: Eclectic Medical Publications, 1994.

Vogel, Virgil J. *American Indian Medicine*. Norman: University of Oklahoma Press, 1970.

Weiss, Rudolf Fritz. *Herbal Medicine*. Beaconsfield: Beaconsfield Publishers LTD, 1988.

Aloe

Chithra, P., G.B. Sajithlal, and Gowri Chandrakasan. "Influence of Aloe Vera on the Glycosaminoglycans in the Matrix of Healing Dermal Wounds in Rats." *Journal of Ethnopharmacology* 59 (1998): 179-186.

D.N. Herndon and J.P. Heggers. "Retardation of Wound Healing by Silver Sulfadiazine is Reversed by Aloe Vera and Nystatin." *Burns* 29 (2003): 834-836.

Seyger, M.M.B., P.C.M. van de Kerkhof, I.M.J.J. van Vlijmen-Willems, E.S.M. de Bakker, F. Zwiers, and E.M.G.J. de Jong. "The Efficacy of a New Topical Treatment for Psoriasis: Mirak." *Journal of the European Academy of Dermatology and Venereology* 11 (1998): 13-18.

Femenia, Antoni, Emma S. Sánchez, Susana Simal, and Carmen Rosselló. "Compositional Features of Polysaccharides from Aloe Vera (Aloe Barbadensis Miller) Plant Tissues." *Carbohydrate Polymers* 39 (1999): 109-117.

Grover, J.K., S. Yadav, and V. Vats. "Medicinal Plants of India with Anti-diabetic Potential." *Journal of Ethnopharmacology* 81 (2002): 81-100.

Kent, Carol Miller. *Aloe Vera*. Arlington: Carol Miller Kent, 1980.

Muller, M.J., M.A. Hollyoak, Z. Moaveni, Tim La H. Brown, T. Reynolds, A.C. Dweck. "Aloe Vera Leaf Gel: A Review Update." *Journal of Ethnopharmacology* 68 (1999): 3-37.

Rodríguez, D. Jasso de, D. Hernández-Castillo, R. Rodríguez-García, and J.L. Angulo-Sánchez. "Antifungal Activity In Vitro of Aloe Vera Pulp and Liquid Fraction Against Plant Pathogenic Fungi." *Industrial Crops and Products* xxx (2004): xxx-xxx.

Sadiq, Yusuf, Agunu Abdulkarim, and Diana Mshelia. "The Effect of Aloe Vera A. Berger (Liliaceae) on Gastric Acid Secretion and Acute Gastric Mucosal Injury in Rats." *Journal of Ethnopharmacology* 93 (2004): 33-37.

Váquez, Beatriz, Guillermo Avila, David Segura, and Bruno Escalante. "Antiinflammatory Activity of Extracts from Aloe Vera Gel." *Journal of Ethnopharmacology* 55 (1996): 69-75.

Verlag, Gustav Fischer. "Antidiabetic Activity of Aloe Vera L. Juice. I. Clinical Trial in New Cases of Diabetes Mellitus." *Phytomedicine* 3, 3 (1996): 241-243.

Antelope Horns

Chiu, F.C. and Watson, T.R. "Conformational Factors in Cardiac Glycoside Activity." *Journal of Medical Chemistry* 28, 4 (1985): 509-515.

Giordani, R., Moulin-Traffort, J., and Regli, P. "Glycosidic Activities of Candida Albicans After Action of Vegetable Latex Saps (Natural Antifungals) and Isoconazole (Synthetic Antifungal)." *Mycoses* 34, 1-2 (1991): 67-73.

Kelley, Bruce D., Glenn D. Appelt, and Jennifer M. Appelt. "Pharmacological Aspects of Selected Herbs Employed in Hispanic Folk Medicine in the San Luis Valley of Colorado, USA: II Asclepias Asperula (Inmortal) and Achillea Lanulosa (Plumajillo)." *Journal of Ethnopharmacology* 22 (1988): 1-9.

Radford, D.J., Gillies, A.D., Hinds, J.A., and Duffy, P. "Naturally Occurring Cardiac Glycosides." *Medical Journal of Australia* 144, 10 (1986): 540-544.

Sady, Michael B. and James N. Seiber. "Chemical Differences Between Species of Asclepias from the Intermountain Region of North America." *Phytochemistry* 30, 9 (1991): 3001-3003.

Seiber, James N., Carolyn J. Nelson, and S. Mark Lee. "Cardenolides in the Latex and Leaves of Seven Asclepias Species and Calotropis Procrea." *Phytochemistry* 21, 9 (1982): 2343-2348.

Beargrass

Mimaki, Y., Takaashi, Y., Kuroda, M., Sashida, Y., and Nikaido, T. "Steroidal Saponins from Nolina Recurvata Stems and their Inhibitory Activity on Cyclic AMP Phosphodiesterase." *Phytochemisty* 42, 6 (1996): 1609-1615.

Bird of Paradise

Andrade, C.T., E.G. Azero, L. Luciano, and M.P. Goncalves. "Solution Properties of the Galactomannans Extracted from the Seeds of Caesalpinia Pulcherrima and Cassia Javanica: Comparison with Locust Bean Gum." *International Journal of Biological Macromolecules* 26 (1999): 181-185.

Heras, B. de las, K. Slowing, J. Benedí, E. Carretero, T. Ortega, C. Toledo, P. Bermejo, I. Iglesias, M.J. Abad, P. Gómez-Serranillos, P.A. Liso, A. Villar, and X. Chiriboga. "Antiinflammatory and Antioxidant Activity of Plants Used in Traditional Medicine in Ecuador." *Journal of Ethnopharmacology* 61 (1998): 161-166.

Krishna, K.V.S. Rama, K. Hara Kishore, and U.S.N. Murty. "Flavanoids from Caesalpinia Pulcherrima." *Phytochemistry* 63 (2003): 789-793.

Muschietti L., V. Martino, G. Ferraro, J. Coussio, L. Segura, C. Cartana, S. Canigueral, and T. Adzet. "The Anti-Inflammatory Effect of some Species from South America." *Phytotherapy Research* 10, 1 (1996): 84-86.

Patil, Ashok D., Alan J. Freyer, R. Lee Webb, Gary Zuber, Rex Reichwein, Mark F. Bean, Leo Faucette, and Randall K. Johnson. "Pulcherrimins A - D, Novel Diterpene Dibenzoates from Caesalpinia pulcherrima with Selective Activity against DNA Repair-Deficient Yeast Mutants." *Tetrahedron* 53, 5 (1997): 1583-1592.

Pavón, Numa P. and Oscar Briones. "Phenological Patterns of Nine Perennial Plants in an Intertropical Semi-arid Mexican Scrub." *Journal of Arid Environments* 49 (2001): 265-277.

Bricklebush

Beck, John J. and Frank R. Stermitz. "Pyrrolizidine Alkaloids from Brickellia Grandiflora and Cryptantha Jamesii." *Biochemical Systematics and Ecology* 30 (2002): 1079-1081.

Perez-Gutierrez, R.M., Perez-Gonzalez, C., Zavala-Sanchez, M.A., Perez-Gutierrez, S. "Hypoglycemic Activity of Bouvardia Terniflora, Brickellia Veronicaefolia, and Parmentiera Edulis." *Salud Publica Mex* 40, 4 (1998): 354-358.

Brittlebush

Proksch, P., M. Breuer, and H. Budzikiewicz. "Benzofuran Derivatives from Two Encelia Species." *Phytochemistry* 24, 12 (1985): 3069-3071.

Proksch, P., U. Politt, E. Wollenweber, V. Wray, and C. Clark. "Epicuticular Flavonoids from Encelia." *Planta Medica* 54, 6 (1988): 542-546.

Proksch, Peter, Aristotelis Mitsakos, Jutta Bodden, and Eckhard Wollenweber. "Benzofurans and Methylated Flavonoids of Geraea (Asteraceae)." *Phytochemistry* 25, 10 (1986): 2367-2369.

Wisdom, Charles and Eloy Rodriguez. "Seasonal Age-Specific Measurements of the Sesquiterpene Lactones and Chromenes of Encelia Farinosa." *Biochemical Systematics and Ecology* 11, 4 (1978): 345-352.

Wisdom, Charles and Eloy Rodriguez. "Quantitative Variation of the Sesquiterpene Lactones and Chromenes of Encelia Farinosa." *Biochemical Systematics and Ecology* 10, 1 (1978): 43-48.

Burrobrush

Balza, F. and G. H. Neil Towers. "Structural Analysis of Sesquiterpene Lactones from Hymenoclea Salsola." *Phytochemlstry* 27, 5 (1988): 1421-1424.

Geissman, T. A. and F. P. Toribio. "Sesquiterpene Lactones. Constituents of Hymenoclea Salsola T. and G." *Phytochemistry* 6 (1967): 1563-1567.

Miyakado, M., T. Kato, N. Ohno, and T. J. Mabry. "Pinocembrin and (+)-B-Nocembrin and Eudesmol from Hymenoclea Monogyra and Baccharis Glutinosa." *Phytochemistry* 15 (1976): 846.

California Poppy

Beck, Mona-Antonia and Hanns Häberlein. "Flavonol Glycosides from Eschscholtzia Californica." *Phytochemistry* 50 (1999): 329-332.
Chaffee, M.A. and C.W. Gale, III. "The California Poppy (Eschscholtzia Mexicana) as a Copper Indicator—A New Example." *Journal of Geochemical Exploration* 5 (1976): 59-63.
Fabre, Nicolas, Catherine Claparols, Suzanne Richelme, Marie-Laure Angelin, Isabelle Fourasté, and Claude Moulis. "Direct Characterization of Isoquinoline Alkaloids in a Crude Plant Extract by Ion-Pair Liquid Chromatography–Electrospray Ionization Tandem Mass Spectrometry: Example of Eschscholtzia Californica." *Journal of Chromatography A* 904, 1 (2000): 35-46.
Paul, Liane D. and Hans H. Maurer. "Studies on the Metabolism and Toxicological Detection of the Eschscholtzia Californica Alkaloids Californine and Protopine in Urine Using Gas Chromatography–Mass Spectrometry." *Journal of Chromatography B* 789 (2003): 43-57.

Caltrop

Lia, Veronica V., Viviana A. Confalonieri, Cecilia I. Comas, and Juan H. Hunziker. "Molecular Phylogeny of Larrea and Its Allies (Zygophyllaceae): Reticulate Evolution and the Probable Time of Creosote Bush Arrival to North America." *Molecular Phylogenetics and Evolution* 21, 2 (2001): 309-320.
Saleh, Nabiel A. M., Mohamed Nabil El-Hadidi, and Ahmed A. Ahmed. "The Chemosystematics of Tribulaceae." *Biochemical Systematics and Ecology* 10, 4 (1982): 313-317.

Camphorweed

Gené, Rosa M., Laura Segura, Tomás Adzet, Esther Marin, and José Iglesias. "Heterotheca Inuloides: Anti-inflammatory and Analgesic Effect." *Journal of Ethnopharmacology* 60 (1998): 157-162.
Lincoln, David E. and Brian M. Lawrence. "The Volatile Constituents of Camphorweed, Heterotheca Subaxillaris." *Phytochemistry* 23, 4 (1984): 933-934.

Canadian Fleabane

Heras, B. de las, K. Slowing, J. Benedía, E. Carretero, T. Ortega, C. Toledo, P. Bermejo, I. Iglesias, M.J. Abad, P. Gómez-Serranillos, P.A. Liso, A. Villar, and X. Chiriboga. "Antiinflammatory and Antioxidant Activity of Plants Used in Traditional Medicine in Ecuador." *Journal of Ethnopharmacology* 61 (1998): 161-166.

Lenfeld, J., O. Motl, and A. Trka. "Antiinflammatory Activity of Extracts from Conyza Canadensis." *Pharmazie* 41, 4 (1986): 268-269.

Todd, Albert M. "Oils of Erigeron and Fireweed." *American Journal of Pharmacy* 59, 6 (1887).

Canyon Bursage

Muschietti, L., V. Martino,G. Ferraro, J. Coussio, L. Segura, C. Cartana, S. Canigueal, and T. Adzet. "The Antiiflammatory Effects of some Species from South America." *Phytotherapy Research* 10, 1 (1996): 84-86.

Wang, P.H., J. XU, and M.Y. WU. "Chemical Constituents of Ragweed (Artemisia Artemisiifolia)." *China Journal of Chinese Materia Medica* 18, 3 (1993): 164-166.

Canyon Walnut

Biancoa, M. A., A. Handajia, and H. Savolainenb. "Quantitative Analysis of Ellagic Acid in Hardwood Samples." *The Science of the Total Environment* 222 (1998): 123-126.

Boelkins, James N., Lloyd K. Everson, and Theodore K. Auyong. "Effects of Intravenous Juglone in the Dog." *Toxicon* 6, 2 (1968): 99-102.

Guarrera, Paolo Maria. "Traditional Antihelmintic, Antiparasitic and Repellent Uses of Plants in Central Italy." *Journal of Ethnopharmacology* 68 (1999): 183-192.

Lopez, A., J.B. Hudson, and G.H.N. Towers. "Antiviral and Antimicrobial Activities of Colombian Medicinal Plants." *Journal of Ethnopharmacology* 77 (2001): 189-196.

Omar, S., B. Lemonnier, N. Jones, C. Ficker, M.L. Smith, C. Neema, Towers, G.H.N., K. Goel, and J.T. Arnason. "Antimicrobial Activity of Extracts of Eastern North American Hardwood Trees and Relation to Traditional Medicine." *Journal of Ethnopharmacology* 73 (2000): 161-170.

Chaste Tree

Böhnert, K. J. "The Use of Vitex Agnus Castus for Hyperprolactinemia." *Quarterly Review of Natural Medicine*, spring (1997): 19-21.

Brown, Donald J. "Vitex Agnus Castus Clinical Monograph from Quarterly Review of Natural Medicine." *Herbal Research Review*, Summer (1994)

Halaška, M., P. Beles, C. Gorkow, and C. Sieder. "Treatment of Cyclical Mastalgia with a Solution Containing a Vitex Agnus Castus Extract: Results of a Placebo-Controlled Double-Blind Study." *The Breast* 8 (1999): 175-181.

Lauritzen, CH., H.D. Reuter, R. Repges, K.J. Böhnert, and U. Schmidt. "Treatment of Premenstrual Tension Syndrome with Vitex Agnus Castus Controlled, Double-Blind Study Versus Pyridoxine." *Phytomedicine* 4, 3 (1997): 183-189.

Lucks, Barbara Chopin. "Vitex Agnus Castus Essential Oil and Menopausal Balance: A Research Update." *Complementary Therapies in Nursing and Midwifery* 8 (2003): 148-154.

Schellenberg, R. "Treatment for the Premenstrual Syndrome with Agnus Castus Fruit Extract: Prospective, Randomized, Placebo Controlled Study." *British Medical Journal* 322 (2001): 134-137.

Chickweed

Pande, Archana, Yogendra N. Shukla, and Arun K. Tripathi. "Lipid Constituents from Stellaria Media." *Phytochemistry* 39, 3 (1995): 709-711

Chinchweed

Downum, K. R., D. J. Keil, and E. Rodriguez. "Distribution of Acetylenic Thiophenes in the Pectidinae." *Biochemical Systematics and Ecology* 13, 2 (1985): 109-113.

Clematis

Buzzini, P. and A. Pieroni. "Antimicrobial Activity of Extracts of Vitalba Clematis Towards Pathogenic Yeast and Yeast-Like Microorganisms." *Fitoterapia* (2003).
Kern, John R. and John H. Cardellina II. "Native American Medicinal Plants. Anemonin from the Horse Stimulant Clematis Hirsutissima." *Journal of Ethnopharmocology* 8 (1983): 121-123.
Li, Rachel W., G. David Lin, Stephen P. Myers, and David N. Leach. "Anti-inflammatory Activity of Chinese Medicinal Vine Plants." *Journal of Ethnopharmacology* 85 (2003): 61-67.

Cocklebur

Malik, Mabgel S., Naresh K. Sangwan, and Kuldip Singh Dhindsa. "Xanthanolides from Xanthium Strumarium." *Phytochemistry* 32, 1 (1993): 206-207.
Omar, Abdallah A., Elsayed M. Elrashidy, Nabila A. Ghazy, Ali M. Metwally, Jurgen Ziesche, and Ferdinand Bohlmann. "Xanthanolides from Xanthium Spinosum." *Phtyochemistry* 23, 4 (1984): 915-916.

Copperleaf

Büssing, A., G.M. Stein, I. Herterich-Akinpelu, and U. Pfüller. "Apoptosis-Associated Generation of Reactive Oxygen Intermediates and Release of Pro-Inflammatory Cytokines in Human Lymphocytes and Granulocytes by Extracts from the Seeds of Acalypha Wilkesiana." *Journal of Ethnopharmacology* 66 (1999): 301-309.
Samy, R. Perumal, S. Ignacimuthu, and D. Patric Raja. "Short Communication Preliminary Screening of Ethnomedicinal Plants from India." *Journal of Ethnopharmacology* 66 (1999): 235-240.
Cáceres, Armando, Beatriz López, Sonia González, Ingeborg Berger, Isao Tada, and Jun Maki. "Plants Used in Guatemala for the Treatment of Protozoal Infections. I. Screening of Activity to Bacteria, Fungi and American Trypanosomes of 13 Native Plants." *Journal of Ethnopharmacology* 62 (1998): 195-202.

Reddy, J. Suresh, P. Rajeswara Rao, and Mada S. Reddy. "Wound Healing Effects of Heliotropium Indicum, Plumbago Zeylanicum and Acalypha Indica in Rats." *Journal of Ethnopharmacology* 79 (2002): 249-251.

Irobia, O.N. and A. Bansob. "Effects of Crude Leaf Extracts of Acalypha Torta Against some Anaerobic Bacteria." *Journal of Ethnopharmacology* 43, 1 (1994): 63-65.

Cottonwood

English, S, W. Greenaway, and F.R. Whatley. "Analysis of Phenolics in the Bud Exudates of Populus Deltoides, P. Fremontii, P. Sargentii and P. Wislizenii by GC-MS." *Phytochemistry* 31, 4 (1992): 1255-1260.

Mattes, Benjamin R., Thomas P. Clausen, and Paul B. Reichardt. "Volatile Constituents of Balsam Popular: The Phenol Glycoside Connection." *Phytochemistry* 25, 5 (1987): 1361-1366.

Pearl, Irwin A. and Stephen F. Darling. "Hot Water Phenolic Extractives of the Bark and Leaves of Diploid Populus Tremuloides." *Phytochemistry* 10 (1971): 483-484.

Tiitto, Julkunen Riitta. "A Chemotaxonomic Survey of Phenolic in Leaves of Northern Salicaceae Species." *Phytochemistry* 25, 3 (1986): 663-667.

Creosote Bush

Anesini, Claudia and Cristina Perez. "Screening of Plants Used in Argentine Folk Medicine for Antimicrobial Activity." *Journal of Ethnopharmacology* 39 (1993): 119-128.

Craigo, Jodi, Michelle Callahan, Ru Chih C. Huang, and Angelo L. DeLucia. "Inhibition of Human Papillomavirus Type 16 Gene Expression by Nordihydroguaiaretic Acid Plant Lignan Derivatives." *Antiviral Research* 47 (2000): 19-28.

Grant, Kathryn L., Leslie V. Boyer, and Boyd E. Erdman. "Chaparral Induced Hepatotoxicity." *Intagrative Medicine* 1, 2 (1998): 83-87.

Hyder, Paul W., E.L. Fredrickson, Rick E. Estell, Mario Tellez, and Robert P. Gibbens. "Distribution and Concentration of Total Phenolics, Condensed Tannins, and Nordihydroguaiaretic Acid (NDGA) in Creosotebush (Larrea Tridentata)." *Biochemical Systematics and Ecology* 30 (2002): 905-912.

Quiroga, Emma Nelly, Antonio Rodolfo Sampietro, and Marta Amelia Vattuone. "Screening Antifungal Activities of Selected Medicinal Plants." *Journal of Ethnopharmacology* 74 (2001): 89-96.

Verástegui, M. Angeles, César A. Sánchez, Norma L. Heredia, and J. Santos García-Alvarado. "Antimicrobial Activity of Extracts of Three Chihuahuan Desert Major Plants from the Chihuahuan Desert." *Journal of Ethnopharmacology* 52 (1996): 175-177.

Crownbeard

Banerjee, Shanta, Jasmin Jakupovic, Ferdinand Bohlmann, Robert M. King, and Harold Robinson. "A Rearranged Eudesmane and Further Verbesindiol Derivatives from Verbesina Eggersii." *Phytochemistry* 24, 5 (1985): 1106-1108.
Eichholzer, John V., Ivor A. S. Lewis, John K. Macleod, Peter B. Oelrichsa, and Peter J. Vallelya. "Galegine and a New Dihydroxyalkylacetamide from Verbesina Enceloiodes." *Phytochemistry* 21, 1 (1982): 97-99.
Glennie, C. W. and S. C. Jaint. "Flavonol 3,7-Diglycosides of Verbesina Encelioides." *Phytochemistry* 19, 1 (1980): 157-158.

Cudweed

Caceresa, Armando, Alma V. Alvareza, Ana E. Ovandoa, and Blanca E. Samayoa. "Plants Used in Guatemala for the Treatment of Respiratory Diseases. 1. Screening of 68 Plants Against Gram-Positive Bacteria." *Journal of Ethnopharmacology* 31, 2 (1991): 193-208.
Rojas, Gabriela, Juan Lévaro, Jaime Tortoriello, and Victor Navarro. "Antimicrobial Evaluation of Certain Plants Used in Mexican Traditional Medicine For the Treatment of Respiratory Diseases." *Journal of Ethnopharmacology* 74 (2001): 97-101.
Villagómez-Ibarra, J. Roberto, Maricruz Sánchez, Ofelia Espejo, Armida Zúniga-Estrada, J. Martín Torres-Valencia, and Pedro Joseph-Nathan. "Antimicrobial Activity of Three Mexican Gnaphalium Species." *Fitoterapia* 72 (2001): 692-694.

Cypress

Homer, K.A., F. Manji, and D. Beighton. "Inhibition of Peptidase and Glycosidase Activities of Porphyromonas Gingivalis, Bacteroides Intermedius and Treponema Denticola by Plant Extracts." *Journal of Clinical Periodontology* 19, 5 (1992): 305-310.
Lopéz, L., M.A. Villavicencio, A. Albores, M. Martínez, J. de la Garza, J. Meléndez-Zajgla, and V. Maldonado. "Cupressus Lusitanica (Cupressaceae) Leaf Extract Induces Apoptosis in Cancer Cells." *Journal of Ethnopharmacology* 80 (2002): 115-120.
Pauly, Ginette, Abdelhamid Yani, Louis Piovetti, and Colette Bernard-Dagen. "Volatile Constituients of the Leaves of Cupressus Sempervirens." *Phytochemistry* 22, 4 (1983): 957-959.
Piovetti, Louis, Abdelhamid Yani, Georges Combaut, and Anne Diara. "Waxes of Cupressus Dupreziana and Cupressus Sempervirens." *Phytochemistry* 20, 5 (1981): 1135-1136.
Ponce-Macotela, M., I. Navarro-Alegria, M.N. Martinez-Gordillo, R. and Alvarez-Chacon. "In Vitro Effect Against Giardia of 14 Plant Extracts." *Revista De Investigacion Clinica* 46, 5 (1994): 343-347.

Dandelion

Grases, F., G. Melero, A. Costa-Bauza, R. Prieto, and J.G. March. "Urolithiasis and Phytotherapy." *International Urology and Nephrology* 26, 5 (1994): 507-511.

Kisiel, W. and B. Barszcz. Further Sesquiterpenoids and Phenolics from Taraxacum Officinale. *Fitoterapia* 71 (2000): 269-273.

Rauwald, Hans-Willi and Jai-Tung Huang. "Taraxacoside, a Type of Acylated ã-Butyrolactone Clycoside from Taraxacum Officinale." *Phytochemutry* 24, 7 (1985): 1557-1559.

Williams, Christine A., Fiona Goldstone, and Jenny Greenham. "Flavonoids, Cinnamic Acids, and Coumarins from the Different Tissues and Medicinal Preparations of Taraxacum Officinale." *Phytochemistry* 42, 1 (1996): 121-127.

Datura

Abena, A.A., L.M. Miguel, A. Mouanga, Th. Hondi Assah, and M. Diatewa. "Evaluation of Analgesic Effect of Datura Fastuosa Leaves and Seed Extracts." *Fitoterapia* 74 (2003): 486-488.

Evens, William C. and Aim-On Somanabandhl. "Alkoloids of Datura Discolor." *Phytochemistry* 13 (1974): 304-305.

Gnanamani, A., K. Shanmuga Priya, N. Radhakrishnan, and Mary Babu. "Antibacterial Activity of Two Plant Extracts on Eight Burn Pathogens." *Journal of Ethnopharmacology* 86 (2003): 59–61.

Griffin, William J. and G. David Lin. "Chemotaxonomy and Geographical Distribution of Tropane Alkaloids." *Phytochemistry* 53 (2000): 623-637.

Miraldia, Elisabetta, Alessandra Masti, Sara Ferri, and Ida Barni Comparini. "Distribution of Hyoscyamine and Scopolamine in Datura Stramonium." *Fitoterapia* 72 (2001): 644-648

Pate, David W. and John E. Averett. "Flavonoids of Datura." *Biochemical Systematics and Ecology* 14, 6 (1986): 647-649.

Priya, K. Shanmuga, A. Gnanamani, N. Radhakrishnan, and Mary Babu. "Healing Potential of Datura Alba on Burn Wounds in Albino Rats." *Journal of Ethnopharmacology* 83 (2002): 193-199.

Rajesh, G.L. Sharma. "Studies on Antimycotic Properties of Datura Metel." *Journal of Ethnopharmacology* 80 (2002): 193-197.

Deerweed

Guillet, Gabriel, André Bélanger, and John Arnason. "Volitile Monoterpenes in Porophyllum Gracile and P. Ruderale (Asteraceae): Identification, Localization and Insecticidal Synergism with á-Terthienyl." *Phytochemistry* 49, 2 (1998): 423-429.

Desert Barberry

Ivanovska, N. and S. Philipov. "Study on the Anti-Inflammatory Action of Berberis Vulgaris Root Extract, Alkaloid Fractions and Pure Alkaloids." *International Journal Of Immunopharmacology* 18,10 (1996): 553-561.

Janbaz, K.H. and A.H. Gilani. "Studies on Preventive and Curative Effects of Berberine on Chemical-Induced Hepatotoxicity in Rodents." *Fitoterapia* 71 (2000): 25-33.

Ji, Xiuhong, Yi Li, Huwei Liu, Yuning Yan, and Jiashi Li. "Determination of the Alkaloid Content in Different Parts of some Mahonia Plants by HPCE." *Pharmaceutica Acta Helvetiae* 74 (2000): 387-391.

Khin-Maung-U and Nwe-Nwe-Wai. "Effect of Berberine on Enterotoxin-Induced Intestinal Fluid Accumulation in Rats." *J Diarrhoeal Dis Res* 10, 4 (1992): 201-204.

Kostalova, D., A. Kardosova, and V. Hajnicka. "Effect of Mahonia Aquifolium Stem Bark Crude Extract and One of its Polysaccharide Components on Production of IL-8." *Fitoterapia* 72 (2001): 802-806.

Sack, R.B. and J.L. Froehlich. "Berberine Inhibits Intestinal Secretory Response of Vibrio Cholerae and Escherichia Coli Enterotoxins." *Infect Immun* 35, 2 (1982): 471-475.

Shamsa, F., A. Ahmadiani, and R. Khosrokhavar. "Antihistaminic and Anticholinergic Activity of Barberry Fruit (Berberis Vulgaris) in the Guinea-Pig Ileum." *Journal of Ethnopharmacology* 64 (1999): 161-166

Sohni, Y.R., P. Kaimal, and R.M. Bhatt. "The Antiamoebic Effect of a Crude Drug Formulation of Herbal Extracts Against Entamoeba Histolytica In Vitro and in Vivo." *Journal of Ethnopharmacology* 45, 1 (1995): 43-52.

Sohni, Youvraj R. and Ranjan M. Bhatt. "Activity of a Crude Extract Formulation in Experimental Hepatic Amoebiasis and in Immunomodulation Studies." *Journal of Ethnopharmacology* 54 (1996): 119-124.

Stermitz, F.R., J. Tawara-Matsuda, P. Lorenz, P. Mueller, L. Zenewicz, and K. Lewis. "5'-Methoxyhydnocarpin-D and Pheophorbide A: Berberis Species Components That Potentiate Berberine Growth Inhibition of Resistant Staphylococcusaureus." *Journal of Natural Products* 63, 8 (2000): 1146-1149.

Stermitz, Frank R., Teresa D. Beeson, Paul J. Mueller, Jen-Fang Hsiang, and Kim Lewis. "Staphylococcus Aureus MDR Effux Pump Inhibitors from a Berberis and a Mahonia (Sensu Strictu) Species." *Biochemical Systematics and Ecology* 29 (2001): 793-798.

Yesilada, Erdem and Esra Küpeli. Berberis Crataegina DC. "Root Exhibits Potent Anti-Inflammatory, Analgesic and Febrifuge Effects in Mice and Rats." *Journal of Ethnopharmacology* 79 (2002): 237-248.

Desert Cotton

Bai, Junping and Yuliang Shi. "Inhibition of T-Type Ca2+ Currents in Mouse Spermatogenic Cells by Gossypol, an Antifertility Compound." *European Journal of Pharmacology* 440 (2002): 1-6.

Coutinho, Elsimar Metzker. "Gossypol: A Contraceptive for Men." *Contraception* 65 (2002): 259-263.

Coutinho, Elsimar M., Célia Athayde, Gabriel Atta, Zhi-Ping Gut, Zhen-Wen Chen, Guo-Wei Sang, Edward Emuveyan, Adeyemi O. Adekunle, Japheth Mati, Joseph Otubu, Marcus M. Reidenberg, and Sheldon J. Segal. "Gossypol Blood Levels and Inhibition of Spermatogenesis in Men Taking Gossypol as a Contraceptive." *Contraception* 61 (2000): 61-67.

Fiorini, Céline, Anne Tilloy-Ellul, Stephan Chevalier, Claude Charuel, and Georges Pointis. "Sertoli Cell Junctional Proteins as Early Targets for Different Classes of Reproductive Toxicants." *Reproductive Toxicology* 18 (2004): 413-421.

Hedin, P. A., A.C. Thompson, R.C. Gueldner, and J.P. Minyard. "Constituents of the Cotton Bud." *Phytochemistry* 10 (1971): 3316-3318.

Lane, Harry C. and Michael F. Schuster. "Condensed Tannins of Cotton Leaves." *Phytochemistry* 20 (1981): 425-427.

Waage, Susan K. and Paul A. Hedin. "Biologically Active Flavonoids from Gossypium Arboreum." *Phytochemistry* 23, 2 (1984): 2509-2511.

Desert Lavender

Pandey, V. N. and N. K. Dubey. "Antifungal Potential of Leaves and Essential Oils from Higher Plants Against Soil Phytopathogens." *Soil Biology and Biochemistry* 26, 10 (1994): 1417-1421.

Kuhnt, M., A. Probstle, H. Rimpler, R. Bauer, and M. Heinrich. "Biological and Pharmacological Activities and Further Constituents of Hyptis Verticellata." *Planta Medica* 61, 3 (1995): 227-232.

Bispo, M.D., R.H.V. Mourao, E.M. Franzotti, K.B.R. Bomfim, M. de F. Arrigoni-Blank, M.P.N. Moreno, M. Marchioro, and A.R. Antoniolli. "Antinociceptive and Antiedematogenic Effects of the Aqueous Extract of Hyptis Pectinata Leaves in Experimental Animals." *Journal of Ethnopharmacology* 76 (2001): 81-86.

Asekun, Olayinka Taiwo, Olusegun Ekundayo, and Bolanle A. Adeniyi. "Antimicrobial Activity of the Essential Oil of Hyptis Suaveolens Leaves." *Fitoterapia* 70 (1999): 440-442.

Rojas, A., Hernandez, L., Pereda-Miranda, R., and Mata, R. "Screening for Antimicrobial Activity of Crude Drug Extracts and Pure Natural Products from Mexican Medicinal Plants." *Journal of Ethnopharmacology* 35, 3 (1992): 275-83.

Desert Milkweed

Chiu, F.C. and T.R. Watson. "Conformational Factors in Cardiac Glycoside Activity." *Journal of Medical Chemistry* 28, 4 (1985): 509-515.

Giordani, R., J. Moulin-Traffort, and P. Regli. "Glycosidic Activities of Candida Albicans After Action of Vegetable Latex Saps (Natural Antifungals) and Isoconazole (Synthetic Antifungal)." *Mycoses* 34, 1-2 (1991): 67-73.

Radford, D.J., A.D. Gillies, J.A. Hinds, and P. Duffy. "Naturally Occurring Cardiac Glycosides." *Medical Journal of Australia* 144, 10 (1986): 540-544.

Sady, Michael B. and James N. Seiber. "Chemical Differences Between Species of Asclepias from the Intermountain Region of North America." *Phytochemistry* 30, 9 (1991): 3001-3003.

Seiber, James N., Carolyn J. Nelson, and S. Mark Lee. "Cardenolides in the Latex and Leaves of Seven Asclepias Species and Calotropis Procrea." *Phytochemistry* 21, 9 (1982): 2343-2348.

Desert Rhubarb

Demirezer, L. Omur, Ayse Kuruuzum-Uza, Isabelle Bergere, H.-J. Schiewe, and Axel Zeeck. "The Structures of Antioxidant and Cytotoxic Agents from Natural Source: Anthraquinones and Tannins from Roots of Rumex Patientia." *Phytochemistry* 58 (2001): 1213-1217.

Fairbairn, J. W. and F. J. El-Muhtadi. "Chemotaxonomy of Anthraquinones in Rumex." *Phytochemistry* 11 (1972): 263-268.

Midiwo, J. Ogweno and G. Muriki Rukunga. "Distrubution of Anthraquinone Pigments in Rumex Species." *Phytochemistry* 24, 6 (1985): 1390-1391.

Saleh, Nabiel A.M., Mohamed N. El-Hadidi and Raafat F.M. Arafa. "Flavonoids and Anthraquinones of some Egyptian Rumex Species (Polygonaceae)." *Biochemical Systematics and Ecology* 21, 2 (1993): 301-303.

VanderJagt, T.J., R. Ghattas, D.J VanderJagt, M. Crossey, and R.H Glew. "Comparison of the Total Antioxidant Content of 30 Widely Used Medicinal Plants of New Mexico." *Life Sciences* 70 (2002): 1035-1040.

Elder

Ahmadiani, A., M. Fereidoni, S. Semnanian, M. Kamalinejad, and S. Saremi. "Antinociceptive and Anti-inflammatory Effects of Sambucus Ebulus Rhizome Extract in Rats." *Journal of Ethnopharmacology* 61 (1998): 229-235.

Bergner, Paul. "Elderberry (Sambucus Nigra, Canadensis)." *Medical Herbalism* 8, 4 (1996-1997).

Buhrmester, Rex A., John E. Ebinger, and David S. Seigler. "Sambunigrin and Cyanogenic Variability in Populations of Sambucus Canadensis L. (Caprifoliaceae)." *Biochemical Systematics and Ecology* 28 (2000): 689-695.

Caceres, Armando, Brenda R. Lopez, Melba A. Giron, and Heidi Logemann. "Plants Used in Guatemala for the Treatment of Dermatophytic Infections. 1. Screening for Antimycotic Activity of 44 Plant Extracts." *Journal of Ethnopharmacology* 31 (1991): 263-276.

Caceres, Armando, Orlando Cano, Blanca Samayoa and Leila Aguilar. "Plants Used in Guatemala for the Treatment of Gastrointestinal Disorders. 1. Screening of 84 Plants Against Enterobacteria." *Journal of Ethnopharmacology* 30 (1990): 55-73.

Hernández, Nancy E., M.L. Tereschuk, and L.R. Abdala. "Antimicrobial Activity of Flavonoids in Medicinal Plants from Tafí del Valle (Tucumán, Argentina)." *Journal of Ethnopharmacology* 73 (2000): 317-322.

Losey, Robert J., Nancy Stenholm, Patty Whereat-Phillips, and Helen Vallianatos. "Exploring the Use of Red Elderberry (Sambucus Racemosa) Fruit on the Southern Northwest Coast of North America." *Journal of Archaeological Science* 30 (2003): 695-707.

McCutcheon, A.R., T.E. Roberts, E. Gibbions, S.M. Ellis, L.A. Babiuk, R.E.W. Hancock, and G.H.N. Towers. "Antiviral Screening of British Columbian Medicinal Plants." *Journal of Ethnopharmacology* 49 (1995): 101-110.

Mormon Tea

Feresin, Gabriela Egly, Alejandro Tapia, Silvia N. López, and Susana A. Zacchino. "Antimicrobial Activity of Plants Used in Traditional Medicine of San Juan Province, Argentine." *Journal of Ethnopharmacology* 78 (2001): 103-107.

Gurni, A. Alberto and Marcelo L. Wagner. "Proanthocyanidins from some Argentine Species of Ephedra." *Biochemical Systematics and Ecology* 12, 3 (1984): 319-320.

Konno, Chohachi, Takashi Taguchi, Misturu Tamada, and Hiroshi Hikino. "Ephedroxane, Anti-Inflammatory Principle of Ephedra Herbs." *Phytochemistry* 18 (1979): 697-698.

Filaree

Saleh, Nabiel A.M., Zeinab A.R. El-Karemy, Ragaa M.A.. Mansour, and Abdel-Aziz A. Fayed. "A Chemosystematic Study of some Geraniaceae." *Phytochemistry* 22, 11 (1983): 2501-2505.

Sroka, Z., H. Rzadkowska-Bodalska, and I. Mazol. "Antioxidative Effect of Extracts from Erodium Cicutarium L." *Z Naturforsch* 49, 11-12 (1994):881-884.

Zielinska-Jenczylik, J., A. Sypula, E. Budko, and H. Rzadkowska-Bodalska. "Interferonogenic and Antiviral Effect of Extracts from Erodium Cicutarium. II. Modulatory Activity of Erodium Cicutarium Extracts." *Arch Immunol Ther Exp (WARSZ)* 36, 5 (1988): 527-36.

Golden Smoke

Abbasoglu, U., B. Sener, Y. Gunay, and H. Temizer. "Antimicrobial Activity of some Isoquinoline Alkaloids." *Archiv Der Pharmazie* 324, 6 (1991): 379-80.

Chang, Cheng-Kuei and Mao-Tsun Lin. "DL-Tetrahydropalmatine May Act Through Inhibition of Amygdaloid Release of Dopamine to Inhibit an Epileptic Attack in Rats." *Neuroscience Letters* 307 (2001): 163-166.

Chernevskaja, N.I., O.A. Krishtal, and A.Y. Valeyev. "Inhibitions of the GABA-Induced Currents of Rat Neurons by the Alkaloid Isocoryne from the Plant Corydalis Pseudoadunca." *Toxicon* 28 (1990): 727-730.

Ito, Chihiro, Toyoko Mizuno, Tian-Shung Wua, and Hiroshi Furukawa. "Alkaloids from Corydalis." *Phytochemistry* 29 (1990): 2044-2045.

Kleber, E., W. Schneider, H.L. Schafer, and E.F. Elstner. "Modulation of Key Reactions of the Catecholamine Metabolism by Extracts from Eschscholtzia Californica and Corydalis Cava." *Arzneimittelforschung* 45, 2 (1995): 127-31.

Lin, Mao-Tsun, Jhi-Joung Wang, and Ming-Shing Young. "The Protective Effect of DL-tetrahydropalmatine Against the Development of Amygdala Kindling Seizures in Rats." *Neuroscience Letters* 320 (2002): 113-116.

Ma, Wei guang, Yukiharu Fukushi, and Satoshi Tahara. "Fungitoxic Alkaloids from Hokkaido Corydalis species." *Fitoterapia* 70 (1999): 25-265.

Hopbush

Amabeoku, G.J., P. Eagles, G. Scott, I. Mayeng, and E. Springfield. "Analgesic and Antipyretic Effects of Dodonaea Angustifolia and Salvia Africana-Lutea." *Journal of Ethnopharmacology* 75 (2001): 117-124.

Getie, M., T. Gebre-Mariam, R. Rietz, C. Hohne, C. Huschka, M. Schmidtke, A. Abate, and R.H.H. Neubert. "Evaluation of the Anti-Microbial and Anti-Inflammatory Activities of the Medicinal Plants Dodonaea Viscosa, Rumex Nervosus and Rumex Abyssinicus." *Fitoterapia* 74 (2003): 139-143.

Heerden, F.R. van, A.M. Viljoen, and B-E. van Wyk. "The Major Flavonoid of Dodonaea Angustifolia." *Fitoterapia* 71 (2000): 602-604.

Rojas, Alejandra, Lourdes Hernandez, Rogelio Pereda-Miranda, and Rachel Mata. "Screening for Antimicrobial Activity of Crude Drug Extracts and Pure Natural Products from Mexican Medicinal Plants." *Journal of Ethnopharmacology* 35, 3 (1992): 275-283.

Sachdev, Kusum and Dinesh K. Kulshreshtha. "Viscosol, a C-3-Prenylated Flavonoid from Dodonaea Viscosa." *Phytochemistry* 25, 8 (1986): 1967-1969.

Wagner, Hildebert, Christine Ludwig, Lutz Grotjahn, and Mohd S.Y. Khan. "Biologically Active Saponins from Dodonaea Viscosa." *Phytochemistry* 26 (1987): 697-701.

Horehound

Rey, Jean-Pierre, Joel Levesque, and Jean Louis Pousset. "Extraction and High-Performance Liquid Chroatographic Methods for the ã-Lactones Parthenolide (Chrysanthemum Parthenium Bernh.), Marrubiin (Marrubium Vulgare L.) and Artemisinin (Artemisia annua L.)." *Journal of Chromatography* 605 (1992): 124-128.

Roman, Ramos R., F. Alarcon-Aguilar, A. Lara-Lemus, and J.L. Flores-Saenz. "Hypoglycemic Effect of Plants Used in Mexico as Antidiabetics." *Archives of Medical Research* 23, 1 (1992): 59-64.

Sahpaz, Sevser, Nancy Garbacki, Monique Tits, and Francois Bailleul. "Isolation and Pharmacological Activity of Phenylpropanoid Esters from Marrubium Vulgare." *Journal of Ethnopharmacology* 79 (2002): 389-392.

VanderJagt, T.J., R. Ghattas, D.J. VanderJagt, M. Crossey, and R.H Glew. "Comparison of the Total Antioxidant Content of 30 Widely Used Medicinal Plants of New Mexico." *Life Sciences* 70 (2002): 1035-1040.

Horsetail

Amarowicz, R., R.B. Pegg, P. Rahimi-Moghaddam, B. Barl, and J.A. Weil. "Free-Radical Scavenging Capacity and Antioxidant Activity of Selected Plant Species from the Canadian Prairies." *Food Chemistry* 84 (2004): 551-562.

Grases, F., G. Melero, A. Costa-Bauza, R. Prieto, and J.G. March. "Urolithiasis and Phytotherapy." *International Urology and Nephrology* 26, 5 (1994): 507-11.

Gurbuz, Iÿlhan, Osman Ustun, Erdem Yesilada, Ekrem Sezik, and Nalan Akyurek. "In Vivo Gastroprotective Effects of Five Turkish Folk Remedies Against Ethanol-Induced Lesions." *Journal of Ethnopharmacology* 83 (2002): 241-244.

Harrison, C.C. "Evidence for Intramineral Macromolecules Containing Protein from Plant Silicas." *Phytochemistry* 41, 1 (1996): 37-42.
Veit, Markus, Cornelia Beckert, Cornelia Hohne, Katja Bauer, and Hans Geiger. "Interspecific and Intraspecific Variation of Phenolics in the Genus Equisetum Subgenus Equisetum." *Phytochemistry* 38, 4 (1995): 881-891.

Jojoba

Boven, M. Van, R. Busson, M. Cokelaere, G. Flo, and E. Decuypere. "4-Demethyl Simmondsin from Simmondsia Chinensis." *Industrial Crops and Products* 12 (2000): 203-208.
Cappillino, Patrick, Robert Kleiman, and Claudia Botti. "Composition of Chilean Jojoba Seeds." *Industrial Crops and Products* 17 (2003): 177-182.
Ham, Roeline, Sabien Vermaut, Gerda Flo, Marnix Cokelaere, and Eddy Decuypere. "Digestive Performance of Dogs Fed a Jojoba Meal Supplemented Diet." *Industrial Crops and Products* 12 (2000): 159-163.
York, David A., Lori Singer, Julian Oliver, Thomas P. Abbott, and George A. Bray. "The Detrimental Effect of Simmondsin on Food Intake and Body Weight of Rats." *Industrial Crops and Products* 12 (2000): 183-192.

Juniper

Adams, Robert P. "Systematics of the One Seeded Juniperus of the Eastern Hemisphere Based on Leaf Essential Oils and Random Amplified Polymorphic DNAs (RAPDs)." *Biochemical Systematics and Ecology* 28 (2000): 529-543.
Adams, Robert P., Ernst Von Rudloff, and Lawrence Hogge. "Chemosystematic Studies of the Western North American Junipers Based on their Volatile Oils." *Biochemical Systematics and Ecology* 11, 3 (1983): 189-193.
Adams, Robert P., Thomas A. Zanoni, and Lawrence Hogge. "Analyses of the Volatile Leaf Oils of Juniperus Deppeana and its Infraspecific Taxa: Chemosystematic Implications." *Biochemical Systemics and Ecoclogy* 12, 1 (1984): 23-27.
Adams, Robert P., Thomas A. Zanoni, Ernst Von Rudloff, and Lawrence Hogge. "The South-Western USA and Northern Mexico One-seeded Junipers: their Volatile Oils and Evolution." *Biochemical Systematics and Ecology* 9, 2/3 (1981): 93-96.
Karaman, I., F. Sahin, M. Güllüce, H. Öğütçü, M. Sengül, and A. Adigüzel. "Antimicrobial Activity of Aqueous and Methanol Extracts of Juniperus Oxycedrus L." *Journal of Ethnopharmacology* 85 (2003): 231-235.
San Feliciano, A., M. Gordaliza, J.M. Miguel del Corral, M.A. Castro, M.D. Garcia-Gravalos, and P. Ruiz-Lazaro. "Antineoplastic and Antiviral Activities of some Cyclolignans." *Planta Med* 59, 3 (1993): 246-249.
Tunón, H., C. Olavsdotter, and L. Bohlin. "Evaluation of Anti-Inflammatory Activity of some Swedish Medicinal Plants. Inhibition of Prostaglandin biosynthesis and PAF-Induced Exocytosis." *Journal of Ethnopharmacology* 48 (1995): 61-76.

Kidneywood

BIBLIOGRAPHY

Alvarez, Laura and Guillermo Delgado. "C- and O-Glycosyl-á-Hydroxydihydrochalcones from Eysenhardtia Polystachya." *Phytochemistry* 50 (1999): 681-687.

Burns, Duncan T., Barry G. Dalgarno, Paul E. Gargan, and James Grimshaw. "An Isoflavone and a Coumestan from Eysenhardtia Polystachya-Robert Boyle's Fluorescent Acid-base Indicator." *Phytochemistry* 23, 1 (1984): 167-169.

Wächtera, Gerald A., Joseph J. Hoffmann, Todd Furbacher, Mary E. Blake, and Barbara N. Timmermann. "Antibacterial and Antifungal Flavanones from Eysenhardtia Texana." *Phytochemistry* 52 (1999): 1469-1471.

Mallow

Billeter, Martin, Beat Meier, and Otto Sticher. "8-Hydroxyflavonoid Glucuronides from Malva Sylvestris." *Phytochemistry* 30, 3 (1991): 987-990.

Classen, B. and W. Blaschek. "High Molecular Weight Acidic Polysaccharides from Malva Sylvestris and Alcea Rosea." *Planta Med* 64, 7 (1998): 640-644.

Giron, Lidia M., Virginia Freire, Aida Alonzo, and Armando Caceres. "Ethnobotanical Survey of the Medicinal Flora Used by the Caribs of Guatemala." *Journal of Ethnopharmacology* 34 (1991): 113-187.

Gonda, R., M. Tomoda, N. Shimizu, and M. Kanari. "Characterization of an Acidic Polysaccharide from the Seeds of Malva Verticillata Stimulating the Phagocytic Activity of Cells of the RES." *Planta Med* 56, 1 (1990): 73-76.

Gonda, Ryoko, Masashi Tomoda, and Noriko Shimizu. "Structure and Anticomplementary Activity of an Acidic Polysaccharide from the Leaves of Malva Sylvestris var. Mauritiana." *Carbohydrate Research* 198 (1990): 323-329.

Grierson, D.S. and A.J. Afolayan. "Antibacterial Activity of some Indigenous Plants Used for the Treatment of Wounds in the Eastern Cape, South Africa." *Journal of Ethnopharmacology* 66 (1999): 103-106.

Schmidgall, J., E. Schnetz, and A. Hensel. "Evidence for Bioadhesive Effects of Polysaccharides and Polysaccharide-Containing Herbs in an ex vivo Bioadhesion Assay on Buccal Membranes." *Planta Med* 66, 1 (2000): 48-53.

Shimizu, N., H. Asahara, M. Tomoda, R. Gonda, and N. Ohara. "Constituents of Seed of Malva Verticillata. VII. Structural Features and Reticuloendothelial System-Potentiating Activity of MVS-I, the Major Neutral Polysaccharide." *Chem Pharm Bull (Tokyo)* 39, 10 (1991): 2630-2632.

Wang, Xing and Greg J. Bunkers. "Potent Heterologous Antifungal Proteins from Cheeseweed (Malva parviflora)." *Biochemical and Biophysical Research Communications* 279 (2000): 669-673.

Manzanita

Dykes, Gary A., Ryszard Amarowicz, and Ronald B. Pegg. "Enhancement of Nisin Antibacterial Activity by a Bearberry (Arctostaphylos Uva-ursi) Leaf Extract." *Food Microbiology* 20 (2003): 211-216.

Grases, F., G. Melero, A. Costa-Bauza, R. Prieto, and J.G. March. "Urolithiasis and Phytotherapy." *International Urology and Nephrology* 26, 5 (1994): 505-511

Marsh Fleabane

Domínguez, Xorge Alejandro and Angeles Zamudio. "b-Amyrin Acetate and Campesterol from Pluchea Odorata." *Phytochemistry* 11 (1972): 1179.

Pérez-García, Francisco, Esther Marín, Salvador Canigueral, and Tomás Adzet. "Anti-Inflammatory Action of Pluchea Sagittalis: Involvemnet of an Antioxidant Mechanism." *Life Sciences* 59, 24 (1996): 2033-2040.

Reyes-Trejo, Benito and Pedro Joseph-Nathan. "Modhephene derivatives from Pluchea Sericea." *Phytochemistry* 51 (1999): 75-78.

Souza, G. Coelho de, A.P.S. Haas, G.L. von Poser, E.E.S. Schapoval, and E. Elisabetsky. "Ethnopharmacological Studies of Antimicrobial Remedies in the South of Brazil." *Journal of Ethnopharmacology* 90 (2004): 135-143.

Mesquite

Adikwu, M.U., O.K. Udeala, and F.C. Ohiri. "Emulsifying Properties of Prosopis African Gum. S.T.P." *Pharma Sciences* 4, 4 (1994): 298-304.

Aqeel, A., Khursheed, A.K., Viqaruddin, A., and Sabiha, Q. "Antimicrobial Activity of Julifloricine Isolated from Prosopis Juliflora." *Arzneimittel Forschung* 39, 6 (1989): 652-655.

Mimosa

Pavón, Numa P. and Oscar Briones. "Phenological Patterns of Nine Perennial Plants in an Intertropical Semi-Arid Mexican Scrub." *Journal of Arid Environments* 49 (2001): 265-277.

Yusuf, Umi Kalsom, Noriha Abdullah, Baki Bakar, Khairuddin Itam, Faridah Abdullah, and Mohd Aspollah Sukari. "Flavonoid Glycosides in the Leaves of Mimosa Species." *Biochemical Systematics and Ecology* 31 (2003): 443-445.

Mountain Marigold

Abdala, Lidia Rosa. "Chemosystematic Interpretations of the Flavonoids Identified in Tagetes Gracilis (Asteraceae)." *Biochemical Systematics and Ecology* (2003).

Abdala, Lidia Rosa. "Flavonoids of the Aerial Parts from Tagetes Lucida (Asteraceae)." *Biochemical Systematics and Ecology* 27 (1999): 753-754.

Heras, B. de las, K. Slowing, J. Benedí, E. Carretero, T. Ortega, C. Toledo, P. Bermejo, I. Iglesias, M.J. Abad, P. Gómez-Serranillos, P.A. Liso, A. Villar, and X. Chiriboga. "Antiinflammatory and Antioxidant Activity of Plants Used in Traditional Medicine in Ecuador." *Journal of Ethnopharmacology* 61 (1998): 161-166.

Kruger, C.L., M. Murphy, Z. DeFreitas, F. Pfannkuch, and J. Heimbach. "An Innovative Approach to the Determination of Safety for a Dietary Ingredient Derived from a New Source: Case Study Using a Crystalline Lutein Product." *Food and Chemical Toxicology* 40 (2002): 1535-1549.

Piccaglia, Roberta, Mauro Marotti, and Silvia Grandi. "Lutein and Lutein Ester Content in Different Types of Tagetes Patula and T. Erecta." *Industrial Crops and Products* 8 (1998): 45-51.

Night Blooming Cereus

Knight, John C. and George R. Pettit. "Arizona Flora: The Sterols of Peniocereus Greggii." *Phytochemistry* 8 (1969): 477-482.

Ocotillo

Domínguez, X. A., J. O. Velasquez, and D. Guerra. "Extractives from the Flowers of Fouquieria Splendens." *Phytochemistry* 11, 9 (1972): 2888.
Jensen, Søren Rosendal and Bent Juhl Nielsen. "Iridoid Glucosides in Fouquieriaceae." *Phytochemistry* 21, 7 (1982): 1623-1629.
Scogin, Ron. "Leaf Phenolics of the Fouquieriaceae." *Biochemical Systematics and Ecology* 6, 4 (1978): 297-298.

Passionflower

Andersen, Lise, Anne Adsersen and Jerzy W. Jaroszewski. "Cyanogenesis of Passiflora Foetida." *Phytochemistry* 47, 6 (1998): 1049-1050.
Carlini, E.A. "Plants and the Central Nervous System." *Pharmacology, Biochemistry and Behavior* 75 (2003): 501-512.
Dhawan, Kamaldeep and Anupam Sharma. "Antitussive Activity of the Methanol Extract of Passiflora Incarnata Leaves." *Fitoterapia* 73 (2002): 397-399.
Dhawan, Kamaldeep and Anupam Sharma. "Prevention of Chronic Alcohol and Nicotine-Induced Azospermia, Sterility and Decreased Libido, by a Novel Tri-Substituted Benzoflavone Moiety from Passiflora Incarnata Linneaus In Healthy Male Rats." *Life Sciences* 71 (2002): 3059-3069.
Dhawan, Kamaldeep, Suresh Kumar, and Anupam Sharma. "Anxiolytic Activity of Aerial and Underground Parts of Passiflora Incarnata." *Fitoterapia* 72 (2001): 922-926.
Dhawan, Kamaldeep, Suresh Kumar, and Anupam Sharma. "Comparative Biological Activity Study on Passiflora Incarnata and P. Edulis." *Fitoterapia* 72 (2001): 698-702.
Dhawan, Kamaldeep, Suresh Kumar, and Anupam Sharma. "Suppression of Alcohol-Cessation-Oriented Hyper-Anxiety by the Benzoflavone Moiety of Passiflora Incarnata Linneaus in Mice." *Journal of Ethnopharmacology* 81 (2002): 239-244.
Jaroszewski, Jerzy W., Elin S. Olafsdottir, Petrine Wellendorph, Jette Christensen, Henrik Franzyk, Brinda Somanadhan, Bogdan A. Budnik, Lise Bolt Jørgensen, and Vicki Clausen. "Cyanohydrin Glycosides of Passiflora: Distribution Pattern, a Saturated Cyclopentane Derivative from P. Guatemalensis, and Formation of Pseudocyanogenic a-hydroxyamides as Isolation Artifacts." *Phytochemistry* 59 (2002): 501-511.

Seigler, David S., Guido F. Pauli, Adolf Nahrstedt, and Rosemary Leen. "Cyanogenic
    Allosides and Glucosides from Passiflora Edulis and Carica Papaya."
    Phytochemistry 60 (2002): 873-882.
Wolfman, Claudia, Hatdee Viola, Alejandro Paladini, Federico Dajas, and Jorge H.
    Medina. "Possible Anxiolytic Effects of Chrysin, a Central Benzodiazepine
    Receptor Ligand Isolated from Passiflora Coerulea." *Pharmacology Biochemistry
    and Behavior* 47 (1994).

Penstemon

Franzyk, Henrik, Soren Rosendal Jensen, and Frank R. Stermitz. "Iridoid Glucosides
    from Penstemon Secundiflorus and Grandiflorus: Revised Structure of 10-
    Hydroxy-8-Epihastatoside." *Phytochemistry* 49, 7 (1998): 2025-2030.
Stermitz, Frank R., Andrei Blokhin, Christina S. Poley and Robert E. Krull. "Iridoid
    Glycosides of Additional Penstemon Species." *Phytochemistry* 37, 5 (1994):
    1283-1286.
Wysokinska, H. and Z. Skrzypek. "Studies on Iridoids of Tissue Cultures of
    Penstemon Serrulatus: Isolation and their Antiproliferative Properties." *J Nat
    Prod* 55, 1 (1992): 58-63.

Peppergrass

Songsak, T. and G.B. Lockwood. "Glucosinolates of Seven Medicinal Plants from
    Thailand." *Fitoterapia* 73 (2002): 209-216.

Periwinkle

Avijit Banerji and Manas Chakrabarty. "Lochvinerine: a New Indole Alkaloid of Vinca
    Major." *Phytochemistry* 13 (1974): 2309-2312.
Avijit Banerji and Manas Chakrabarty. "Majvinine: a New Indole Alkaloid of Vinca
    Major." *Phytochemistry* 16 (1977): 1124-1125.
Rahman, Atta-ur, Abida Sultana, Farzana Nighat, M. Khalid Bhatti, Semra Kurucu,
    and Murat Kartal. "Alkaloids from Vinca Major." *Phytochemistry* 38, 4 (1995):
    1057-1061.

Plantain

Samuelsen, Anne Berit. "The Traditional Uses, Chemical Constituents and Biological
    Activities of Plantago Major L." *Journal of Ethnopharmacology* 71 (2000): 1-21.
Samuelsen, Anne Berit, Berit Smestad Paulsen, Jens Kristian Wold, Svein H.
    Knutsen, and Haruki Yamada. "Characterization of a Biologically Active
    Arabinogalactan from the Leaves of Plantago Major L." *Carbohydrate Polymers*
    35 (1998): 145-153.
Taskova, Rilka, Nedjalka Handjieva, Ljubka Evstatieva, Simeon Popov. "Iridoid
    Glucosides from Plantago Cornuti, Plantago Major and Veronica Cymbalaria."
    Phytochemistry 52 (1999): 1443-1445.

Plumbago

Abdul, Kamal Mohammed and Rao Pinninti Ramchender. "Modulatory Effect of Plumbagin (5-Hydroxy-2-Methyl1-1,4-Naphthoquinone) on Macrophage Functions in BALB/c Mice. 1. Potentiation of Macrophage Bactericidal Activity." *Immunopharmacology* 30 (1995): 231-236.

Ahmad, Iqbal, Zafar Mehmood, and Faiz Mohammad. "Screening of Some Indian Medicinal Plants for their Antimicrobial Properties." *Journal of Ethnopharmacology* 62 (1998): 183-193.

Bhattacharyya, J. and Vicente R. De Carvalho. "Epi-Isoshinanolone from Plumbago Scandens." *Phytochemistry* 25, 3 (1986): 764-765.

Reddy, J. Suresh, P. Rajeswara Rao, and Mada S. Reddy. "Wound Healing Effects of Heliotropium Indicum, Plumbago Zeylanicum and Acalypha Indica in Rats." *Journal of Ethnopharmacology* 79 (2002): 249-251.

Solomon, F. Emerson, A.C. Sharada, and P. Uma Devi. "Toxic Effects of Crude Root Extract of Plumbago Rosea (Rakta chitraka) on Mice and Rats." *Journal of Ethnopharmacology* 38 (1993): 79-84.

Prickly Pear

Budinsky, A., R. Wolfram, A. Oguogho, Y. Efthimiou, Y. Stamatopoulos, and H. Sinzinger. "Regular Ingestion of Opuntia Robusta Lowers Oxidation Injury." *Prostaglandins, Leukotrienes and Essential Fatty Acids* 65, 1 (2001): 45-50.

Bwititi, P., C.T. Musabayane, and C.F.B. Nhachi. "Effects of Opuntia Megacantha on Blood Glucose and Kidney Function in Streptozotocin Diabetic Rats." *Journal of Ethnopharmacology* 69 (2000): 247-252.

Frati-Munari, A.C., R. Licona-Quesada, C.R. Araiza-Andraca, R. Lopez-Ledesma, and A. Chavez-Negrete. "Activity of Opuntia Streptacantha in Healthy Individuals With Induced Hyperglycemia." *Archivos de Investigacion Medica* 21, 2 (1990): 99-102.

Fernandez-Lopez, Jose A., Luis Almela. "Application of High-Performance Liquid Chromatography to the Characterization of the Betalain Pigments in Prickly Pear Fruits." *Journal of Chromatography A*, 913 (2001): 415-420.

Galati, E.M., M.M. Tripodo, A. Trovato, N. Miceli, and M.T. Monforte. "Biological Effect of Opuntia Ficus Indica (L.) Mill. (Cactaceae) Waste Matter Note I: Diuretic Activity." *Journal of Ethnopharmacology* 79 (2002): 17-21.

Galati, E.M., S. Pergolizzi, N. Miceli, M.T. Monforte, and M.M. Tripodo. "Study on the Increment of the Production of Gastric Mucus in Rats Treated with Opuntia Ficus Indica (L.) Mill. Cladodes." *Journal of Ethnopharmacology* 83 (2002): 229-233.

Loro, J.F., I. del Rio, L. Pérez-Santana. "Preliminary Studies of Analgesic and Anti-inflammatory Properties of Opuntia Dillenii Aqueous Extract." *Journal of Ethnopharmacology* 67 (1999): 213-218.

Meckes-Lozoya, M. and R. Ibanez-Camacho. "Hypoglycemic Activity of Opuntia Streptacantha Throughout Its Annual Cycle." *American Journal of Chinese Medicine* 17, 3-4 (1989): 221-224.

Medina-Torres, L., E. Brito-De La Fuente, B. Torrestiana-Sanchez, and R. Katthain. "Rheological Properties of the Mucilage Gum (Opuntia Ficus Indica)." *Food Hydrocolloids* 14 (2000): 417-424.

Park, E.-H. and M.-J. Chun. "Wound Healing Activity of Opuntia Ficus-Indica." *Fitoterapia* 72 (2001): 165-167.

Park, Eun-Hee, Ja-Hoon Kahng, Sang Hyun Lee, Kuk-Hyun Shin. "An Anti-Inflammatory Principle from Cactus." *Fitoterapia* 72 (2001): 288-290.

Pimienta-Barrios, Eulogio, María Eugenia González del Castillo-Aranda, and Park S. Nobel. "Ecophysiology of a Wild Platyopuntia Exposed to Prolonged Drought." *Environmental and Experimental Botany* 47 (2002): 77-86.

Roman-Ramos, R., J.L. Flores-Saenz, and F.J. Alarcon-Aguilar. "Anti-hyperglycemic Effect of some Edible Plants." *Journal of Ethnopharmacology* 48 (1995): 25-32.

Prickly Poppy

Bandoni, A.L., F.R. Stermitz, R.V.D. Rondina, and J.D. Coussio. "Alkaloidal Content of Argentine Argemone." *Phytochemistry* 14, 8 (1975): 1785-1788.

Stermitz, F.R., R.J. Ito, S.M. Workman and W.M. Klein. "Alkaloids of Argemone Fruticosa and A. Echinata." *Phytochemistry* 12, 2 (1973): 381-382.

Husain, Sajid, R. Narsimha, and R. Nageswara Rao. "Separation, Identification and Determination of Sanguinarine in Argemone and Other Adulterated Edible Oils by Reversed-Phase High-Performance Liquid Chromatography." *Journal of Chromatography* A, 863 (1999): 123-126.

Shenolikar, I.S., C. Rukmini, K.A.V.R. Krisnamachari, and K. Satayanarayana. "Sanguinarine in the Blood and Urine of Cases of Epidemic Dropsy." *Food and Cosmetics Toxicology* 12, 5-6 (1974): 699-702.

Stermitz, Frank R., Don K. Kim and Kenneth A. Lamon. "Alkaloids of Argemone Albiflora, A. Revicornuta, and A. Turnerae." *Phytochemistry* 12, 6 (1973): 1355-1357.

Stermitz, Frank R., Joseph R. Stermitz, Thomas A. Zanoni, and John Gillespie. "Alkaloids of Argemone Subintegrifolia and A. Munita." *Phytochemistry* 13, 7 (1974): 1151-1153.

Verma, S.K., G. Dev, A.K. Tyagi, S. Goomber, and G.V. Jain. "Argemone Mexicana Poisoning: Autopsy Findings of Two Cases." *Forensic Science International* 115 (2001): 135-141.

Puncturevine

Achenbach, Hans, Harald Hübner, Wolfgang Brandta, and Melchior Reitera. "Cardioactive Steroid Saponins and other Constituents from the Aerial Parts of Tribulus Cistoides." *Phytochemistry* 35, 6 (1994): 1527-1543.

Ali, N.A. Awadh, W.-D. Jülich, C. Kusnick, and U. Lindequist. "Screening of Yemeni medicinal plants for antibacterial and Cytotoxic Activities." *Journal of Ethnopharmacology* 74 (2001): 173-179.

Anand, R., G.K. Patnaik, D.K. Kulshreshtha, and B.N. Dhawan. "Activity of Certain Fractions of Tribulus Terrestris Fruits Against Experimentally Induced

Urolithiasis in Rats." *Indian Journal of Experimental Biology* 32, 8 (1994): 548-552.

Bhutani, S. P., S. S. Chibber, and T.R. Seshadri. "Flavonoids of the Fruits and Leaves of Tribulus Terrestris: Constitution of Tribuloside." *Phytochemistry* 8, 1 (1969): 299-303.

Gauthaman, K., P.G. Adaikan, and R.N.V. Prasad. "Aphrodisiac Properties of Tribulus Terrestris Extract (Protodioscin) in Normal and Castrated Rats." *Life Sciences* 71 (2002): 1385-1396.

Kirby, Andrew J. and Richard Schmidt. "The Antioxidant Activity of Chinese Herbs for Eczema and of Placebo Herbs." *Journal of Ethnopharmacology* 56 (1997): 103-108.

Lin, Zhi Xiu, J.R.S. Hoult, and Amala Raman. "Sulphorhodamine B Assay for Measuring Proliferation of a Pigmented Melanocyte Cell Line and its Application to the Evaluation of Crude Drugs Used in the Treatment of Vitiligo." *Journal of Ethnopharmacology* 66 (1999): 141-150.

Saleh, Nabiel A.M., Ahmed A. Ahmed, and Mohamed F. Abdalla. "Flavonoid Glycosides of Tribulus Pentandrus and T. Terrestris." *Phytochemistry* 21, 8 (1982): 1995-2000.

Sangeeta, D., H. Sidhu, S.K. Thind, and R. Nath. "Effect of Tribulus Terrestris on Oxalate Metabolism in Rats." *Journal of Ethnopharmacology* 44, 2 (1994): 61-66.

Wu, Tian-Shung, Li-Shian Shi, and Shang-Chu Kuo. "Alkaloids and Other Constituents from Tribulus Terrestris." *Phytochemistry* 50 (1999): 1411-1415.

Wang, B., L. Ma, and T. Liu. "406 Cases of Angina Pectoris in Coronary Heart Disease Treated with Saponin of Tribulus Terrestris." *Chung His I Chien Ho Tsa Chih Chinese Journal Of Modern Developments* 10, 2 (1990): 68, 85-87.

Wu, G., S. Jiang, F. Jiang, D. Zhu, H. Wu, and S. Jiang. "Steroidal Glycosides from Tribulus terrestris." *Phytochemistry* 42, 6 (1996): 1677-1681.

Purple Gromwell

Grases, F., G. Melero, A. Costa-Bauza, R. Prieto, and J.G. March. "Urolithiasis and Phytotherapy." *International Urology and Nephrology* 26, 5 (1994): 507-511.

Krenn, L., H. Wiedenfeld, and E. Roeder. "Pyrrolizidine Alkaloids from Lithospermum Officinale." *Phytochemistry* 37, 1 (1994): 275-277.

Singh, Fiza, Dayuan Gao, Mark G. Lebwohl, and Huachen Wei. "Shikonin Modulates Cell Proliferation by Inhibiting Epidermal Growth Factor Receptor Signaling in Human Epidermoid Carcinoma Cells." *Cancer Letters* 200 (2003): 115-121.

Weng, X.C., G.Q. Xiang, A.L. Jiang, Y.P Liu, L.L. Wu, X.W. Dong, and S. Duan. "Antioxidant Properties of Components Extracted from Puccoon (Lithospermum Erythrorhizon Sieb. et Zucc.)." *Food Chemistry* 69 (2000): 143-146.

Ratany

Achenbach, Hans, Wolfgang Utz, Humberto Sánchez V., Elsa M. Guajardo Touché, Juia Verde S., and Xorge A. Domínguez. "Neolignans, Nor-neolignans and Other

Compounds from Roots of Krameria Grayi." *Phytochemistry* 39, 2 (1995): 413-415.

Guevara, J.M., J. Chumpitaz, and E. Valencia. "The In Vitro Action of Plants on Vibrio Cholerae." *Revista de Gastroenterologia del Peru* 14, 1 (1994): 27-31.

Scholz, E. and H. Rimpler. "Proanthocyanidins from Krameria Triandra Root." *Planta Medica* 55, 4 (1989): 379-384.

Rayweed

Chhabra, B.R., J.C. Kohli, and R.S. Dhillon. "Three Ambrosanolides from Parthenium Hysterophorus." *Phytochemistry* 52 (1999): 1331-1334.

Coates, Wayne, Ricardo Ayerza, and Damian Ravetta. "Guayule Rubber and Latex Content – Seasonal Variations Over Time in Argentina." *Industrial Crops and Products* 14 (2001): 85-91.

Maatooq, Galal T., Ali A. H. El Gamal, Todd R. Furbacher, Tracy L. Cornuelle, and Joseph J. Hoffmann. "Triterpenoids from Parthenium Argentatum x P. Tomentosa." *Phytochemistry* 60 (2002): 755-760.

Proksch, Peter, H. Mohan Behl, and Eloy Rodriguez. "Detection and Quantification of Guayulins A and B in Parthenium Argentatum (Guayule) and F, Hybrids by High-Performance Liquid Chromatography." *Journal of Chromatography* 2, 13 (1981): 345-348.

Rodriguez, Eloy, Hirosuke Yoshioka, and Tom J. Mabry. "The Sesquiterpene Lactone Chemistry of the Genus Parthenium (Compositae)." *Phytochemistry* 10 (1971): 1145-1154.

Sage

Al-Yousuf, M.H., A.K. Bashir, B.H. Ali, M.O.M. Tanira, and G. Blunden. "Some Effects of Salvia Aegyptiaca L. on the Central Nervous System in Mice." *Journal of Ethnopharmacology* 81 (2002): 121-127.

Baricevic, D., S. Sosa, R. Della Loggia, A. Tubaro, B. Simonovska, A. Krasna, and A. Zupancic. "Topical Anti-Inflammatory Activity of Salvia Officinalis L. Leaves: The Relevance of Ursolic Acid." *Journal of Ethnopharmacology* 75 (2001): 125-132.

Gali-Muhtasib, Hala, Christo Hilan, and Carla Khater. "Traditional Uses of Salvia Libanotica (East Mediterranean Sage) and the Effects of its Essential Oils." *Journal of Ethnopharmacology* 71 (2000): 513-520.

Vardar-Unlu, Gülhan, Moschos Polissiou, and Atalay Sokmen. "Antimicrobial and Antioxidative Activities of the Essential Oils and Methanol Extracts of Salvia Cryptantha (Montbret et Aucher ex Benth.) and Salvia Multicaulis (Vahl)." *Food Chemistry* 84 (2004): 519-525.

Lu, Yinrong and L. Yeap Foo. "Polyphenolics of Salvia—A Review." *Phytochemistry* 59 (2002): 117-140.

Miliauskas, G., P.R. Venskutonis, and T.A. van Beek. "Screening of Radical Scavenging Activity of some Medicinal and Aromatic Plant Extracts." *Food Chemistry* 85 (2004) 231-237.

Perry, Nicolette S.L., Chloe Bollen, Elaine K. Perry, and Clive Ballard. "Salvia for Dementia Therapy: Review of Pharmacological Activity and Pilot Tolerability Clinical Trial." *Pharmacology, Biochemistry and Behavior* 75 (2003): 651-659.

Radulescu, Valeria, Silvia Chiliment, and Eliza Oprea. "Capillary Gas Chromatography–Mass Spectrometry of Volatile and Semi-Volatile Compounds of Salvia Officinalis." *Journal of Chromatography A*, 1027 (2004): 121-126.

Savelev, S., E. Okello, N.S.L. Perry, R.M. Wilkins, and E.K. Perry. "Synergistic and Antagonistic Interactions of Anticholinesterase Terpenoids in Salvia Lavandulaefolia Essential Oil." *Pharmacology, Biochemistry and Behavior* 75 (2003): 661-668.

Tepe, Bektas, Dimitra Daferera, Atalay Sokmen, Munevver Sokmen, and Moschos Polissiou. "Antimicrobial and Antioxidant Activities of the Essential Oil and Various Extracts of Salvia Tomentosa Miller (Lamiaceae)." *Food Chemistry* (2003).

Tepe, Bektas, Erol Donmez, Mehmet Unlu, Ferda Candan, Dimitra Daferera, N.T.J. Tildesley, D.O. Kennedy, E.K. Perry, C.G. Ballard, S. Savelev, K.A. Wesnes, and A.B. Scholey. "Salvia Lavandulaefolia (Spanish Sage) Enhances Memory in Healthy Young Volunteers." *Pharmacology, Biochemistry and Behavior* 75 (2003): 669-674.

Wake, George, Jennifer Court, Anne Pickering, Rhiannon Lewis, Richard Wilkins, and Elaine Perry. "CNS Acetylcholine Receptor Activity in European Medicinal Plants Traditionally Used to Improve Failing Memory." *Journal of Ethnopharmacology* 69 (2000): 105-114.

Sagebrush

Gunawardena, K., S.B. Rivera, and W.W. Epstein. "The Monoterpenes of Artemisia Tridentata ssp. Vaseyana, Artemisia Cana ssp. Viscidula and Artemisia Tridentata ssp. Spiciformis." *Phytochemistry* 59 (2002): 197-203.

Kelley, B.D., J.M. Appelt, and G.D. Appelt. "Artemisia Tridentata (Basin Sagebrush) in the Southwestern United States of America: Medicinal Uses and Pharmacologic Implications." *International Journal of the Addictions* 27, 3 (1992): 347-366.

McCutcheon, A.R., S.M. Ellis, R.E.W. Hancock, and G.H.N. Towers. "Antifungal Screening of Medicinal Plants of British Columbian Native Peoples." *Journal of Ethnopharmacology* 44, 3 (1994): 157-169.

Smith, Bruce N., Thomas A. Monaco, Clayton Jones, Robert A. Holmes, Lee D. Hansen, E. Durant McArthur, and D. Carl Freeman. "Stress-Induced Metabolic Differences Between Populations and Subspecies of Artemisia Tridentata (Sagebrush) from a Single Hillside." *Thermochimica Acta* 394 (2002): 205-210.

Senna

Barbosa, Francisco G., Maria da Conceicao F. de Oliveira, Raimundo Braz-Filho, and Edilberto R. Silveira. "Anthraquinones and Naphthopyrones from Senna Rugosa." *Biochemical Systematics and Ecology* 32 (2004): 363-365.

Djozan, DJ and Y. Assadi. "Determination of Anthraquinones in Rhubarb Roots, Dock Flowers and Senna Leaves by Normal-Phase High Performance Liquid Chromatography." *Talanta* 42, 6 (1995): 861-865.

Fairbairn, J. W. and A.B. Shrestha. "The Distribution of Anthraquinone Glycosides in Cassia Senna L." *Phytochemistry* 6 (1967): 1203-1207.

Snakeweed

Ferdinand Bohlmann, Christa Zdero, Robert M. King, and Harold Robinson. "Gutierrezial and Further Diterpenes from Gutierrezia Sarothrae." *Phytochemistry* 23, 9 (1984): 2007-2012.

Soapberry

Lal, J., S. Chandra, V. Raviprakash, and M. Sabir. "In Vitro Anthelmintic Action of some Indigenous Medicinal Plants on Ascardia Galli Worms." *Indian J Physiol Pharmacol* 20, 2 (1976) 64-68

Albiero, Adriana L. Meyer, Jayme Antonio Aboin Sertié, and Elfriede Marianne Bacchi. "Antiulcer Activity of Sapindus Saponaria L. in the Rat." *Journal of Ethnopharmacology* 82 (2002): 41-44.

Spanish Needles

Alvarez, A., F. Pomar, M.A. Sevilla, and M.J. Montero. "Gastric Antisecretory and Antiulcer Activities of an Ethanolic Extract of Bidens Pilosa L. var. Radiata Schult. Bip." *Journal of Ethnopharmacology* 67 (1999): 333-340.

Alarcon de la Lastra, C., M.J. Martin, C. La Casa, and V. Motilva. "Antiulcerogenicity of the Flavonoid Fraction from Bidens Aurea: Comparison With Ranitidine and Omeprazole." *Journal of Ethnopharmacology* 42, 3 (1994): 161-168.

Brandao, M.G.L., A.U. Krettli, L.S.R. Soares, C.G.C. Nery, and H.C. Marinuzzi. "Antimalarial Activity of Extracts and Fractions from Bidens Pilosa and Other Bidens Species (Asteracea) Correlated With the Presence of Acetylene and Flavonoid Compounds." *Journal of Ethnopharmacology* 57 (1997): 131-138.

Cano, Juan Hernández and Gabriele Volpato. "Herbal Mixtures in the Traditional Medicine of Eastern Cuba." *Journal of Ethnopharmacology* xxx (2004): xxx–xxx.

Dimo, Théophile, Silver Rakotonirina, René Kamgang, Paul V. Tan, Albert Kamanyi, and Marc Bopelet. "Effects of Leaf Aqueous Extract of *Bidens Pilosa* (Asteraceae) on KCl- and Norepinephrine-Induced Contractions of Rat Aorta." *Journal of Ethnopharmacology* 60 (1998): 179-182.

Dimo, Théophile, Silvere V. Rakotonirina, Paul V. Tan, Jacqueline Azay, Etienne Dongo, and Gérard Cros. "Leaf Methanol Extract of Bidens Pilosa Prevents and Attenuates the Hypertension Induced by High-fructose Diet in Wistar Rats." *Journal of Ethnopharmacology* 83 (2002): 183-191.

Geissberger, P. and U. Sequin. "Constituents of Bidens Pilosa L.: Do the Components Found So Far Explain the Use of this Plant in Traditional Medicine?" *Acta Tropica* 48, 4 (1991): 251-261.

Khan, M.R., M. Kihara, and A.D. Omoloso. "Anti-Microbial Activity of Bidens Pilosa, Bischofia Javanica, Elmerillia Papuana and Sigesbekia Orientalis." *Fitoterapia* 72 (2001): 662-665.

Pereira, Rachel L.C., Tereza Ibrahim, Leonardo Lucchetti, Antonio Jorge R. da Silva, and Vera Lucia Goncalves de Moraes. "Immunosuppressive and Anti-Inflammatory Effects of Methanolic Extract and the Polyacetylene Isolated from Bidens pilosa L." *Immunopharmacology* 43 (1999): 31-37.

Rivera, D. and C. Obón. "The Ethnopharmacology of Madeira and Porto Santo Islands, a Review." *Journal of Ethnopharmacology* 46 (1995): 73-93.

Sarg, T.M., A.M. Ateya, N.M. Farrag, and F.A. Abbas. "Constituents and Biological Activity of Bidens Pilosa L. Grown in Egypt." *Acta Pharmaceutica Hungarica* 61, 6 (1991): 317-323.

Tan, Paul V., Théophile Dimo, and Etienne Dongo. "Effects of Methanol, Cyclohexane and Methylene Chloride Extracts of Bidens Pilosa on Various Gastric Ulcer Models in Rats." *Journal of Ethnopharmacology* 73 (2000): 415-421.

Sumac

Homer, K.A., F. Manji, and D. Beighton. "Inhibition of Protease Activities of Periodontopathic Bacteria by Extracts of Plants Used in Kenya as Chewing Sticks (Mswaki)." *Archives of Oral Biology* 35, 6 (1990): 421-424.

Saxena, G., A.R. McCutcheon, S. Farmer, G.H.N. Towers, and R.E.W. Hancock. "Antimicrobial Constituents of Rhus Glabra." *Journal of Ethnopharmacology* 42 (1994) 95-99.

Zalacain, A., M. Prodanov, M. Carmona, and G.L. Alonso. "Optimization of Extraction and Identification of Gallotannins from Sumac Leaves." *Biosystems Engineering* 84, 2 (2003): 211-216.

Syrian Rue

Abdel-Fattah, Abdel-Fattah Mohamed, Kinzo Matsumoto, Hatim Abdel-Khalik Gammaz, and Hiroshi Watanabe. "Hypothermic Effect of Harmala Alkaloid in Rats: Involvement of Serotonergic Mechanism." *Pharmacology Biochemistry and Behavior* 52, 2 (1995): 421-426

El-Saad, El-Rifaie. "Peganum Harmala: Its Use in Certain Dermatoses." *International Journal of Dermatology* 19, 4 (1980): 221-222.

Kartal, M., M.L. Altun, and S. Kurucu. "HPLC Method for the Analysis of Harmol, Harmalol, Harmine and Harmaline in the Seeds of Peganum Harmala L." *Journal of Pharmaceutical and Biomedical Analysis* 31 (2003): 263-269.

Prashanth, D. and S. John. "Antibacterial Activity of Peganum Harmala." *Fitoterapia* 70 (1999): 438-439.

Tamarisk

Nawwar, Mohamed A.M. and Sahar A.M. Hussein. "Gall Polyphenolics of Tamarix Aphylla." *Phytochemistry* 36, 4 (1994): 1035-1037.

Souliman, Ahmed M.A., Heba H. Barakat, Amani M.D El-Mousallamy, Mohamed
S.A. Marzouk, and Mohamed A.M. Nawwar. "Phenolics from the Bark of Tamarix
Aphyua." *Phytochemistry* 30, 11 (1991): 3763-3766.

Sultanova, N., T. Makhmoor, Z.A. Abilov, Z. Parween, V.B. Omurkamzinova, Atta-ur-
Rahman, and M. Iqbal Choudhary. "Antioxidant and Antimicrobial Activities of
Tamarix Ramosissima." *Journal of Ethnopharmacology* 78 (2001): 201-205.

Tarbush

M. M. Rao, D.G.I. Kingston and T.D. Spittler. "Flavonoids from Flourensia Cernua."
Phytochemistry 9 (1970): 227-228.

Mata, Rachel, Robert Bye, Edelmira Linares, Martha Macías, Isabel Rivero-Cruz,
Olga Pérez, and Barbara N. Timmermann. "Phytotoxic Compounds from
Flourensia Cernua." *Phytochemistry* 64 (2003): 285-291.

Richard E. Estell, Kris M. Havstad, Eddie L. Fredrickson, and Jorge L. Gardea-
Torresdey. "Secondary Chemistry of the Leaf Surface of Flourensia cernua."
Biochemical Systematics and Ecology 22, 1 (1994): 73-77.

Tobacco

P.A. Steenkamp, F.R. van Heerden, and B.-E. van Wyk. "Accidental Fatal Poisoning
by Nicotiana Glauca: Identification of Anabasine by High Performance Liquid
Chromatography/Photodiode Array/Mass Spectrometry." *Forensic Science
International* 127 (2002): 208-217.

Tree of Heaven

Hitotsuyanagi, Yukio, Akira Ozeki, Chee Yan Choo, Kit Lam Chan, Hideji Itokawa,
and Koichi Takeya. "Malabanones A and B, Novel Nortriterpenoids from
Ailanthus Malabarica DC." *Tetrahedron* 57 (2001): 7477-7480.

Takeya, Koichi, Hideyuki Kobata, Akira Ozeki, Hiroshi Morita, and Hiden Itokawa.
"Quassinoids from Ailanthus Vilmoriniana." Phytochemistry 48, 3 (1998): 565-
568.

Trumpet Flower

Binutu, O.A. and B.A. Lajubutu. "Antimicrobial Potentials of some Plant Species of
the Bignoniaceae Family." *African Journal of Medicine and Medical Sciences* 23,
3 (1994): 269-273.

Dickinson, E.M. and G. Jones. "Pyrindane Alkaloids from Tecoma Stans." *Tetrahedron*
25, 7 (1969): 1523-1529.

Hammouda, Y. and N. Khalafallah. "Stability of Tecomine, the Major Antidiabetic
Factor of Tecoma Stans (Juss.) F. Bignoniaceae." *Journal of Pharmaceutical
Sciences* 60, 8 (1971): 1142-1145.

Harris, G.H., E.C. Fixman, F.R. Stermitz, and L. Castedo. "(-)-Delta-N-Normethylskytanthine from Tecoma Arequipensis." *Journal of Natural Products* 51, 3 (1988): 543-548.

Kunapuli, Satya P. and C.S. Vaidyanathan. "Indole-Metabolizing Enzyme Systems in Tropical Plants." *Phytochemistry* 24, 5 (1985): 973-975.

Lins, Arlete Paulino and Joana D'Arc Felicio. "Monoterpene Alkaloids from Tecoma Stans." *Phytochemistry* 34, 3 (1993): 876-878.

Lozoya-Meckes, M. and V. Mellado-Campos. "Is the Tecoma Stans Infusion an Antidiabetic Remedy?" *Journal of Ethnopharmacology* 14, 1 (1985): 1-9.

Meckes-Lozoya, M. and R. Ibáñez-Camacho. "Hepatic Gycogenolysis Produced by Intraperitoneal Administration of Total Extract of Tecoma Stans in Rats." *Archivos de Investigacion Medica* 16, 4 (1985): 387-393.

Okarter, Temple U., Paul L. Schiff Jr. , Joseph E. Knapp and David J. Slatkin. "Lipid and Phenolic Constituents of Tecoma Radicans." *Phytochemistry* 15, 3 (1976): 436.

Prakash, E.O. and J.T. Rao. "A New Flavone Glycoside from the Seeds of Tecoma Undulata." *Fitoterapia* 70 (1999): 287-289.

Qureshi, S., M.K. Rai, and S.C. Agrawal. "In Vitro Evaluation of Inhibitory Nature of Extracts of 18-Plant Species of Chhindwara Against 3-keratinophilic Fungi." *Hindustan Antibiotics Bulletin* 39, 1-4 (1997): 56-60.

Roman-Ramos, R., J.L. Flores-Saenz, G. Partida-Hernandez, A. Lara-Lemus, and F. Alarcon-Aguilar. "Experimental Study of the Hypoglycemic Effect of some Antibiabetic Plants." *Archivos de Investigation Medica* 22,1 (1991): 87-93.

Shapiro, Karen and William C. Gong. "Natural Products Used for Diabetes." *Journal of the American Pharmaceutical Association* 42, 2 (2002): 217-226.

Verbena

Hernández, Nancy E., M.L. Tereschuk, and L.R. Abdala. "Antimicrobial Activity of Flavonoids in Medicinal Plants from Tafí del Valle (Tucumán, Argentina)." *Journal of Ethnopharmacology* 73 (2000): 317-322.

Kawashty, S.A. and I.A. El-Garf. "The Favonoid Chemosystematics of Egyptian Verbena Species." *Biochemical Systematics and Ecology* 28 (2000): 919-921.

Western Black Willow

Chrubasik, Sigrun, Elon Eisenberg, Edith Balan, Tuvia Weinberger, Rachel Luzzati, and Christian Conradt. "Treatment of Low Back Pain Exacerbations with Willow Bark Extract: A Randomized Double-Blind Study." *The American Journal of Medicine* 109 (2000): 9-14.

Orians, Colin M., Megan E. Griffiths, Bernadette M. Roche, and Robert S. Fritz. "Phenolic Glycosides and Condensed Tannins in Salix Sericea, S. Eriocephala and their F1 Hybrids: Not All Hybrids are Created Equal." *Biochemical Systematics and Ecology* 28 (2000): 619-632.

Tunón, H., C. Olavsdotter, and L. Bohlin. "Evaluation of Anti-Inflammatory Activity of some Swedish Medicinal Plants. Inhibition of Prostaglandin Biosynthesis and PAF-Induced Exocytosis." *Journal of Ethnopharmacology* 48 (1995): 61-76.

Western Mugwort

Bork, Peter M., M. Lienhard Schmitz, Michaela Kuhnt, Claudia Escher, and Michael Heinrich. "Sesquiterpene Lactone Containing Mexican Indian Medicinal Plants and Pure Sesquiterpene Lactones as Potent Inhibitors of Transcription Factor NF-B." *FEBS Letters* 402, 1 (1997): 85-90.
Jakupovic, J., R.X. Tan, F. Bohlmann, P.E. Boldt, and Z.J. Jia. "Sesquiterpene Lactones from Artemisia Ludoviciana." *Phytochemistry* 30, 5 (1991): 1573-1577.
Juteau, Fabien, Veronique Masotti, Jean Marie Bessiere, Michel Dherbomez, and Josette Viano. "Antibacterial and Antioxidant Activities of Artemisia Annua Essential Oil." *Fitoterapia* 73 (2002): 532-535.
Lee, K.H. and T.A. Geissman. "Sesquiterpene Lactones of Artemisia Constituents of A. Ludoviciana ssp. Mexicana." *Phytochemistry* 9, 2 (1970): 403-408.
Liu, Yong-Long and T.J. Mabry. "Flavonoids from Artemisia Ludoviciana var. Ludoviciana." *Phytochemistry* 21, 1 (1982): 209-214.
Ruiz-Cancino, Alejandro, Arturo E. Cano, and Guillermo Delgado. "Sesquiterpene Lactones and Flavonoids from Artemisia Ludoviciana ssp. Mexicana." *Phytochemistry* 33, 5 (1993): 1113-1115.

Western Peony

Papandreou, Vasiliki, Prokopios Magiatis, Ioanna Chinou, Eleftherios Kalpoutzakis, Alexios-Leandros Skaltsounis, and Anthony Tsarbopoulos. "Volatiles with Antimicrobial Activity from the Roots of Greek Paeonia Taxa." *Journal of Ethnopharmacology* 81 (2002): 101-104
Ikuta, Akira, Kohei Kamiya, Toshiko Satake, and Yasuhisa Saiki. "Triterpenoids from Callus Tissue Cultures of Paeonia Species." *Phytochemistry* 38, 5 (1995): 1203-1207.

Wild Licorice

Fukai, Toshio, Kazue Satoh, Taro Nomura, and Hiroshi Sakagami. "Antinephritis and Radical Scavenging Activity of Prenylflavonoids." *Fitoterapia* 74 (2003): 720-724.
Fukai, Toshio, Ai Marumo, Kiyoshi Kaitou, Toshihisa Kanda, Sumio Terada, and Taro Nomura. "Anti-Helicobacter Pylori Flavonoids from Licorice Extract." *Life Sciences* 71 (2002): 1449-1463.
Fukai, Toshio, Kazue Satoh, Taro Nomura, and Hiroshi Sakagami. "Preliminary Evaluation of Antinephritis and Radical Scavenging Activities of Glabridin from Glycyrrhiza Glabra." *Fitoterapia* 74 (2003): 624-629.

Amarowicz, R., R.B. Pegg, P. Rahimi-Moghaddam, B. Barld, and J.A. Weil. "Free-Radical Scavenging Capacity and Antioxidant Activity of Selected Plant Species from the Canadian Prairies." *Food Chemistry* 84 (2004): 551-562.

Yellowdock

Fairbairn, J. W. and F.J. El-Muhtadi. "Chemotaxonomy of Anthraquinones in Rumex." *Phytochemistry* 11 (1972): 263-268.

Saleh, Nabiel A.M., Mohamed N. El-Hadidi, and Raafat F.M. Arafa. "Flavonoids and Anthraquinones of some Egyptian Rumex Species (Polygonaceae)." *Biochemical Systematics and Ecology* 21, 2 (1993): 301-303.

Yucca

Hussain, I., A.M. Ismail, and P.R. Cheeke. "Effects of Feeding Yucca Schidigera Extract in Diets Varying in Crude Protien and Urea Contents on Growth Performance and Cecum and Blood Urea and Ammonia Concentrations of Rabbits." *Animal Feed Science Technology* 62, (1996): 121-129.

Hussain, I. and P.R. Cheeke. "Effect of Dietary Yucca Schidigera Extract on Rumen and Blood Profiles of Steers Fed Concentrate or Roughage-Based Diets." *Animal Feed Science and Technology* 51 (1995): 231-242.

Wang, Y., T.A. McAllister, C.J. Newbold, L.M. Rode, P.R. Cheeke, and K-J. Cheng. "Effects of Yucca Schidigera Extract on Fermentation and Degradation of Steroidal Saponins in the Rumen Simulation Technique (RUSITEC)1." *Animal Feed Science and Technology* 74 (1998): 143-153.

INDEX

ORDERING INFORMATION

Wholesaler/Distributor list

Treasure Chest Books/PO Box 5250
Tucson AZ 85703/800-969-9558

Baker and Taylor Books/PO Box 8888
Momence IL 60954

Books West/5757 Arapahoe Ave. Unit D
Boulder CO 80303/303-449-5995

Integral Yoga/Rt. 1 Box 1379
Buckingham VA 23921/434-969-1049

Quality Books/1003 Pines Road
Oregon IL 61061/815-732-4450

Brodart, Co/500 Arch Street
Williamsport, PA 17701/800-233-8467

Midwest Library Service/1143 St. Charles Rock Road
Bridgeton MO 63044-2789/314-739-2999

...and
Available at your local bookstore

.

If interested in applying for Charles Kane's 5 month program, Studies in Western
Herbal Medicine, or to schedule an office visit, he can be reached at 520-731-3379
or PO Box 57304 Tucson, AZ 85732. For more information go to
www.tcbmed.com.

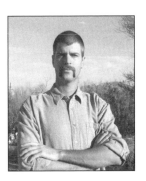

As a boy Charles Kane was introduced to plant usage through his grandfather. As director of the Tucson Clinic of Botanical Medicine he combines traditional and modern herbal uses, western physiology, with constitutional diagnosis. He personally collects and prepares the majority of plants he dispenses. Charles is an active lecturer/teacher in the field of western herbal medicine. Annually he offers a course of study focusing on medicinal plants of the American West. He is veteran of the war on terrorism and lives with his wife Christy in the desert surrounding Tucson.

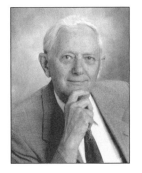

Frank S. Rose was born 1927 in Bryn Athyn, Pennsylvania, the ninth child of Don and Marjorie Rose. He began painting in his teens. He served for 51 years as an ordained clergyman in Europe, Canada and the United States, doing painting on the side. He is a signature member of the Southern Arizona Watercolor Guild and the Western Federation of Watercolor Societies. Since his retirement in 2003, he has devoted himself to his art, combining it with an interest in botany. His art work is available in Tucson from El Presidio Gallery. He lives in Tucson with his wife, Louise.